D1598874

HANDBOOK OF NUTRITION AND IMMUNITY

HANDBOOK OF NUTRITION AND IMMUNITY

Edited by

M. ERIC GERSHWIN, MD

*Division of Rheumatology, Allergy, and Clinical Immunology,
University of California School of Medicine, Davis, CA*

PENELOPE NESTEL, PhD

Micronutrient Global Leadership Project, Washington, DC

CARL L. KEEN, PhD

Department of Nutrition, University of California, Davis, CA

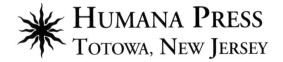

HUMANA PRESS
TOTOWA, NEW JERSEY

Production Editor: Tracy Catanese

Cover design by Patricia F. Cleary.

This publication is printed on acid-free paper. ∞
ANSI Z39.48-1984 (American National Standards Institute) Permanence of Paper for Printed Library Materials.

Printed in the United States of America. 10 9 8 7 6 5 4 3 2 1

1-59259-790-4 (e-book)

Library of Congress Cataloging-in-Publication Data

Handbook of nutrition and immunity / edited by M. Eric Gershwin, Penelope Nestel, Carl L. Keen.
    p. ; cm.
  Includes bibliographical references and index.
  ISBN 1-58829-308-4 (alk. paper)
    1. Immunity--Nutritional aspects--Handbooks, manuals, etc. 2. Nutrition--Handbooks, manuals, etc.
3. Malnutrition--Immunological aspects--Handbooks, manuals, etc. 4. Diet therapy--Handbooks, manuals, etc.
    [DNLM: 1. Nutrition--Handbooks. 2. Immunity--Handbooks. QU 39 H23578 2004] I. Gershwin, M. Eric,
1946- II. Nestel, Penelope. III. Keen, Carl L.
  QR182.2.N86H36 2004
  613.2--dc22
                                                                           2003027639

PREFACE

Several years ago, two of us published a full-length textbook entitled *Nutrition and Immunology: Principles and Practice*. The book was academically successful and well received by our peers. Our colleagues commented that while the book was eminently suitable for a library, there was still an intellectual need for a more concise volume on nutrition and immunology for health care providers and scientists working at the interface of delivering therapeutic and/or preventive health care. We agreed and decided that a book focused on issues relevant to laboratory workers and to developing countries would be valuable. We invited well-known experts in their fields to contribute a chapter each and asked that they err on the short rather than the long side and update cited review articles rather than original papers wherever possible. *The Handbook of Nutrition and Immunity* is the culmination of that process. Our intention is that the book will grow over time and new editions will fill identified voids that meet the changing needs of health care providers and scientists interested in the practical aspects related to evaluating nutrition and immunology in the field. *The Handbook of Nutrition and Immunity* is for those people working in both adult and child nutrition throughout the world. It is also of relevance to those in the pharmaceutical and the food industry who are interested in developing ways to evaluate both the efficacy and effectiveness of their products.

The goal of this handbook is to make available a short text replete with useful information. It is not intended to replace our large textbook, but rather to serve as a fundamental source of practical information that is immediately useful and that can be updated every few years. As with any text, there will be errors in omission; the responsibility for these belong to the editors.

Finally, we express our gratitude to Nikki Phipps, who was so gracious in the international communication required and in helping us assemble the final product.

M. Eric Gershwin, MD
Penelope Nestel, PhD
Carl L. Keen, PhD

v

CONTENTS

CONTRIBUTORS

AFTAB A. ANSARI, PhD, *Department of Pathology, Emory University School of Medicine, Atlanta, GA*

ANDREA T. BORCHERS, PhD, *Division of Rheumatology, Allergy, and Clinical Immunology, University of California School of Medicine, Davis, CA*

PHILIP C. CALDER, PhD, *Institute of Human Nutrition, University of Southampton, Southampton General Hospital, Southampton, England*

CHRISTOPHER CHANG, MD, PhD, *Pacific Coast Allergy, Crescent City, CA*

CARLOTA DOBAÑO, PhD, *Center for International Health, University of Barcelona, Barcelona, Spain*

JODI L. ENSUNSA, MS, *Department of Nutrition, University of California, Davis, CA*

KENT L. ERICKSON, PhD, *Department of Cell Biology and Human Anatomy, University of California School of Medicine, Davis, CA*

WAFAIE FAWZI, MBBS, PhD, *Departments of Nutrition and Epidemiology, Harvard School of Public Health, Boston, MA*

SUZANNE FILTEAU, PhD, *Centre for International Child Health, Institute of Child Health, London, England*

M. ERIC GERSHWIN, MD, *Division of Rheumatology, Allergy, and Clinical Immunology, University of California School of Medicine, Davis, CA*

RACHEL GITAU, PhD, *Centre for International Child Health, Institute of Child Health, London, England*

LAURENCE S. HARBIGE, PhD, *School of Chemical and Life Sciences, University of Greenwich, Medway, Kent, England*

MICHAEL K. HENDRICKS, MD, *Child Health Unit, School of Child and Adolescent Health, University of Cape Town, Cape Town, South Africa*

NEIL E. HUBBARD, PhD, *Department of Cell Biology and Human Anatomy, University of California School of Medicine, Davis, CA*

GREG HUSSEY, MD, *Child Health Unit, School of Child and Adolescent Health, University of Cape Town, Cape Town, South Africa*

PIETRO INVERNIZZI, MD, PhD, *Division of Internal Medicine, San Paolo School of Medicine, University of Milan, Milan, Italy*

ALAN A. JACKSON, MD, *Institute of Human Nutrition, University of Southampton, Southampton General Hospital, Southampton, England*

CARL L. KEEN, PhD, *Department of Nutrition, University of California, Davis, CA*

DARSHAN S. KELLEY, PhD, *Western Human Nutrition Research Center, Animal Resources Service, United States Department of Agriculture, Davis, CA*

ANNAMARIA KIURE, MD, SM, *Departments of Nutrition and Epidemiology, Harvard School of Public Health, Boston, MA*

CLARA MENÉNDEZ, MD, PhD, *Center for International Health, University of Barcelona, Barcelona, Spain*

RITU NALUBOLA, PhD, *South Shafer Drive, Tempe, AZ*

PENELOPE NESTEL, PhD, *Micronutrient Global Leadership Project, Washington, DC*

KAREN OLOGOUDOU, BS, *Nutrition and Health Sciences Program, Graduate Division of Biological and Biomedical Sciences, Emory University, Atlanta, GA*

USHA RAMAKRISHNAN, PhD, *Department of International Health, Rollins School of Public Health, Emory University, Atlanta, GA*

IAN D. RILEY, MD, *Australian Centre for International and Tropical Health and Nutrition, School of Population Health, University of Queensland, Australia*

CARLO SELMI, MD, PhD, *Division of Rheumatology, Allergy, and Clinical Immunology, University of California School of Medicine, Davis, CA*

DOUGLAS L. TAREN, PhD, *Mel and Enid Zuckerman Arizona College of Public Health, University of Arizona, Tucson, AZ*

JANET Y. URIU-ADAMS, PhD, *Department of Nutrition, University of California, Davis, CA*

AMY L. WEBB, BS, *Nutrition and Health Sciences Program, Graduate Division of Biological and Biomedical Sciences, Emory University, Atlanta, GA*

MASSIMO ZUIN, MD, *Division of Internal Medicine, San Paolo School of Medicine, University of Milan, Milan, Italy*

VALUE-ADDED EBOOK/PDA

This book is accompanied by a value-added CD-ROM that contains an eBook version of the volume you have just purchased. This eBook can be viewed on your computer, and you can synchronize it to your PDA for viewing on your handheld device. The eBook enables you to view this volume on only one computer and PDA. Once the eBook is installed on your computer, you cannot download, install, or e-mail it to another computer; it resides solely with the computer to which it is installed. The license provided is for only one computer. The eBook can only be read using Adobe® Reader® 6.0 software, which is available free from Adobe Systems Incorporated at www.Adobe.com. You may also view the eBook on your PDA using the Adobe® PDA Reader® software that is also available free from Adobe.com.

You must follow a simple procedure when you install the eBook/PDA that will require you to connect to the Humana Press website in order to receive your license. Please read and follow the instructions below:

1. Download and install Adobe® Reader® 6.0 software
   You can obtain a free copy of the Adobe® Reader® 6.0 software at www.adobe.com

Note: If you already have the Adobe® Reader® 6.0 software installed, you do not need to reinstall it.

2. Launch Adobe® Reader® 6.0 software
3. Install eBook: Insert your eBook CD into your CD-ROM drive
   PC: Click on the "Start" button, then click on "Run"
   At the prompt, type "d:\ebookinstall.pdf" and click "OK"

Note: If your CD-ROM drive letter is something other than d: change the above command accordingly.

   MAC: Double click on the "eBook CD" that you will see mounted on your desktop.
   Double click "ebookinstall.pdf"

4. Adobe® Reader® 6.0 software will open and you will receive the message "This document is protected by Adobe DRM" Click "OK"

Note: If you have not already activated the Adobe® Reader® 6.0 software, you will be prompted to do so. Simply follow the directions to activate and continue installation.

Your web browser will open and you will be taken to the Humana Press eBook registration page. Follow the instructions on that page to complete installation. You will need the serial number located on the sticker sealing the envelope containing the CD-ROM.

If you require assistance during the installation, or you would like more information regarding your eBook and PDA installation, please refer to the eBookManual.pdf located on your CD. If you need further assistance, contact Humana Press eBook Support by e-mail at ebooksupport@humanapr.com or by phone at 973-256-1699.

*Adobe and Reader are either registered trademarks or trademarks of Adobe Systems Incorporated in the United States and/or other countries.

1 Evaluation of the Immune Function in the Nutritionally At-Risk Patient

CARLO SELMI, PIETRO INVERNIZZI, MASSIMO ZUIN,
AFTAB A. ANSARI, AND M. ERIC GERSHWIN

CONTENTS

KEY POINTS

- Impaired or inadequate nutriture is prevalent throughout the world, and frequently accompanies a number of medical and social conditions.
- It is important in clinical practice to determine whether the patient is malnourished to avoid consequences such as increased susceptibility to disease owing to poor immune function.
- Many underlying causes of malnutrition can be treated effectively and promptly. Therefore, it is recommended that health care workers prevent, rather than treat, possible immune dysfunctions.
- Malnutrition can lead to impaired immune function at the cellular, tissue, and whole body level, and can compromise an individual's ability to resist infections.
- Both innate and acquired immune functions, including mucosal barriers and white blood cells and their products such as cytokines/chemokines,

From: *Handbook of Nutrition and Immunity*
Edited by: M. E. Gershwin, P. Nestel, and C. L. Keen © Humana Press, Totowa, NJ

can be negatively influenced by a lack of specific nutrients and/or insufficient energy intake.

- The immune status of a malnourished individual or population can be assessed by taking a careful history, conducting a physical examination, and conducting laboratory tests.
- The type of laboratory tests carried out depends on general conditions and the infrastructure available at the site where the immunological evaluations take place, the availability of materials, and the capabilities of personnel available.
- A flexible system that can adapt to a variety of situations, but still achieve the goal of obtaining reliable and useful immunological information, should be used.
- A practical approach for both nutrition and immunity might include a tiered system, applying increasingly sophisticated analysis of materials as one moves from remote isolated villages to large urban city centers.

Introduction

Nutrition and immunity have been linked to each other for centuries. In the last decade, systematic studies have confirmed that nutrient deficiencies can alter the immune response and lead to a higher incidence of infections resulting in increased mortality, especially in children. Protein-energy malnutrition is widespread in developing countries and results in an altered number of T-cells, phagocytic cells, and secretory immunoglobulin (Ig) A antibody response, as well as reduced levels of several complement components. Other impairments of immune function have been reported for moderate deficiencies of trace minerals and vitamins. The interactions between nutrition and the immune system have clinical, practical, and public health importance *(1,2)*. This chapter focuses on the conditions in which malnutrition can lead to different grades of immunodeficiency, the methods to assess the immune competence, and the options for detecting the latter in particular settings. Specific influences of nutrients on immune function are summarized for generic nutritional depletion (*see* Table 1), vitamins (*see* Table 2), trace elements and minerals (*see* Table 3), and antioxidants (*see* Table 4).

Nutrients and Immunity in Specific Conditions

Inadequate nutriture because of insufficient food intake is found in patients of all ages (especially children) in developing countries, whereas isolated or combined dietary deficiencies/excesses of one or more nutrients are important factors that accompany a number of physiologic and pathologic conditions in developed countries. It is important to consider and/or recognize these risks because these physiologic and pathologic conditions can be reversed with the

Table 1
Immunologic Consequences
of Nutritional Impairment from Food and Macronutrient Intake

Nutrient	Decrease in	Increase in
Food deficit	• Immunocompetence (at <60% age-corrected body weight) • CD4$^+$/CD8$^+$ ratio • Plasma complement	• Circulating B-cells and antibodies
Energy deficit (rodents)	• Tumor virus expression and malignancies • Proliferation of autoreactive B1-cells • Pro-inflammatory and Th1 cytokines	• T-cell proliferative response
Severe protein and protein -energy deficit	• Humoral and cell-mediated response	• Oxidative stress
Protein deficit (mice)	• Delayed-type hyper-sensitivity • Circulating IgG • Tissue repair mechanisms • Macrophage function	• Th2 tolerance • Oxidative stress • Splenic suppressor T-cells
Amino acid deficit (particularly Arg and Gln)	• Immune competence: impairment of T-cell development and growth (Arg), thymic integrity (Arg), leukocytes energy source (Gln)	
Nucleic acid deficit	• Natural killer activity • Recovery in sepsis • Cell-mediated immune response	
Fatty acid supple-mentation	• Inflammation (n-3 fatty acids) • Composition and fluidity of cell membranes	• Immunosuppression (mostly saturated fatty acid)

Source: Ref. *3*

Table 2
The Role of Vitamins in Immunity

Vitamin A

- Deficiency reduces leukocytes number, lymphoid tissue weight, complement, T-cell function, tumor resistance, NK cell number, Ag-specific IgG and IgE, Th2 cytokines
- Deficiency increases IFN-γ synthesis
- Supplementation increases lymphocytes proliferation, tumor resistance, graft rejection, and cytotoxic T-cell activity
- Excess intake has adjuvant effects, possibly by apoptosis inhibition
- Physiologically, maintains intact epithelial membranes

Vitamin B complex

- Pyridoxine (B_6) deficiency reduces lymphocytes number and proliferative response, lymphoid tissue weight, graft rejection, IL-2 production, DTH response, Ab response
- Pyridoxine supplementation protects against UV-B induced immunosuppression
- B_{12} deficiency depresses phagocyte functions, DTH response, T-cells proliferation
- Biotin (H) deficiency reduces thymic weight, Ab response, lymphocytes proliferation
- Pantothenic acid deficiency reduces Ab responses
- Thiamin (B_1) deficiency reduces thymic weight, Ab response, PMN motility
- Riboflavin (B_2) deficiency decreases Ab responses, thymic weight, circulating lymphocytes number

Vitamin C

- Deficiency lowers phagocytes activity, tumor resistance, DTH reactions, graft rejection, and slows wound repair
- Antioxidant function protects phagocytes

Vitamin D

- Stimulates monocytes and macrophages development and phagocytosis
- Selectively suppresses Th1, and not Th2 or CD8$^+$ cells activity

Vitamin E

- Deficiency reduces lymphocytes proliferation, phagocytes functions, tumor resistance
- Supplementation increases lymphocytes proliferation, Ab levels, DTH reaction, IL-2 production, phagocytosis, Th1 activity, and reduces PGE_2 synthesis

Source: Ref. *3*

Table 3
The Role of Trace Elements and Minerals in Immunity

Copper

- Deficiency reduces antibody production, phagocytic activity, IL-2 production, T-cell proliferation, and neutrphils respiratory burst and anti-Candida activity in rodents; decreases T-cells proliferation in humans; increases B-cell number
- Involved in complement function, cell membrane integrity, Cu-Zn superoxide dismutase (SOD), Ig structure

Iron

- Deficiency reduces DTH reaction, graft rejection, and cytotoxic activity of phagocytes
- Low plasma iron selectively inhibits proliferation of Th1, and not Th2, cells
- High plasma iron interferes with IFN-γ
- Important in the formation of reactive oxygen and radicals during respiratory burst
- Component of metalloenzymes

Magnesium

- Deficiency increases thymic cellularity, eosinophils, IL-1, IL-6, TNF-α and histamine levels; reduces acute-phase protein and complement activity
- Influences cytotoxicity of CTL through interactions with ATP and adhesion molecules
- Component of metalloenzymes

Selenium

- Deficiency reduces thymic cellularity, eosinophils, cytokines synthesis, cell-mediated cytotoxicity, lymphocytes proliferation
- A component of antioxidant enzyme glutathione peroxidase

Zinc

- Important for thymocyte development, T-cell function, and thymic integrity; component of many proteins including transcription factors, SOD, MHC I
- Deficiency causes reduction in T-cell development, thymic hormone release, T-cell function

Source: Ref. *3*

Table 4
The Role of Antioxidants in Immunity

- Defenses include antioxidant vitamins and trace elements compounds of antioxidant enzymes
- Dietary oils oxidized by heating or frying may compromise antioxidant defenses
- Kwashiorkor is characterized by oxidative stress
- CD8⁺ T-cells may be more susceptible to oxidant damage than CD4⁺ cells
- As cell-mediated immune responses produce reactive oxygen and radical species, the Th1 cell may be an important focus for feedback inhibition by products of inflammation

---

Source: Ref. 3

proper use of micronutrient supplements. In most cases, such supplementation stimulates the immune response resulting in fewer infections, particularly in the elderly, low-birth-weight infants, and critically ill patients in hospitals.

Aging (4)

Assessing the nutritional status of the elderly is an important component of their medical examination. The early recognition of malnutrition in a patient is important because its prevention may influence the incidence of infectious diseases and restore immunocompetence, in addition to preventing deficiency diseases and increasing longevity.

Energy intake and energy needs are generally thought to decrease proportionally with age. This perception, however, ignores the wide variations in both energy intakes and needs among the healthy, sick, or institutionalized elderly. Nutritional requirements also depend on many social and physiological factors. For these reasons health care providers must recognize that dietary requirements for the elderly are qualitatively grossly comparable to those for middle-aged adults. However, the elderly are particularly at-risk of marginal deficiencies of vitamins and trace elements; thus, questions need to be asked to ascertain whether this risk exits and, if so, advice given about the appropriate use of pharmaceutical supplements and increasing the intakes of fruits and vegetables. Particular attention must be dedicated to investigating the risk of protein-energy malnutrition in the elderly. Such condition, in fact, is more common in the ageing population (because of chronic diseases and/or social factors) and may be held resposible for the high frequency of recurrent or severe infections in these patients, mostly regarding the upper and lower airways. In the respiratory system, besides causing immunity impairment, malnutrition can modify muscle structure and decrease respiratory function and ventilatory drive. The resulting disease, in turn, can easily complicate the mosaic of nutrients deficits resulting from diverse dietary inadequacies. In a similar fashion, iron deficiency must be ruled out as this common condition can cause impaired immune function and increased morbidity, together with an anemia (4).

The elderly, therefore, need to be encouraged to optimize the total amount of food and energy they consume; lose weight in the case of obesity; decrease blood lipid levels; and increase calcium and iron intakes, while ensuring a good nutritional status is maintained.

Low-Birth-Weight Infants (5)

Low-birth-weight infants have a prolonged impairment of cell-mediated immunity that can be partly restored by providing extra dietary zinc through the use of fortified formula, although other deficiencies need to be ruled out.

Critically Ill Patients (6)

The nutritional and immunological state of the critically ill patient depends on a number of factors including the patient's age and the presence of chronic conditions. As up to 50% of patients admitted to intensive-care units can be malnourished, it is essential to assess regularly the nutritional and biochemical status of the individual because multiple nutrient supplementation is usually recommended and given with total parenteral or enteral nutrition. Obtaining enteral access and providing sufficient micro- or macronutrients early on in the hospital-stay can improve a patient's outcome through the progression of the disease process. Failure to use enteral feeding can promote a proinflammatory state, which exacerbates disease severity and worsens morbidity. Enteral feeding, when indicated, also provides a conduit for the delivery of immune stimulants and can be considered as an effective prophylactic tool against stress-induced gastrointestinal problems.

Obesity (7)

A long-standing positive imbalance between energy intake and requirements leads to obesity, and immune responses mediated by both humoral and cell-mediated mechanisms can be impaired. However, limited and often controversial data exist comparing immunological fitness in obese and nonobese subjects as well as the associated mechanisms of potential dysfunction implicated in the former condition. Clinical and epidemiological data support the view that the incidence and severity of specific types of infections are higher, but antibody responses to antigens are poorer, in obese people compared with lean individuals. The hormone leptin is now recognized as the best candidate as a key factor in the link between nutritional status and T-cell function.

Alcoholism (8)

The association between alcohol exposure and the risk of developing an alcohol-related immunodeficiency is multifactorial. Moreover, variables such as age, gender, smoking habits, dietary intake, and exercise are also involved. The evaluation of the host cellular and humoral immune responses has shown that alcohol may induce some benefits when consumption is moderate (alcohol intake below 10–12 g/d and 20–24 g/d for women and men, respectively). Alcoholic beverages such as red wine contain antioxidants that may protect against immune cell damage.

Among alcoholics particular attention must be paid to specific vitamin deficiencies that can be caused by generic or specific malnutrition. The most common cause of thiamine (vitamin B_1) deficiency in developed countries is alcoholism. Thiamine diphosphate—the active form of thiamine—is a cofactor for several enzymes involved primarily in carbohydrate catabolism. Alcohol affects thiamine uptake and other aspects of thiamine utilization, and these effects may contribute to the prevalence of thiamine deficiency in alcoholics.

Eating Disorders (9)

Despite the serious undernourishment observed in patients with anorexia and bulimia nervosa, aspects of the immune system that are otherwise impaired in more typical types of undernutrition, such as protein-energy malnutrition, are still being debated. In general, adaptative mechanisms appear to become activated, for example, cytokines, the acute phase response to infection, and the hormones cortisol and leptin thereby limiting the impairment of the immune function during prolonged periods. However, cell-mediated immunity is usually altered as reflected by changes in lymphocyte subset counts and the response to skin tests, a measure of the delayed hypersensitivity response. The duration of the eating disorder and the time before appropriate treatment is started are thought to be the most likely factors that contribute to the alteration of the helper/cytotoxic T-cell ratio. Despite these findings, it is worth noting that anorexic patients seem to present a low incidence of common viral infections until the most advanced stages of undernutrition.

Gastrointestinal Diseases (10)

A number of gastrointestinal conditions can result in impaired nutrient absorption either primarily (through inflammatory processes) or secondarily (after surgical resection, short-bowel syndrome). Crohn disease most commonly involves the ileum, resulting in the malabsorption of a variety of elements that may result from extensive inflammation, resected small bowel, or both. In patients with Crohn disease levels of biotin, folate, iron, β-carotene, and vitamins A, C, D, B_1, B_6, and B_{12} need to be carefully monitored. Untreated celiac disease can be associated with severe iron deficiency, vitamin D deficiency, and hypocalcemia; thus concentrations of these nutrients need to be montoried. Where disaccharidase deficiencies exist (sucrase-isomaltase, lactase, primarily involving children), it is important to prevent or treat insufficient absorption of carbohydrates, folate, calcium, iron, and electrolytes.

Clinical Evaluation of the Patient With Suspected Immunodeficiency

Impaired immunity, or immunodeficiency, whether congenital or acquired (including conditions resulting from malnutrition or infections such as HIV), must always be suspected and promptly recognized in order to initiate treatment and prevent the associated major complications from not only infections, but also autoimmune diseases and malignancies.

The conditions under which immune evaluations are carried out vary widely. In developing countries physicians may have a very narrow spectrum of feasible technical options. In this situation decisions will have to be based on simple and reliable tests or samples refered to larger clinical centers for further analysis. The physician will also have to pay careful attention to the local prevalence of infectious diseases, sanitation and public health conditions, use and/or misuse of herbal medicines and over-the-counter drugs, social sensitivities, historical details, and physical findings. A tentative screening evaluation protocol for suspected immunodeficiencies is shown in Table 5.

History and Physical Examination

A careful history and physical examination will usually indicate whether the major problem involves the antibody-complement-phagocyte system or cell-mediated immunity. A history can provide very useful facts; for example, referred presence of dermatitis owing to contact with poison ivy indicates intact cellular immunity, whereas persistent candidiasis usually provides suggestive evidence of a deficiency of this type of immunity. During the physical examination particular attention must be given to a proper evaluation of the lymph nodes because the absence of palpable nodes associated with lymphopenia may be an important findings, whereas diffuse lymphoid hyperplasia can be found in patients with profound immunodeficiency.

Recurrent Infections

The study of recurring infectious diseases is a powerful investigative tool. A major cause of recurrent infections is excessive exposure of individuals (mostly infants or children) to infectious agents in settings with low hygiene standards.

Table 5
Screening Evaluation for Immunodeficiencies

History

- Medications and treatments
- Relatedness of parents, umbilical stump separation, age of onset, dental history
- Previous/recurrent infectious diseases: frequency, severity, distribution, causative agents
- Vaccination history, type of vaccines

Physical examination

- Weight and height
- Hair: sheen, pigmentation
- Abdomen: organomegaly
- Skin: dystrophic scars, telangiectasias, eczema
- Oropharynx: thrush, ulcers, gingivitis, secondary tooth eruption
- Skeleton: kyphoscoliosis, fractures

Routine laboratory tests

- Complete blood count
- Differential: lymphopenia, neutropenia, eosinophilia
- Peripheral smear: giant granules, specific granules
- Platelet count: thrombocytopenia
- Erythrocyte sedimentation rate
- Chemistry
- Serum calcium and uric acid
- Liver function tests
- Immunoglobulins
- IgA, IgM, IgG, IgE
- Iso-hemagglutinins
- Antibody titers (tetanus, pneumococcus, and so on)
- Complement
- Total hemolytic complement (CH50)

Radiographs

- Plain chest films: kyphoscoliosis, pneumatoceles, scarring

Source: Ref. 11

In most cases, however, an underlying immunodeficiency status must be ruled out (*see* Table 6).

Patients with defects in humoral immunity have recurrent or chronic sino-pulmonary infection, meningitis, and bacteremia, most commonly caused by pyogenic bacteria such as *Hemophilus influenza*, *Streptococcus pneumonia*, and staphylococci. These and other pyogenic organisms also cause frequent infections in individuals who have either neutropenia or a deficiency of some components of complement (especially C3). The collaboration of antibody, complement, and phagocytes in host defense against pyogenic organisms makes it important to assess all three systems in individuals with unusual susceptibility to bacterial infections.

Antibody-deficient patients, in whom cell-mediated immunity is intact, may present a unique response to viral diseases. The clinical course of a primary infection in these cases, unless complicated by other infections, does not differ significantly from that of noncompromised individuals. However, as long-lasting immunity often fails to develop, recurrence of diseases such as chickenpox or measles may occur in such patients. As a rule, the occurrence of an unusually serious infection, for example, *H. influenza* meningitis in an older child or adult, as well as recurrent bacterial pulmonary or intestinal infection by *Giardia lamblia*, are conditions that warrant consideration of humoral immune deficiency.

Abnormalities of cell-mediated immunity may lead to disseminated virus infections, particularly by latent viruses such as herpes simplex, varicella zoster, and cytomegalovirus. In addition, patients may develop mucocutaneous candidiasis and frequently acquire systemic fungal infections. Pneumonia caused by *Pneumocystis carinii* and severe enteritis caused by *Cryptosporidium* infection are also common. In all these cases, however, infection by HIV needs to be ruled out. T-cell deficiency is commonly accompanied by some degree of abnormality in antibody responses, although this may not be reflected by hypogammaglobulinemia. This explains partly why patients with primary T-cell defects are also subject to overwhelming bacterial infection.

Finally, individuals with defects of both humoral and cell-mediated immunity are susceptible to the whole range of infectious agents including otherwise common nonpathogenic organisms.

Laboratory Evaluation

Most immunodeficiencies can be diagnosed using tests available in many clinical laboratories. More precise evaluation of immunologic function and treatment may require referral to specialized centers. Table 7 presents possible approaches to laboratory investigations on immune status. The assays suggested as an initial screening tool, together with a careful acquisition of history and a physical exam, will identify the vast majority of patients with immunodeficiencies. In most cases, for example, deficiency of humoral immunity is accompanied by diminished serum concentration of one or more classes of immunoglobulins; in these settings, whenever feasible, determining the fre-

Table 6

Evaluation of Suspect Immunodeficiency

Suspected abnormality	Clinical finding	Initial tests	More advanced tests
Antibody	Sinopulmonary and systemic infections (pyogenic bacteria)	Immunoglobulin levels (IgG, IgM, IgA)	B-cell enumeration
	Enteric infections (enterovirus, other viruses, *Giardia* sp.)	Antibody titers to protein antigens (diphtheria, tetanus)	Immunofixation
	Autoimmune disease	Antibody titers to poly-saccharide antigens (2-yr-old child) before and after immunization (pneumococcal poly-saccharide vaccine)	IgG subclass levels
Cell-mediated immunity	Pneumonia (pyogenic bacteria, fungi, *Pneumocystis carinii*, viruses)	Total lymphocyte counts	T-cell enumeration and subsets (CD3, CD4, CD8)
	Gastroenteritis (viruses, *Giardia* sp. *Cryptosporidium* sp.)	HIV ELISA/Western blot	In vitro T-cell proliferation to mitogens, antigens, or allogeneic cells
	Dermatitis/mucositis (fungi)	Delayed-type hypersen-sitivity skin test (*Candida* sp., tetanus toxoid, mumps, *Trichophyton* sp.)	Chest radiography for thymic hyplasia

Antibody and cell-mediated immunity	See above	See above	See above
Phagocytosis	Cutaneous infections, abscesses, lymphadenitis (staphylococci, enteric bacteria, fungi, mycobacteria), poor wound healing	WBC/neutrophil count and morphology	Nitroblue tetrazolium (NBT) tes Chemotactic assay Phagocytic and bacterial assay
Spleen	Bacteremia/hematogenous infection (pneumococcus, other streptococci, Neisseria sp.)	Peripheral blood smears for Howell-Jolly bodies Hemoglobin electrophoresis (HbSS)	Technetium-99 spleen scan
Complement	Bacterial sepsis, autoimmune disease (lupus, glomerulonephritis), angioedema, pyogenic infection, encapsulated bacterial infections (i.e., Neisseria sp.)	CH50 (total hemolytic complement)	Alternative pathway assays Individual component assays

Source: Refs. 1 and 12

13

Table 7
Laboratory Tests for Screening Evaluation of Immunodeficiencies

Initial Screening Assays
- Complete blood count with differential smear
- Serum immunoglobulin levels: IgM, IgG, IgA, IgD, IgE

Other Readily Available Assays
- *Quantification of blood mononuclear cell populations* by immunofluorescence assays employing monoclonal antibody markers
  - T-cells: CD3, CD4, CD8, TCR, TCR
  - B-cells: CD19, CD20, CD21, Ig
  - NK cells: CD16/CD56
  - Monocytes: CD15
  - Activation markers: HLA-DR, CD25, CD80 (B-cells), CD154 (T-cells)
- *T-cell functional evaluation*
  - Delayed hypersensitivity skin tests (PPD, Candida, histoplasmin, tetanus toxoid)
  - Proliferative response to mitogens (anti-CD3 antibody, phytohemagglutinin, concanavalin A) and allogeneic cells (mixed lymphocyte response)
  - Cytokine production
- *B-cell functional evaluation*
  - Natural or commonly acquired antibodies: isohemagglutinins; antibodies to common viruses (influenza, rubella, rubeola) and bacterial toxins (diphtheria, tetanus)
  - Response to immunization with protein (tetanus toxoid) and carbohydrate (pneumococcal vaccine, *H. influenzae* B vaccine) antigens
  - Quantitative IgG subclass determinations
- *Complement*
  - CH50 assays (classic and alternative pathways)
  - C3, C4, and other components
- *Phagocyte function*
- Reduction of nitroblue tetrazolium
- Chemotaxis assays
- Bactericidal activity

Source: Ref. *14*

quency and absolute numbers of peripheral B-cells using specific monoclonal antibodies can provide useful information.

Because antibody deficiency may be mimicked clinically by deficiency of complement components, measurement of total hemolytic complement (CH50) should be a part of the evaluation of host defense; measurement of C3 alone, instead, is not suggested for screening purposes, because of its low sensitivity.

T-cells can be enumerated by their expression of surface markers as the TCR/CD3 complex, the CD4 molecule in helper T-cells, and the CD8 molecule in cytotoxic T-cells.

Normal levels of serum immunoglobulins and antibody responsiveness are considered to indicate intact helper T-cell function. T-lymphocyte function can also be assessed directly by delayed hypersensitivity skin tests using a variety of antigens to which the majority of older children and adults have been either immunized and/or naturally sensitized. These include intradermally injected antigens such as tetanus toxoid, purified protein derivative (PPD), mumps antigen, and extracts of Candida.

In vitro methods to estimate T-lymphocyte function include studying the capacity of cells to proliferate in response to (1) antigens to which the patient has been sensitized, (2) lymphocytes from an unrelated donor (allogeneic rsponse), (3) a number of polyclonal mitogens, or (4) other stimuli (by measurement of incorporation of radioactive thymidine into newly synthesized DNA). Last, the production of cytokines (or interleukins) by activated T-cells, the ability of T-cells activated in culture to lyse target cells, and defects in T-cell surface receptors and specific elements of their signal transduction pathways can all be analyzed.

In most developing country situations, the above tests will not be feasible. In these cases, the materials and personnel needed to obtain and interpret the acquired information might be the limiting factors. A flexible system capable of adapting to different situations to achieve the goal of proper immunological investigation has been proposed and organized in tiers.

The Tier System

The feasibility and appropriateness of the methods available for evaluating immunity will by necessity depend on the actual environment, the capabilities of the health care personnel, the particular conditions of the population, and the available resources. Table 8 describes a tiered system for health care that can be applied to most working environments *(1)*. By establishing a communication network that connects tier centers, biological samples can be sent to a higher tier facility where tests can be carried out in a more controlled environment or additional immunologic parameters can be determined using techniques otherwise not feasible in the original location. For the tier system to be effective a number of factors must be clearly delineated, including the practicality of preserving and transporting samples, which depends on the distance between tier sites; the condition of roads, boats, or airfields; the efficiency of the temperature-controlled storage (the cold chain and cryopreservation); and ways to communicate and share information. Although isolated sites may have airfields and airplanes nearby, their use will be expensive and therefore limited. Nevertheless, a number of methods for evaluating immunity—including

Table 8
Suggested Tier System for Immunity Assessment

Tier	Characteristics	Methods
One	Absence of permanent public health facility	• Hematology • Dermatologic hypersensitivity tests
Two	Rural medical clinic	• Immunodiffusion, ELISA, and electrophoresis • Short-term cell culture for chemotaxis, phagocytosis, antibody production Immunofluorescence staining with fluorescent microscopy for cell phenotyping
Three	Medical center	• Flow cytometry for cytokine analysis, cell phenotyping, cell cycle analysis • *In situ* hybridization and RT-PCR for cytokine analysis • Longer-term cell culturing for cytotoxicity, proliferation, antigen presentation

Source: Ref. *1*

laboratory tests—are feasible even under conditions that preclude sophisticated analyses, thereby considerably limiting the number of referrals to higher tier facilities.

Tier 1

The first tier is a setting in which no permanent or a very basic health facility exists. Health care personnel may need to do outreach and travel into rural or undeveloped areas and be required to perform evaluations in temporary environments. In these situations the availability of water or electricity cannot be taken for granted.

Careful history assessments, physical examinations, skin tests, and blood smears are usually feasible. Skin tests investigate contact hypersensitivity to various immunologic stimuli and tuberculin-type assays. Subsequent skin testing can be used as an overall measure of the immunologic response. Immunodeficiencies may be indicated by an altered (both in magnitude or latency) or nonresponse to antigens. It must be emphasized, however, that antibody IgE-mediated "immediate hypersensitivity" will be evident in minutes while cell-mediated "delayed hypersensitivity" must be followed over several days. Blood smears can also be performed in most tier one scenarios, allowing staining and microscopic analysis of blood cells for hematologic counts.

Tier 2

The tier-2 scenario can be represented by a clinic located in a rural setting. Running water (possibly with portable filtering devices and the ability to boil) and electricity (usually fairly dependable but subject to occasional outages with a potential to utilize diesel/battery powered electric power and solar powered refrigeration units as back ups) are present, but the availability and maintenance of sterile conditions can be problematic. A tier two facility is unlikely to have an air-conditioned workroom and it will almost never have an ultracold freezer for storage or a cold room. Equipment such as fluorescent microscopes and enzyme-linked immunosorbent assay (ELISA) readers may be present, but performing assays using radioactivity will not be possible.

In addition to the tests described for tier one, immunodiffusion assays and ELISA probably constitute the least complicated and least expensive ways to determine the presence of antigen and/or antibody and the classes of antibodies from peripheral blood. Assuming the necessary reagents and scientific equipment are available, both methods can be used in a rural setting. While complement proteins can be measured by ELISA, the determination of their activity may be problematic because the shelf-life of most reagents is limited. The study of phagocytic and chemotactic activity, the quantitation of antigen-specific B-lymphocytes, and the staining of cells (using fluorescent antibodies and counting by fluorescent microscope) are also feasible assays in tier two settings.

Tier 3

The third tier represents a medical center in a large urban center, for example, the national, state, or provincial/district capital. This facility has the personnel, materials, storage facilities, and laboratory equipment needed for highly specialized immunological tests. In such centers, the proliferative capacity of lymphocytes (by either the mixed leukocyte reaction or mitogen stimulation), the cytotoxic capacity of peripheral blood T-lymphocytes and NK cells (demonstrated on live target cells) may be measured. Assays using radioactive labels can also be performed.

Conclusions

In this chapter, we described how malnutrition can lead to impaired immunity among specific groups of people and how health care providers can evaluate these changes in different clinical settings. We explained a three-tier system that can be used to study nutrition-immunology in resource limited areas. This system is flexible to adapt to most situations and still achieve the goals of a proper immunological evaluation. A system that facilitates the collection of blood samples in rural areas, before and after dietary supplementation, represents an ideal method to study a population's response to common infections, thereby enabling the monitoring and evaluation of preventive strategies. The rapid growth of techniques for assessing immunological status and function, best represented by the increasing variety of available recombinant antigen, raises hope for the improvement of one or two tier scenarios.

References

1. Gershwin M.E., Borchers, A.T., and Keen, C.L. (2000)Phenotypic and functional considerations in the evaluation of immunity in nutritionally compromised hosts. *J. Infect. Dis.* **182**, **Suppl 1**, S108–S114.
2. Chandra, R.K. (1999) Nutrition and immunology: from the clinic to cellular biology and back again. *Proc. Nutr. Soc.* **58**, 681–683.
3. Powell, J., Borchers, A.T., Yoshida, S., and Gershwin, M.E. (2000) Evaluation of the immune system in the nutritionally at-risk host, in *Nutrition and Immunology: Principles and Practice*, (Gershwin, M.E., German, J.B., Keen, C.L., eds.) Humana, Totowa, NJ, pp. 21–31.
4. Schlienger, J.L., Pradignac, A., and Grunenberger, F. (1995) Nutrition of the elderly: a challenge between facts and needs. *Horm. Res.* **43**, 46–51.
5. Ziegler, E. E., Thureen, P. J., and Carlson, S.J. (2002) Aggressive nutrition of the very low birthweight infant. *Clin. Perinatol.* **29**, 225–244.
6. Mechanick, J.I. and Brett, E.M. (2002) Nutrition support of the chronically critically ill patient. *Crit. Care Clin.* **18**, 597–618.
7. Marti, A., Marcos, A., and Martinez, J.A. (2001) Obesity and immune function relationships. *Obes. Rev.* **2**, 131–140.
8. Diaz, L.E., Montero, A., Gonzalez-Gross, M., Vallejo, A.I., Romeo, J., and Marcos, A. (2002) Influence of alcohol consumption on immunological status: a review. *Eur. J. Clin. Nutr.* **56**, **Suppl. 3**, S50–S503.
9. Nova, E., Samartin, S., Gomez, S., Morande, G., and Marcos, A. (2002) The adaptive response of the immune system to the particular malnutrition of eating disorders. *Eur. J. Clin. Nutr.* **56**, **Suppl. 3**, S34–S37.
10. Kastin, D.A. and Buchman, A.L. (2002) Malnutrition and gastrointestinal disease. *Curr. Opin. Clin. Nutr. Metab. Care* **5**, 699–706.
11. Holland, S.M. and Gallin, J.I. (2000) Evaluation of the patient with suspect immunodeficiency, in *Principles and Practice of Infectious Diseases*, (Mandell, G.L., Bennett, J.E., and Dolin, R., eds.) Churchill Livingstone, Philadelphia, PA.
12. Rosen, F.S., Cooper, M.D., and Wedgwood, R.J. (1995) The primary immunodeficiencies. *N. Engl. J. Med.* **333**, 431–440.
13. Shyur, S.D. and Hill, H.R. (1996) Recent advances in the genetics of primary immunodeficiency syndromes. *J. Pediatr.* **129**, 8–24.
14. Cooper, M.D. and Schroeder, H.W.J. (2001) Primary immune deficiency diseases, in *Harrison's Principle of Internal Medicine*, (Braunwald, E., Fauci, A.S., Kasper, D.L., eds.) McGraw-Hill Professional, New York.

2 The Field Assessment of Nutrition

Michael K. Hendricks and Greg Hussey

Contents

Key Points

- Undernutrition contributes globally to more than 50% of deaths among children below the age of 5 yr.
- Nutritional assessment is the cornerstone of comprehensive child health care and should be implemented at all levels of care.
- Clinical, dietary, and anthropometric measurements are the main components of nutritional assessment.
- Different methods are available for assessing dietary intake, and each has its strengths and limitations. All, however, require the use of well-trained and experienced personnel.
- Growth monitoring and the use of clinical signs based on the World Health Organization's (WHO) Integrated Management of Childhood Illness strategy can identify children in need of nutrition intervention, especially at the primary care level.
- Underweight, wasting, and stunting based on the WHO Z-score cutoff values are recommended for screening individuals and populations. They are also useful for monitoring the effectiveness of nutrition interventions.
- Although limited quantitatively, body mass index and skinfold thickness measurements can be used to screen for obesity at both the individual and population level.

From: *Handbook of Nutrition and Immunity*
Edited by: M. E. Gershwin, P. Nestel, and C. L. Keen © Humana Press, Totowa, NJ

- Deuterium dilution, dual energy X-ray absorptiometry, and bioelectrical impedance more accurately determine body composition than equations based on skinfold thickness, but their use is limited in resource-poor settings.
- Biochemical tests are used to assess the micronutrient status of individuals and/or populations. However, some indicators, such as ferritin, zinc, and retinol, are acute phase reactants; thus they may not reflect status in the presence of subclinical or clinical infections.

Introduction

Malnutrition in early childhood interacts synergistically with infectious disease resulting in increased morbidity, mortality, and impaired cognitive development (1). Every year, 10.8 million under-5-yr-old children die in developing countries. Ninety percent of these deaths, which are mainly caused by neonatal disorders, diarrhea, pneumonia, malaria, and HIV/AIDS, occur in 42 countries. Undernutrition contributes to over 50% of childhood deaths, and the risk of mortality is directly associated with the degree of underweight (2). Changes in weight-for-age are significantly associated with changes in child mortality independent of socioeconomic and other health-related changes. Child and under-5 mortality rates could be reduced by 30% and 13%, respectively, with a 5% improvement in weight-for-age by 2005 (2). In both developing and developed countries the prevalence of obesity is increasing. This is significant because obesity leads to an increase in nutrition-related noncommunicable disease and ultimately contributes to high adult mortality rates (3).

Assessing malnutrition—both under and overnutrition—is important at both the individual and population level for developing strategies to improve health. This chapter provides an overview of nutritional assessment and its practical application in children and adolescents.

Assessing Nutritional Status

Nutritional status can be determined clinically, from dietary data, and/or from anthropometric measurements. Indicators of body composition and nutritional biochemistry are also important, but their measurement is not always feasible. Age-related changes in dietary requirements, growth patterns, body composition, and disease epidemiology complicate the nutritional assessment of children.

Medical History (4,5)

A detailed medical history is obtained from the mother/caregiver for all children presenting at a health facility. This includes information about any underlying illness such as diarrhea, nausea and vomiting, intestinal parasites, malaria, cough, symptoms of HIV/AIDS, tuberculosis, or measles, as well as any previous illnesses or exposure to chronic illness such as tuberculosis. The child's immunization status is checked and special attention given to any reported changes in the child's weight and the direction of his or her growth curve on the Road to Health Card. It is important to ask about family circumstances including type of housing, access to water and sanitation, and the availability of cooking fuel as well as maternal age and education, family size, income, and emotional and social support.

Dietary Intake (4,5)

For children under 2 yr old, whether the child is exclusively breastfed or formula fed and whether the child is receiving complementary food is recorded. Where formula or complementary food are used, the type, amount, frequency of feeding, brand, and method of preparation is also noted. For children 2 yr and older, the type, quantity, and frequency of foods and liquids consumed daily are recorded. For all children, appetite, food aversions, and dietary restrictions, as well as the use of any drugs including vitamin and mineral supplements, are noted.

Dietary intake is recorded using a 24-h dietary recall, a food frequency questionnaire, a food record diary, or a dietary history. The strengths and limitations of these methods are shown in Table 1. Data collection requires input from a dietitian or nutritionist trained in the different methods. Irrespective of the method used, the mother/caregiver will provide data for infants and young children, but older children and adolescents must also report what they ate as food is often eaten outside the home.

In a 24-h recall the respondent recalls and provides a detailed description of all food and drink consumed, including cooking methods and brand names (where possible), on the previous day. Food quantities are measured using household measures or food models. Because of day-to-day variation in food intake, a single 24-h recall is not appropriate for assessing the usual food or nutrient intake of individuals. At the population level, it is also not appropriate for young children because there is too much intra- and interindividual variation.

The food frequency questionnaire asks about the frequency (daily, weekly, monthly, or yearly) of consumption of major foods. Quantitative data are not usually provided.

In the food record diary method the respondent records at the time of consumption all the foods and beverages eaten—using household measures or by weighing—over a specified period. The foods eaten are described in detail, as is their method of preparation and cooking.

Table 1
Strengths and Limitations of Dietary Assessment Methods

Method	Strengths	Limitations
24-hour recall	• Relatively easy to administer • Inexpensive • Provides detailed information on foods consumed • Low respondent burden • Can be used in clinical and epidemiological studies • Can be used to quantify nutrient intake • More objective than dietary history	• A single recall may not be representative of usual intake • Under or over reporting possible • Relies on memory and motivation of respondent • Omissions can result in low energy intake estimates • Data entry and analysis is time consuming
Food frequency questionnaire	• Can be self-administered if subjects are iterate • Moderate response burden • Inexpensive • Can be used in epidemiological studies • Can be used to assess associations between diet and disease	• May not represent seasonal foods • Portion sizes not determined • With single listings dietary intake data may be compromised • Cannot use to determine nutrient intake

Food record
- Not memory-dependent
- Provides information about eating habits
- More representative of actual intake
- Reasonably valid up to 5 d

- Requires good cooperation
- High response burden
- Subject must be literate
- Time consuming
- Diet may alter with need to record
- Analysis is expensive and labour intensive

Diet History
- Can detect seasonal changes

- Time consuming
- Skilled interviewers needed
- Difficult and expensive to code
- Can overestimate intake
- Need good cooperation
- Not good for large surveys
- Provides qualitative rather than quantitative data

Source: Adapted from refs. 4, 5

23

The dietary history assesses the individual's dietary intake over a month or year. In addition to a 24-h recall on actual intake, respondents are asked about their general eating pattern, both at meal times and between meals. This includes information on the foods, their frequency of consumption, and usual portion sizes in household measures.

Food consumption data are converted into nutrient intake using food composition tables and reported as percentage of the recommended daily allowances.

Clinical Assessment

The clinical assessment of any child presenting at a health facility is based on the Integrated Management of Childhood Illness strategy. First, the child is checked for general danger signs such as an inability to drink or breastfeed, persistent vomiting, convulsions, lethargy, or loss of consciousness. The presence of any danger sign requires urgent assessment, specific management, and referral to the nearest hospital. After asking about the main problem(s) such as cough or difficulty breathing, diarrhea, fever, or an ear problem, the nutritional status of the child is determined (6).

Physical Examination

Severe wasting over the shoulders, arms, ribs, buttocks, and thighs indicates marasmus, whereas edema over the dorsum of both feet is an early indicator of kwashiorkor (see Chapter 4). Other signs of kwashiorkor include hepatomegaly; changes in the hair, skin, and mucous membranes; apathy; and anemia (see Table 2) (7–9). Children with undernutrition or severe undernutrition (marasmus and kwashiorkor) are at high risk of mortality (10). All children must be examined for clinical signs and symptoms of vitamin A deficiency (see Table 2), fever or hypothermia, and underlying infection such as pneumonia, tuberculosis, and HIV/AIDS (11).

An examination of the conjunctivae and palms for pallor or a finger-prick hemoglobin (Hb) test will identify anemia. Severe palmar pallor or a Hb below 70 g/L indicates severe anemia, while palmar pallor and a Hb below 110 g/L in children 6 mo to 5 yr, below 115 g/L in children 5–11 yr, below 120 g/L in children 12–13 yr and adolescent girls, and below130 g/L in boys 13+ yr indicates anemia (12).

Children's thyroids are checked for visible signs of goiter that may indicate iodine deficiency.

Table 2
Clinical Features of Undernutrition and Micronutrient Deficiency

Parameter	Clinical features
Skin	• Pallor especially palms (anemia from iron or folate deficiency) • Ecchymoses (vitamin K deficiency) • Hypo or hyperpigmentation, desquamation, ulceration (zinc or protein deficiency) • Hyperpigmentation exposed areas (niacin deficiency) • Perifollicular hyperkeratosis (vitamin A deficiency)
Eye	• Night blindness, xerotic conjunctivae, xerotic cornea, Bitot's spots, keratomalacia, corneal scars (vitamin A deficiency) • Conjunctival pallor (anemia from iron or folate deficiency)
Hair	• Depigmentation, easy pluckability, sparsity (kwashiorkor)
Nails	• Koilonychia (iron deficiency)
Mouth	• Cheilosis, glossitis, loss of papillae, magenta tongue (riboflavin deficiency) • Glossitis, scarlet tongue (niacin deficiency) • Bleeding gums (vitamin C deficiency)
Subcutaneous tissue	• Reduced subcutaneous tissue and fat (energy deficiency) • Odema (sodium and potassium disturbances, hypoalbuminemia)
Muscle bulk	• Muscle wasting, weakness (undernutrition)
Bones	• Craniotabes, prominent costochondral junctions, widening of metaphyses (wrists and ankle), frontal bossing, wide anterior fontanelle, rickety rosary, delayed dentition, bow legs (vitamin D deficiency) • Bony tenderness, pseudoparalysis (vitamin C deficiency) • Inadequate bone mass or osteoperosis (calcium)
Abdomen	• Hepatomegaly (kwashiorkor)
Central nervous	• Apathy (kwashiorkor, iron deficiency) system • Peripheral neuropathy (thiamin or pyridoxine deficiency)
Cardiac	• Cardiac failure or enlargement (thiamin deficiency)
Thyroid	• Goiter (iodine deficiency)

Source: Adapted from refs. *7–9.*

Table 3
Advantages and Limitations of Using Anthropometric Measurements

Advantages	Limitations
• Unskilled personnel can be easily trained • Reproducible • Reflects recent or longstanding nutritional changes	• Affected by non-nutritional factors • Does not indicate specific nutrient deficiencies

Anthropometry (4,5,13)

All children presenting at a health facility need to be weighed and their weight plotted on their weight-for-age chart or Road to Health Card. A child is categorised as having good growth (growth curve following the percentile curves), growth faltering or failure (growth curve flat or dropping below the percentile curves), underweight-for-age (weight 60–80% expected weight without edema), kwashiorkor (weight 60–80% expected weight with edema) or marasmus (weight below 60% expected weight without edema).

Anthropometric measures include physical measurements of weight, height, head circumference, mid upper arm circumference, and skin fold thickness that are compared to reference values. The first three assess growth while the latter two can be used to estimate body composition. The strengths and limitations of using these measurements are shown in Table 3. A single measurement generally indicates cumulative growth, while repeated measurements show whether growth is proceeding normally.

Head Circumference

Head and brain growth is maximal during the first two years of life, after which growth is very slow. Head circumference is measured with the infant or child seated on the caregiver's lap. A nonstretchable measuring tape is positioned just above the eyebrows and over the occiput. Measurement is read to the nearest 0.1 cm.

Length or Height (Stature)

Two people are always needed to take length or height measurements. Children below 2 yr of age, or less than 85 cm, are measured in the supine position using a measuring board with a fixed headboard and a moveable footboard that is perpendicular to the headboard. One person positions the child's head against the headboard and aligns the body centrally keeping shoulders and buttocks against the backboard. The head is positioned in the Frankfurt horizontal plane, which is a line joining the lowest point of the margin of the orbit and the tragion (the notch above the tragus) with the face positioned upwards. The other person straightens the legs and brings the footboard up to the heels. Children over 2 yr old, or more than 85 cm tall, are measured standing up using a portable anthropometer, a non-stretchable tape attached to a wall, or a stadiometer. The child stands with the heels together, knees straight, and heels, buttocks, and shoulders touching the vertical surface of the anthropometer, wall, or stadiometer with the head positioned in the Frankfurt plane and arms hanging loosely by the sides. Both length and height are recorded to the nearest 0.1 cm. Length measurements are 0.5–1.5 cm greater than height measurement. If length is measured in children over 2 yr old, or greater than 85 cm tall, it is recommended that that 1 cm be subtracted from the length measurement before comparing it with the reference.

WEIGHT

Ideally, a spring, beam balance, or electronic scale is used to measure weight. Bathroom scales are not accurate and should be avoided. Scales must be calibrated regularly with a known set of weights and always zeroed before weighing the child. Children are weighed naked or with minimal clothing, and care must be taken to ensure the child is not touching any person or surrounding objects while being weighed. Weight is recorded to the nearest 0.1 kg, and plotted on the growth chart.

MID-UPPER-ARM CIRCUMFERENCE (MUAC)

MUAC measurements reflect the amount of subcutaneous fat and muscle, and changes correlate positively with changes in weight. A decrease in MUAC indicates a reduction in one or both of these tissues. MUAC measurements are made using a flexible, nonstretchable tape. Measurement is done with the subject standing erect and the arms hanging by the sides. The midpoint of the upper arm is first located by flexing the right elbow to a 90° angle with the palm facing upward. Using a measuring tape, the observer identifies and marks the midpoint between the lateral tip of the acromion and the distal tip of the olecranon processes. With the arm extended and hanging by the side just away from the trunk with the palm towards the thigh, the tape measure is placed around the arm at the marked midpoint. The tape is pulled snug around the arm and the circumference is recorded to the nearest 0.1 cm.

SKINFOLD THICKNESS

Skinfold thickness measurements can provide an estimate of the amount of subcutaneous fat and total body fat. The commonly used skinfolds include triceps, biceps, subscapular, suprailiac, and midaxillary. Measurements from at least two sites are needed and it is recommended that a limb (for example, triceps) and body (for example, subscapular) skinfold measurement are used as these correlate best with measures of body fat. Lange or Holtain calipers are needed to measure skinfold thickness. To measure triceps skinfold thickness, the subject stands erect with the arms hanging by the side. The midpoint of the upper arm is first identified as for MUAC. A vertical fold of skin and subcutaneous tissue is then picked up between the thumb and index finger 1 cm proximal to the marked midarm level and the tip of the callipers applied perpendicular to the skinfold. The biceps skinfold is measured over the anterior aspect of the arm over the belly of the muscle opposite to the triceps skinfold site. The site for measuring the subscapular skinfold is below the inferior angle of the left scapula along a 45° diagonal to the horizontal plane. With the subject standing erect and the arms relaxed by the side, a pinch of skin and subcutaneous tissue is taken at a point 1 cm above and medial to the site. The suprailiac skinfold is measured above the suprailiac crest in the midaxillary line with the subject standing. The skinfold is picked up obliquely just posterior to the midaxillary line and parallel to the cleavage lines of the skin. The midaxillary skinfold is picked up horizontally in the midaxillary line at the level of the xiphoid process. Three readings are taken at each site and the mean used as the measure. Skinfold thickness are recorded to the nearest 0.5 mm using Lange callipers and 0.2 mm using Holtain callipers.

Use and Interpretation of Anthropometric Indices

The main anthropometric measurements and indices are listed in Table 4.

HEAD CIRCUMFERENCE-FOR-AGE (4)

Chronic undernutrition in early infancy or intrauterine growth retardation may affect brain development and result in a low head circumference. Head circumference-for-age can be used as an indicator of chronic undernutrition in children under 2 yr old. Microcephaly is a head circumference below the third percentile and may be due to a prenatal or perinatal cerebral insult. Macrocephaly is a head circumference above the 97th percentile and may be due to hydrocephalus.

WEIGHT-FOR-AGE, WEIGHT-FOR-HEIGHT, HEIGHT-FOR-AGE (4,13)

The weight or height of an individual is compared against a known reference of the same age or height. The most widely used reference is that of the US National Centre for Health Statistics (CDC/NCHS/WHO). Anthropometric indices are reported using three different systems namely Z-scores, percentiles, or percentage of the median.

The Z-score or standard deviation (SD) unit is the difference between the value for an individual and the median value of the reference population for the same age divided by the SD of the reference population

$$Z\text{-}score = \frac{(observed\ value) - (median\ of\ the\ reference\ population)}{SD\ of\ the\ reference\ population.}$$

The advantage of this index is that the curves are normally distributed and a fixed Z-score interval corresponds to a fixed weight or height difference for children of a given age. Additionally, summary statistics such as means and standard deviations can be calculated for a population.

Percentiles rank individuals according to a reference distribution and are useful in clinical settings because their interpretation is straightforward. They are not, however, useful for assessing the nutritional status of a population because they are not normally distributed and the same percentile interval may correspond to different changes in weight and height according to the part of the distribution concerned.

The percentage of the median is the ratio of an individual's measured value to the median value of the reference population for the same age or height for the specific sex, expressed as a percentage. The percentage of the median can be used to calculate population summary statistics. The main disadvantage is that a fixed point of the distribution may not be uniform across different ages.

Because of the limitations of percentiles and the percentage of the median, the WHO recommends that Z-scores be used; thus, the focus is on these indices.

- Stunting is defined as a height-for-age Z-score below –2 SD and indicates long-term undernutrition. Severe stunting is a Z-score below –3 SD.
- Underweight is defined as a weight-for-age Z-score below –2 SD and may reflect either recent or long-term undernutrition as it is dependent on both attained weight and height. Severe underweight is a Z-score below –3 SD.
- Wasting is defined as weight-for-height Z-score below –2 SD and reflects recent failure to gain weight or loss of weight. Severe underweight is a Z-score below –3 SD.

Although the CDC/NCHS/WHO growth reference is widely used and recommended, four technical issues limit its use (13,15,16). First, the growth reference was developed from two different data sets. The longitudinal weights and lengths of formula fed children from the Fels Research Institute Longitudinal Study were used for children under 2 yr old, while data from three representative surveys that included standing heights were used for children over 2 yr old. Because length measurements are greater than those for height for a given child, a discrepancy exists before and after 2 yr of age. Also, the children in the Fel's study were taller than those in the three surveys. The use

Table 4

Anthropometric Measurements and Indicators Used in Nutritional Assessment

Measurement	Indicators and indices	Age groups	Usefulness	Disadvantages	Explanation
Weight	Underweight: Wt/age Z-score <−2 SD	All	• Basic measure of nutrition status • Only when related to age or height • Trends over time better than a single measure • Used for growth monitoring	• Need accurate scales and age • Related to height and weight-for-height	• Underweight reflects acute and chronic undernutrition
Height	Stunting: Ht/age Z-score <−2 SD	All	• Related to long-term nutritional status • Serial measures more useful than a single measure	• Influenced by non-nutrition factors, for example, genetic and hormonal factors	• Stunting reflects long-term changes in nutritional status
Weight-for-height (wt/ht)	Wasting: Wt/ht Z-score <−2 SD	Girls ≤137 cm Boys ≤145 cm	• Age independent • Index of body proportion • Can be used in epidemiological surveys	• Not easy to calculate by hand	• Wasting reflects acute under-nutrition

Measure	Cut-off values	Age group	Advantages	Disadvantages
Head circumference	Microcephaly: <3rd percentile Macrocephaly: >97th percentile	0–2 years	• Simple to measure	• Affected by non-nutrition factors • Not useful for assessing nutrition status • May reflect intrauterine growth restriction and/or early childhood undernutrition
Mid upper arm circumference-for-age	Moderate wasting: Z-score <−2 SD Severe wasting: Z score <−3 SD	All	• Simple • Can use in rapid surveys	• No limits for over-nutrition • No standards for adults • Small errors have big implications • Proxy for weight-for-height
Body mass index (BMI)	Thinness <5th percentile Overweight ≥85th percentile Obesity ≥85th percentile BMI and ≥90th percentile skinfold thickness	Older children Adolescents Adults	• Requires simple measurements • Can be used in epidemiological surveys	• Cannot use in younger children because varies with age • Does not differentiate fat from lean body mass • Not easy to calculate by hand • Indirect measure of body composition

Source: Adapted from refs. 7, 14.

of this reference standard can underestimate height status in children under 24 mo old and overestimate that in children over 24 mo old. Second, in population-based studies the 24-mo disjunction can result in variations in the prevalence of low weight-for-age when the nutritional status of children with a range of ages is assessed. Third, the weight-for-age curves are skewed toward the high end, which can result in misclassifying overweight children as normally nourished children. Fourth, the growth pattern of infants living under optimal conditions and fed according to the WHO recommendations differs from that of the CDC/NCHS/WHO reference population.

The limitations of the CDC/NCHS/WHO growth reference can lead to misinterpretation of growth patterns and result in the too early introduction of complementary food to infants who should be exclusively breastfed. This can adversely affect the health and nutritional status of these infants especially in poor communities. An international growth reference based on a representative, geographically diverse population of healthy children from birth to adolescence, who have no constraints on their growth is currently being developed *(17)*.

MUAC *(4,18)*

MUAC increases by about 2 cm between 6 and 59 mo of age. There are also sex specific differences for children below 24 mo of age. A combined MUAC-for-age reference using the US National Health and Examination Surveys has been developed, which can be used in determining the MUAC Z-scores for age. A MUAC Z-score below –2 SD can be used as a proxy for low weight-for-height (wasting) while a Z-score below –3 SD reflects severe wasting.

BODY MASS INDEX (BMI) *(4,8,13)*

BMI is an indirect measure of body composition and is calculated by dividing weight in kg by height in m². Because it is correlated with both lean mass and fat mass, BMI does not distinguish between the two. Cutoff values are available for children in determining overweight and obesity and these are discussed in more detail below.

Application of Anthropometry

NEWBORN INFANTS *(13)*

Intrauterine growth restriction (IUGR) is not easy to measure and birth weight is often used as a proxy. However, birth weight is affected by intrauterine growth and gestation duration. WHO uses weight-for-gestational age at birth to categorize newborn infants as small-for-gestational age (SGA), appropriate-for-gestational age (AGA), or large-for-gestational age (LGA). Using an appropriate sex-specific international reference, SGA is defined as a birth weight below the 10th percentile, AGA a birth weight between the 10th and 90th percentiles, and LGA a birth weight above the 90th percentile.

SGA is not necessarily the same as IUGR because some SGA infants fall in the lower tail of the normal fetal growth distribution curve. Classification of an infant as IUGR should be based on a specific cutoff for SGA. Generally, the greater the prevalence of SGA the more likely this is as result of IUGR. For population-based studies, low birth weight (LBW) (below 2500 g), which can be measured with good precision and validity, is used as a proxy for SGA.

The criteria defining newborn nutrition as being of public health significance and warranting intervention are a SGA rate greater than 20%, LBW rate above 15%, and a very low LBW rate above 2%.

Fetal growth restriction can be further classified as symmetric or stunted, in which all body dimensions are proportionally small, or asymmetric or wasted, in which the fetus has a low ponderal index or BMI owing to a lack of fat and sometimes lean tissue. Symmetric growth restriction may reflect undernutrition throughout pregnancy while asymmetric growth restriction results from inadequate nutrition late in pregnancy when fat deposition is most rapid. Disproportionate IUGR infants tend to be more severely growth retarded and at greater risk of mortality.

INFANTS AND CHILDREN *(13,19)*

Anthropometry is used for both individual and population-based nutritional screening and for program monitoring and evaluation.

The use of anthropometry to screen and monitor the nutritional status of individual infants and children is shown in Table 5. Primary health care or community-based growth monitoring and promotion (GMP) programs track changes in a child's physical development, by regular weighing and sometimes measurement of length, to identify infants and children in need of health and nutrition interventions. The essential components in a GMP program include taking preventive action before undernutrition occurs; effective communication with the mother/caregiver to change behavior; and taking cognizance of the health, nutrition, environmental and social factors that influence each child's growth. GMP is a component of primary health care and is linked to health interventions such as breastfeeding promotion and support, timing and selection of complementary feeding, identification of underlying disease such as tuberculosis and HIV/AIDS, and treatment of disease such as diarrhea and respiratory tract infections. Adequate weight gain is the main indicator for effective GMP but, where possible, attained weight-for-age, height-for-age, and weight-for-height should be assessed.

Table 5

The Use of Anthropometry in Screening and Monitoring Responses to Interventions in Individual Infants and Children

Target group and setting	Recommended measurements	Indices for screening	Cut-offs	Indices for monitoring response to interventions	Criteria
Infants and children with poor growth who need support through: • Breastfeeding • Counseling • Prevention and treatment of disease, e.g., diarrhea	Children under 5 yr attending primary health care centers for growth monitoring	• Weight • Age • Gender • If possible, height/length every 3 mo	Deviation from weight-for-age curve Attained: • Wt/age • Ht/age • Wt/ht	• Direction of curve • Z-scores <–2 SD • No growth >2 visits • <3rd centile on growth chart	Wt/age curve Attained: • Wt/age • Ht/age • Wt/ht	• Direction of curve • Positive Z-score trend
Selection of infants and children for supplementary feeding	Children <5 years attending growth monitoring	• Weight • Height/length • MUAC • Age • Gender	• Wt/ht • MUAC/age	• <–2 SD wt/ht or MUAC/age	Wt/age curve Attained: • Wt/age • Wt/ht	• Direction of curve • Positive Z-score trend
Selection of infants and children for therapeutic feeding	• Attendees at nutrition rehabilitation centers	• Clinical signs of severe under-nutrition	• Wt/ht • MUAC/age • Clinical signs of severe	• Clinical signs • <–3 SD wt/ht or MUAC/age	Wt/age curve Attained: • Wt/age • Wt/ht	Z-score >–2SD wt/ht

Population group	Setting	Measurements	Indicators	Criteria	Indices for change	Desired outcome
	• or hospitals • Children in refugee camps or emergency settings	• Weight • Height/length • MUAC • Age	under-nutrition			• Clinical signs
Infants and children with organic disease or failure to thrive	Children attending: • Paediatric clinics • Hospitals	• Weight • Height/length • Age • Gender	Deviation of curves of: • Wt/age • Ht/age Change in: • Wt/ht	• Direction of curve • Z-scores <−2 SD • No growth >2 visits	• Wt/age • Ht/age Change in: • Wt/age • Ht/age • Wt/ht	• Satisfactory growth pattern
Overweight infants and children	Children attending: • Special clinics • Hospitals • Schools	• Weight • Height/length • Skinfold • Age • Gender	• Wt/ht • Skinfold	• Wt/ht >2+ Z-scores	• Wt/ht • Skinfold measures	• Reduction wt/ht Z-score

Source: Adapted from ref. 13.

Weight-for-height and MUAC-for-age are useful indicators for screening children for enrollment into a supplementary program as these indices predict benefits from the intervention. The identification of severely undernourished children for therapeutic feeding is based on indices of severe wasting, (weight-for-height below –3 Z-scores), clinical signs of severe undernutrition, or low MUAC-for-age. Weight-for-age, weight-for-height, and clinical signs of severe undernutrition can also be used to monitor the response to supplementary feeding.

When a child fails-to-thrive, because of organic reasons, both the screening for and response to the intervention is based on weight and height indicators as well as serial measurements of growth. Weight-for-height can also be used to screen for overweight, using a cutoff value of +2 Z-scores and monitoring the reduction in weight-for-height or weight-for-age.

In assessing the prevalence of undernutrition in communities, and the response to interventions, a representative sample must be selected to enable comparisons to be made between populations. The nature of the intervention determines which indicators to use, as shown in Table 6. For example, height-for-age reflects cumulative growth, long-term nutrition, socioeconomic status, and overall health and development of communities and can be used to measure the response to an intervention. The WHO has proposed prevalence ranges for wasting, underweight, and stunting that define the extent to which undernutrition is a public health problem (*see* Table 7).

ADOLESCENTS *(13,20)*

The nutritional status of an individual or a population of adolescents can be assessed using height-for-age based on the NCHS/WHO reference, BMI-for-age, and subscapular or triceps skinfold thickness (*see* Table 8). For BMI, the reference data published by Must et al. *(20)* are recommended because the percentiles have been smoothed mathematically across age groups. Maturational status with age-specific means and medians adjusted for rates of maturation in relation to the reference population need to be factored in when assessing growth of adolescents *(13)*.

Body Composition (21–25)

Body composition is defined as the ratio of fat to fat-free mass and is usually expressed as the percentage of body fat. Measuring body composition in children is important for quantifying the prevalence of childhood obesity, determining fluid and energy requirements (linked to fat-free mass) in sick children requiring hospitalization, and to assess and treat growth disorders.

Two models have been proposed for measuring body composition. The two-component model, in which the body is divided into fat mass (adipose tissue)

Table 6
The Use of Anthropometry in Screening
and Monitoring Responses to Interventions in Populations of Infants and Children

	Target group and setting	Recommended measurements	Indices for screening	Cut-offs	Indices for monitoring response to interventions	Criteria
Infants and children in need of targeted interventions, e.g., breastfeeding support, supplementation of mothers, etc.	Nutrition surveys of representative sample of children under 5 yr in need of intervention	• Weight • Height/length • Age • Gender • One measurement	• Wt/age • Ht/age • Wt/ht	• Prevalence <−2 Z-scores • Difference in mean Z-scores	• Wt/age • Ht/age • Wt/ht	Significant difference in growth velocity, e.g., between intervention and control groups
Determining the severity of a disaster or emergency and the need for food aid	Rapid assessment surveys	• Weight • Height • MUAC • Clinical signs of severe undernutrition	• Wt/ht • MUAC/age (children 1–5 yr) • Clinical signs of severe undernutrition	• Prevalence <−2 Z-scores • Difference in mean Z-scores	• Wt/ht • Clinical signs of severe undernutrition	Reduction in prevalence of wasting using cutoffs for wt/ht and MUAC
Areas for targeting interventions in reducing food and fat consumption	Representative surveys	• Weight • Height/length • Height/length • Age • Gender • One measurement	• Wt/ht	• Prevalence >2+ Z-scores	• Wt/ht	Reduction in prevalence of wt/ht Z-score >+2 SD

Source: Adapted from ref. 13.

Table 7
Severity Index in Children Under 5 yr Based
on Indices for Wasting, Stunting and Underweight, and Mean wt/ht Z-Score

| Prevalence | Prevalence (% children below –2 SD Z-scores) | | |
	Stunting	Underweight	Wasting
Low/Acceptable	<20	<10	<5
Medium/Poor	20–29	10–19	5–9
High/Serious	30–39	20–29	10–14
Very high/Critical	≥40	≥30	≥5
			Mean wt/ht Z-score
Acceptable	—	—	–0.40
Poor	—	—	–0.40 to –0.69
Serious	—	—	–0.70 to –0.99
Critical	—	—	≤–1.00

Source: Ref. 13.

Table 8
Recommended Cutoff Values for Anthropometric Indices in Adolescents

Indicator	Anthropometric variable	Cut-off value
Stunting	Height-for-age	<3rd percentile or <–2 Z-score
Thinness or low BMI-for-age	BMI-for-age	<5th percentile
At risk of overweight	BMI-for-age	≥85th percentile
Obese	BMI-for-age	≥85th percentile
	Triceps skinfold-for-age	≥90th percentile
	Subscapular skinfold-for-age	≥90th percentile

Source: Ref. 13.

and fat-free mass (muscle, bone, water, and tissues devoid of fat/lipid), and the four-component model, in which the body comprises water, protein, mineral, and fat. The different methods for assessing body composition and their advantages and limitations are outlined in Table 9. Skinfold thickness, BMI and densitometry, bioelectrical impedance, and total body electrical conductivity measure body composition based on the two-component model. Neutron activation analysis, isotope dilution, and dual-energy X-ray absorptiometry measure body composition based on the four-component model, but can also be used to measure fat mass and fat-free mass.

Skinfold thickness measurements can be used to quantify the percent body fat using equations. However, because of inaccuracies in the equations, this method may underestimate fatness in children.

Densitometry measures the body density through hydrostatic or underwater weighing. It is based on Archimedes principle whereby the volume of a submerged object is equal to the volume of the water displaced. An individual's density is determined from the mass and volume measurements, after which it is used to calculate the percent body fat and fat free mass (FFM). Because the densities of fat and fat-free mass are assumed constant, the proportion of these compartments can be calculated using a known value for body density. This technique, however, has limited value in children because it is not always safe to submerge children in water.

Total body water (TBW) can be measured indirectly by dilution using a tracer substance given either orally or parentally that disperses uniformly throughout the water space. Isotopes of hydrogen such as deuterium or tritium and oxygen (^{18}O) are used. Tritium cannot be used in children and women of reproductive age because of its radioactivity; whereas deuterium and ^{18}O are stable and are ideal. The concentration of the tracer in a sample of the subject's blood, urine, or saliva is analyzed and TBW is measured using a formula. Disease states can alter the total body water resulting in inaccuracies in the estimation of the fat-free mass.

More than 90% of potassium in the body is in the fat-free mass; thus, fat-free mass can be estimated from the total amount of body potassium obtained from a whole body counter. This, however, assumes that the fat-free mass contains a constant amount of potassium.

Neutron activation analysis can estimate the body's content of sodium, chloride, phosphorous, carbon, and nitrogen. A beam of neutrons is delivered to the subject, which interacts with the specific elements and emits gamma radiation that is picked up by detectors. Measurements of total body nitrogen and carbon can be used to determine the total amount of body protein and fat, respectively. Bone mineral content can be determined through the measurement of total body calcium.

Fat-free mass has a better electrical conductivity than fat because of the higher concentration of electrolytes, which are capable of conducting electricity. In bioelectrical impedance analysis (BIA) an electronic instrument generates an alternating current, which is passed through the body and a measurement of the resistance (impedance) to the current is used to calculate TBW, fat-free mass, and percent body fat. BIA equations were previously based on the two-component model. Recently, using a multicomponent model, sex-specific and race-combined BIA equations using pooled data from white and black subjects between 12 and 94 yr old from different centers were developed. The equations were validated and cross-validated for TBW and FFM and found to have good precision and accuracy. The equations were more valid for white people than black people, where they tended to under predict TBW and FFM. The authors advise caution when applying the equations to children between

Table 9
Strengths and Limitations of Body Composition Methods

Method	Strengths	Limitations
Skinfold thickness	• Inexpensive • Quick • Measures correlate well with underwater weighing	• Interindividual variation in skinfold compressibility • Variation in the contribution of skin to skinfold thickness measurement • Variation in subcutaneous skinfold thickness between sites • Subcutaneous fat may not correlate with internal fat
Densitometry	• Standard procedure for determining body density and percent fat	• Skilled measurers required • Cannot be used for large studies • Dependent on subject cooperation • Requires special equipment • Requires experience • Assumes constant density of fat-free mass
Isotope dilution	• Isotopes of deuterium and oxygen are stable and safe to use	• Cost of the equipment • Time-consuming • Radioactivity of tritium limits its use in children and women of reproductive age • Water content in fat-free tissue can vary especially in fat subjects

Method	Advantages	Disadvantages
Total body potassium	• Good precision	• Expensive • Overestimation of fat content in the obese
Neutron activation analysis	• Good precision • Noninvasive • Not based on fixed ratios of body compartments	• Exposure to ionizing radiation • Expensive • Requires skilled operators • Units not mobile
Bioelectrical impedance	• Good precision for calculations of total body water • Safe and non-invasive • Portable • Quick	• Assumes normal hydration • Expensive
Dual-energy X-ray absorptiometry	• Low radiation dose • Quick (20–20 min) • Requires little cooperation • Results correlate well with other methods	• Affected by hydration status • Results affected by part being scanned

Source: Refs. *5, 8, 22.*

41

12 yr and maturity as maturational development could influence the results. Despite this, the equations have been recommended for use in large epidemiological studies that describe normal levels of body composition.

Dual-energy X-ray absorptiometry (DEXA) is useful for measuring fat and lean tissue. Estimates of percent body fat using DEXA correlate well with those of underwater weighing.

The two-component model relies on the assumption that properties such as hydration and density of FFM are constant. However, FFM can vary between individuals of the same age and sex, with age and in disease states involving overhydration, underhydration, muscle wasting, mineral loss, or edema. All of these can reduce the validity of the measurements. Inter individual variations can be overcome by using appropriate reference values or techniques such as isotope dilution, which provides a more accurate assessment of body composition based on the two-component model. The use of multicomponent models of body composition, which quantify the sources of variability, may be more appropriate in disease states than two-component models.

Another shortcoming in reporting body composition relates to fat mass (FM) expressed as a percentage of body weight when no adjustment is made for FFM based on size. Percent body fat is dependent on both FM and FFM. Individuals who differ in percent fat may do so because they have differences in FM, but identical FFM or because they have the same FM but differences in FFM. Similarly, disease states may modify FM and FFM and these changes will not be detected in the individual using percent body fat. It is recommended that FM and FFM are normalized for height dividing by height squared and that age- and sex-specific reference data are developed. Body composition can be used to evaluate the prevalence of obesity and to monitor interventions.

Nutritional Biochemistry (4,5,26,27)

Laboratory investigations are not routinely used to assess nutritional status because of the absence of a single laboratory test or a group of tests or indicators that can be used reliably to measure nutritional status. Moreover, the equipment required for most of laboratory tests is not readily available in situations where they are most needed and where undernutrition is common. Nevertheless, biochemical markers are important in some situations and should be regarded as an adjuvant tool to clinical assessment, anthropometric measurement, and dietary intake assessment that are currently regarded as the best methods for assessing overall nutritional status. Table 10 summarises the usefulness of some laboratory tests that can be used in nutritional assessment.

Nutritional biochemistry can be conveniently and arbitrarily divided into static and functional tests. Static tests are a direct measurement of a nutrient or related metabolite in the blood or other body fluids. However, blood levels

Table 10

Usefulness of Selected Laboratory Tests for the Assessment of Nutritional Status

Nutrient	Test	Usefulness	Availability*	Comments
Protein	Serum protein and albumin	Poor	Available	Reduced in liver and renal disease
	Transferrin and transthyretin	Good	Limited	Reduced in infections
	Nitrogen balance	Good	Research tool	
Vitamin A	Serum retinol	Poor	Limited	Reduced with acute phase response
	Retinol binding protein	Poor	Limited	
Vitamin D	Plasma calcium and phosphate	Good	Available	May be first sign of deficiency
	25 OH Vitamin D	Good	Limited	
	1,25 Di OH Vitamin D	Good	Limited	
Folate	Serum folate	Good	Available	Reflects recent uptake
	Red cell folate	Good	Available	Reflects whole body status
Iron	Serum ferritin	Good	Available	Reduced with acute phase response
	Bone marrow iron	Good	Limited	
	Serum iron and total iron binding capacity	Poor	Available	Reduced with acute phase response
Zinc	Plasma zinc	Good	Available	Increased with acute infections
	Plasma alkaline phosphatase	Poor	Available	
Copper	Plasma copper	Good	Limited	
Iodine	Thyroid function tests	Good	Limited	

Adapted from refs. 26 and 27.

*Most of these tests are not available in primary care situations and will generally be available in regional hospitals. However, in many developing countries they may only be available in specialist centres.

43

frequently do not reflect true tissue stores. For example, albumin and calcium declines late in the course of protein deficiency or rickets, respectively. Other factors also influence test results including the presence of fever owing to acute and chronic infections, concomitant medical conditions, general nutritional status, interaction with drugs, sample collection procedures, and the assay used. Examples of static tests include measurement of serum albumin, calcium, potassium, vitamin A, ferritin.

Functional or indirect tests measure a specific physiological or biochemical reaction. These tests are less affected by recent changes in food and fluid intake. However, they are usually influenced by a number of nutrient abnormalities. Functional tests include dark adaptation to measure vitamin A status and immunological tests.

In general, nutritional biochemistry is used at the individual level: to assess macro and micronutrient status; as a prognostic indicator for morbidity and mortality; to identify specific metabolic abnormalities frequently associated with systemic disorders; and to monitor specific therapeutic interventions. At a population level, nutritional biochemistry is used to screen for micronutrient deficiencies such as vitamin A and iron and to monitor specific population-based interventions.

Whereas laboratory tests for nutritional biochemistry may not be practical in most situations, other laboratory tests are extremely useful for excluding a chronic infection such as tuberculosis, HIV, or parasitic infestation in children who are failing to thrive. These tests are also useful as a diagnostic aid to exclude hypoglycemia in a sick infant or child who presents with convulsions (finger-prick dextrostix); identify children with severe anemia (finger-prick hemoglobin); and exclude urinary tract infections in febrile undernourished children (dipsticks).

Conclusion

Nutritional assessment is the cornerstone in comprehensive child health care. The presence of general danger signs or signs of severe undernutrition (severe wasting and bipedal edema) and severe anemia (severe palmar pallor) can be used at the primary care level to determine whether children need referral for hospitalization. At a population level, clinical signs of undernutrition and micronutrient deficiencies need to be supported by anthropometric and biochemical data when deciding about nutrition interventions.

The most useful anthropometric indices are weight-for-age, height-for-age, and weight-for-height that indicate underweight, stunting, and wasting, respectively. Fixed cutoff values exist for each indicator and they can be used for screening as well as monitoring the effect of interventions. WHO recommends the three indices are presented as Z-scores in epidemiological surveys because this allows summary statistics to be computed. MUAC too reflects acute undernutrition and is particularly useful in rapid surveys. Age- and sex-specific graphs or tables rather than fixed cutoff values should be used to assess undernutrition using MUAC.

The CDC/NCHS/WHO growth reference is widely used although it has limitations. A new growth reference is being developed by WHO that will reflect the growth of children from diverse geographical and cultural backgrounds fed according to the WHO feeding recommendations.

BMI-for-age and triceps and subscapular skinfold thickness percentiles can be used to screen for obesity, although there are limitations in measuring fat mass in quantitative terms. Measurements of body composition using deuterium dilution and DEXA are more accurate. The accuracy and precision of techniques such as bioelectrical impedance has been improved using revised equations, and have been recommended for epidemiological studies. However, cost needs to be considered before such techniques can be recommended widely for epidemiological use.

Nutritional biochemistry can be used at the individual and population level to determine nutrition and micronutrient deficiencies. Static tests that measure concentrations of serum retinol, zinc, calcium, and albumin, for example, do not necessarily reflect tissue stores because they are acute phase reactants and respond to underlying infection. There are, however, other tests that have practical importance such as finger-prick dextrostix or hemoglobin. Ideally, biochemical investigations should serve as an adjuvant in the clinical and anthropometric assessment of children and adolescents.

References

1. Pelletier, D.L. and Frongillo, E.A. (2003) Changes in child survival are strongly associated with changes in malnutrition in developing countries. *J. Nutr.* **133**, 107–109.
2. Black, R.E., Morris, S.S., and Bryce. J. (2003) Where and why are 10 million children dying every year? *Lancet* **361**, 2226–2234.
3. Popkin, B. (2002) An overview of the nutrition transition and its implications: the Bellagio meeting. Pub Hlth Nutr **5**, 93–103.
4. Gibson, R.S. (1990) *Principles of Nutritional Assessment.* Oxford University Press, New York.
5. Lee, R.D. and Nieman, D.C. (1996) *Nutritional Assessment.* 2nd Ed. Library of Congress Cataloging in Publication Data, Mosby, St. Louis, MI.
6. World Health Organization: Division of Child Health and Development/UNICEF. Integrated Management of Childhood Illness: sick child age 2 months to 5 years. South African IMCI guideline chartbooklet, 2002.

7. McLaren, D. and Burman, D. (1982) *Textbook of Paediatric Nutrition.* 2nd ed., Churchill Livingstone, New York.
8. Khoshoo, V. (1997) Nutritional assessment in children and adolescents. *Curr. Opin. Pediat.* **9**, 502–507.
9. Wittenberg, D.F. and Hansen, J.D.L. (1998) Nutritional disorders in *Paediatrics and Child Health: A Manual for Health Professionals in the Third World,* 4th ed. (Coovadia, H.M. and Wittenberg, D.F, eds.), Oxford University Press, Cape Town, South Africa.
10. Bern, C., Zucker, J.R., Perkins, B.A., Otieno, J., Oloo, A.J., and Yip, R. (1997) Assessment of potential indicators for protein-energy malnutrition in the algorithm for integrated management of childhood illness. *Bull. World Htlh. Organ.* **75(suppl. 1)**, 87–96.
11. World Health Organization. Management of severe malnutrition: a manual for physicians and other senior health workers. Geneva, Switzerland, WHO, 1999.
12. United Nations Children's Fund, United Nations University, World Health Organization. Iron deficiency anemia: assessment, prevention, and control. A guide for program managers. Geneva, Switzerland, WHO, 2001 (WHO/NHD/01.3).
13. World Health Organization. The use and interpretation of anthropometry; report of the WHO expert committee on physical status. Geneva, Switzerland, WHO, 1995. (WHO Tech. Rep. Series, 854).
14. Poskitt, E.M.E. (1988) Practical paediatric nutrition. Butterworth, London, U.K.
15. De Onis, and Habicht, J.P. (1996) Anthropometric reference data for international use: recommendations from a World Health Organization Expert Committee. *Am. J. Clin. Nutr.* **64**, 650–658.
16. World Health Organization Working group on infant growth: the use and interpretation of anthropometry in infants. (1995) *Bull. World Hlth. Organ.* **73**, 165–174.
17. De Onis, M., Garza, C., and Habicht, J.P. (1997) Time for a new growth reference. *Pediatr.* **100**, E8.
18. De Onis, M., Yip, R., and Mei, Z. (1997) The development of MUAC-for-age reference data recommended by WHO Expert Committee. *Bull. World Hlth. Organ.* **75**, 11–18.
19. Beaton, G., Kelly, A., Kevany, J., Martorell, R., and Mason, J. (1990) Appropriate uses of anthropometric indices in children. Nutrition Policy Discussion Paper, No. 7. Geneva, Switzerland, United Nations ACC/SCN.
20. Must, A., Dallal, G.E., and Dietz, W. (1991) Reference data for obesity: 85th and 95th percentiles of body mass index (wt/ht^2) and triceps skinfold thickness. *Am. J. Clin. Nutr.* **53**, 839–846.
21. Wells, J.C.K., Fuller, N.J., Dewit, O., Fewtrell, M.S., Elia, M., and Cole, T.J. (1999) Four-component model of body composition in children: density and hydration of fat-free mass and comparison with simpler models. *Am. J. Clin. Nutr.* **69**, 904–112.
22. Deurenberg, P., Pieters, J.J.L., and Hautvast, J.G.A. (1990) The assessment of body fat percentage by skinfold thickness measurements in childhood and adolescence. *Br J Nutr* **63**, 293–303.

23. Lukaski, H.C. (1987) Methods for assessment of human body composition: traditional and new. Am J Clin Nutr **46**, 537–556.
24. Sun, S.S., Chumlea, W.C., Heymsfield, S.B., Lukasi, H.C., Schoeller, D., et al. (2003) Development of bioelectrical impedance analysis prediction equations for body composition with the use of multicomponent model for use in epidemiologic surveys. *Am. J. Clin. Nutr.* **77**, 331–340.
25. Wells, J.C.K. (2001) A critique of the expression of paediatric body composition. *Arch. Dis. Child* **85, 67–72.**
26. Gidden, F. and Shenkin, A. (2000) Laboratory support for the clinical nutrition service. *Clin. Chem. Lab. Med.* **38**, 693–714.
27. Selberg, O. and Sel, S. (2001) The adjunctive value of routine biochemistry in nutritional assessment of hospitalised patients. *Clin. Nutr.* **20**, 477–485.

3 The Pregnant and Lactating Woman

RACHEL GITAU AND SUZANNE FILTEAU

CONTENTS

KEY POINTS

- Nutritional and immune status during pregnancy and lactation affect the health of both mother and child.
- The postpartum period is an especially vulnerable, but frequently overlooked, time.
- Assessment of nutritional and immune status in pregnant and lactating women differs from other adults:
  - Higher requirements of some nutrients.
  - Altered immunity during pregnancy to prevent rejection of the fetus.
  - Need to account for the weight gain and hemodilution of pregnancy.
  - Additional biological samples are available: placenta, cord blood, and breast milk.
- Nutritional status affects immune function, and immune activation can complicate the assessment of nutritional status.
- Micronutrients of particular concern during pregnancy and lactation are iron, zinc, iodine, and vitamins A, C, D, and E.
- Neopterin and acute phase proteins are useful nonspecific measures of immune system activation.

From: *Handbook of Nutrition and Immunity*
Edited by: M. E. Gershwin, P. Nestel, and C. L. Keen © Humana Press, Totowa, NJ

- Subclinical mastitis, defined as raised breast milk sodium, is a nonspecific indicator of morbidity unique to the lactating woman.
- Low technology methods for measuring some aspects of nutritional status have been standardized across laboratories and correlated with both high technology methods and with maternal and infant health outcomes, but similar validation is less available for measures of immune status.

Introduction

During pregnancy and lactation, a woman's nutritional and immune status affects both her own health and that of her child. This chapter considers how the assessment of nutritional and immune status in pregnant and lactating women differs from other adults, and how adjustments often need to be made (e.g., the effect of pregnancy on plasma retinol and α-tocopherol). Suggestions on collecting and utilizing the additional biological samples available—placenta, cord blood, and breast milk—are made. The micronutrients of particular concern during pregnancy and lactation are focused on, and techniques for assessing these and for evaluating immune function are suggested. An overview is provided on subclinical mastitis, and its role as a nonspecific indicator of morbidity unique to the lactating woman.

Nutrition and Immunology During Pregnancy and Postpartum

The health and nutrition of pregnant and lactating women have always been a matter of concern. Besides affecting her own health, a woman's nutritional status and immune function affects the growth and health of her offspring during pregnancy through the placenta and during lactation by delivery of energy, nutrients, and immune factors through breast milk. The assessment of maternal nutritional status is an essential component of prenatal care (1). Several nutrients are required in increased amounts during gestation, but the magnitude of the increase varies from nutrient to nutrient (2). Lactation is more nutritionally demanding for a woman than pregnancy; and it is also a vulnerable time for her infant.

The pregnant woman has an altered immune status that provides a favorable environment not only for fetal growth but also for the emergence of certain infections, for example, malaria. Malaria infection is of particular risk to primigravid women, predisposing them to maternal anemia and low birth weight infants (3). As a consequence of delivery practices, morbidity and mortality are more common postpartum than during pregnancy/parturition (4), but postpartum women typically receive less care than during their pregnancy/parturition. Lactating women are also at risk of local infections in the mammary gland.

In addition to their independent importance for maternal health, nutrition and immunity interact and this too can be important. Adequate nutritional status is necessary for optimal immune function. Measuring aspects of the immune system and its active state can help interpret serum concentrations of the micronutrients that are affected by acute phase responses *(5)*.

Many of the analyses of nutritional status and immune function for pregnant and lactating women are similar to those for other adults. However, adjustments often need to be made for weight gain and hemodilution during pregnancy. The availability of biological samples specific to reproduction— placenta, cord blood, and breast milk—broadens the range of potential investigations.

Sample Collection for Investigations in Pregnant and Lactating Women
Blood Samples

Venepuncture blood collection is well defined and is the standard for most studies. For some analytes the type of anticoagulant, if any, is important (*see* Table 1). Venous blood collection is unacceptable in some populations and alternatives are important. Capillary blood is increasingly being used as laboratory assays requiring smaller volumes of sample become available. Capillary blood collection from, for example, finger-prick samples may be more practical in difficult field conditions and can be done by minimally trained nonclinical personnel. A capillary blood sample from a finger-prick can be collected into an appropriate tube, or a drop can be spotted onto filter paper and dried. Many analytes are stable at ambient temperature in such blood spots and filter papers can be easily sent, even by post, to a distant laboratory for analysis. However, both collection of finger-prick blood, which may include variable amounts of extracellular fluid depending on the collection technique, and spotting onto filter paper where spreading of the sample is not completely uniform, tend to increase the variability of analyses from these samples *(6)*. Consequently, blood spots are most useful for qualitative analyses, such as the presence or absence of a specific antibody, or semiquantitative analyses where large differences are expected between normal and abnormal levels, for example, thyroid stimulating hormone.

Cord blood can be collected using a needle and syringe from the cord artery or vein after delivery. Cord blood samples are more associated with the infant's circulation than the mother, although there is a high correlation between many analytes in maternal and cord blood, for example, micronutrients *(7)*. Thus, information can be gained without invasive blood sampling of either the mother or the neonate. Dried blood spot samples can also be prepared from cord blood.

Placenta

A placenta can be collected noninvasively at delivery. Placental histology is considered the most sensitive method for the diagnosis of malaria in pregnancy

Table 1
Characteristics of Micronutrient and Immune Activity Tests and Normal Concentrations in Pregnancy and Lactation

Test	Sample and collection tube	Storage requirements and stability	Assay	Normal levels in pregnancy and lactation
Hemoglobin	Whole venous or capillary blood	Fresh whole blood, before clotting; do not freeze	Cyanmethemoglobin Hemocue	>105 g/L (pregnancy) >120 g/L (lactation)
Ferritin	Serum or heparin plasma	Store frozen <−20°C, approx 6 mo	ELISA	>20 µg/L
Retinol[a]	Serum or heparin plasma	Store frozen −70°C, >7 yr in plasma; protect from light	HPLC for retinol and modified relative dose response; retinol binding protein by ELISA, RIA	>1.05 µmol/L (plasma)
Breast milk				>1.05 µmol/L or 8 µg/g fat (milk)
α-tocopherol[a]	Serum or heparin plasma	Store frozen −70°C, approx 6 mo; protect from light	HPLC	>11.6 µmol/L >2.2 µmol/mmol cholesterol (lactation) (pregnancy may be higher)
Iodine	Serum or heparin plasma Urine (20 mL univeral tube)	Store frozen <−20°C, 1 mo (hormones); iodine indefinitely	Thyroxine, thyroid stimulating hormone by ELISA, RIA Urine Iodine by spectrophometry	>50 µg I/g creatinine (lactation) (pregnancy urine I may be higher)

	Sample	Storage	Method	Reference value
Vitamin D	Serum or plasma (EDTA or heparin)	Store frozen <−20°C, yr	25-Hydroxy vitamin D3 by RIA	>30 nmol/L
Zinc[b]	Serum or heparin plasma (do not use EDTA)	Store frozen <−20°C, yr in serum/plasma	Atomic absorption spectroscopy	>10 μmol/L
Neopterin	Serum or EDTA plasma; Urine (20 mL universal tube)	2–8°C, <72 h; <−20°C, approx 6 mo; protect from light	ELISA	< 10 nmol/L (serum)
CRP	Serum or heparin plasma,	Store frozen <−20°C, approx 6 mo	ELISA	<5 mg/L
α1-anti-chymotrypsin	Serum or bloodspot (filter paper)	Store frozen <−20°C, approx 6 mo	Turbidimetry, ELISA	<0.6 g/L
α1-acid glycoprotein	Serum or heparin plasma	Store frozen <−20°C, approx 6 mo	Turbidimetry, ELISA	<1.0 g/L
Sodium potassium ratio	Whole breast milk (12 mL universal tube)	Store frozen <−20°C, yr	Flame photometry, ion specific electrodes	<1.0

[a]Certified reference standards in plasma (SRM 968b) are available from NIST, Gaithersburg, MD.
[b]Certified zinc controls are available (for example, Bio-Rad, Anaheim, CA; or NIST, Gaithersburg, MD), HPLC, high-performance liquid chromatography; RIA, radioimmunoassay; CRP, c-Reactive Protein.
Source: Ref. 55.

and can detect active and past infection *(8)*. The presence of histological chorioamnionitis is the standard postpartum indicator of intrauterine infection. However, a delivered placenta differs greatly from a placenta during pregnancy as a result of the large local inflammatory response that is a normal part of delivery, and this can affect assessment of immune functions. Any placental samples should only be collected following the routine examination to check the placenta is complete.

Urine

Urine samples are readily collected and can be used to measure analytes such as neopterin and urinary iodine, as well as for routine clinical tests during pregnancy and lactation. Clean plastic, polystyrene, or cardboard cups can be used for midstream sample collection, and the sample transferred into screw-top sample tubes, tightly sealed to prevent leakage and exposure to air. Anti-bacterial agents such as thymol may be added as a preservative.

Breast Milk

Breast milk collection is less invasive and often more acceptable than blood drawing. An additional advantage is that for many assays, milk does not require further processing at the point of collection. Consequently, there has been considerable interest in the use of breast milk, for example, in the assessment of vitamin A status. In our experience, however, the greater technical difficulties of analysing the more complex matrix of breast milk compared with plasma, and of standardizing the results obtained, offset most of the benefits gained at the sample collection stage. We generally analyse breast milk only when interested in it *per se* and not as an alternative to similar measurements in blood samples.

Milk samples can be manually expressed, or collected using a breast pump into sterile plastic screw-top containers. Some components of breast milk vary between breasts (for example, sodium and some immune factors) and it may be necessary to collect from both breasts into separate containers *(9)*. Breast milk can be frozen whole or first separated into aqueous, fat, and cellular components. Care is needed when collecting a standardized cellular fraction because milk macrophages are activated and tend to stick to the walls of the collection tube. Milk macrophages also contain large amounts of lipid and may float in the fat layer rather than sink with the cell pellet during centrifugation. In addition to variations between breasts, breast milk composition varies with time of day and time since the infant was last fed *(9)*. The main source of this variability is in the relative proportions of the fat and aqueous phases. This is a serious concern when analyzing compounds such as fat-soluble vitamins that are found in the milk lipid fraction. Although great efforts can be made to standardize collection methods to control for milk fat, it is usually much easier to standardize results *post hoc* by expressing them per gram milk fat. Commercial assays are available for triglycerides but an alternative is a simple crematocrit "obtained using a hematocrit centrifuge" that correlates well with milk triglycerides *(10)*.

For some analytes, for example, cytokines, the milk fraction in which they are found is unknown. Whole milk is more difficult to work with than the aqueous phase, but it is recommended that the lipid layer be retained until preliminary work confirms that the cytokine or other component of interest is in the aqueous phase. If the analyte is found in the lipid phase, additional steps may be required in the treatment and analysis of the samples in order to measure the component reliably, for example, disruption of the fat globules by the addition of an equal volume of 12 mmol/L bile salts *(11)*.

Technology Considerations

Nutritional status and immune function can be measured using low or high technology methods; the choice depends on both the purpose of the assessment and the facilities available. Methods for assessing the nutritional status of an individual in clinical care may differ from those for assessing the status of a population. For example, zinc status is difficult to determine at the individual level but serum zinc can be used for population assessment (*see* later). Once a population has been identified as being deficient in a nutrient, it is not necessary to measure each individual's status before intervening.

Some laboratory assays are only possible in centers with secure power supplies and access to specialized equipment and personnel to service it. However, it is often possible to collect and prepare samples for shipment to a central facility for assay and have the results sent back to the site of origin. For some measures of nutritional status, for example, body composition and vitamin A status, low technological methods have been validated against the more expensive or complex techniques. Moreover, reference standards are available for interlaboratory comparisons. These types of validation are much less well established for many immunological assays. However, new immunological assays for both well-equipped and more basic laboratories are constantly being developed and their association with important maternal and infant outcomes need to be determined.

Evaluation of Nutritional Status
Overall Nutritional Status

Anthropometric evaluation of overall nutritional status is complicated during pregnancy because of the related weight gain that is very variable. During lactation, standard methods such as body mass index (weight (kg)/height (m)^2)

can be used *(12)*. Despite interpretation difficulties, anthropometry is recommended because it is easy, cheap, and meaningful: both prepregnancy weight and weight gain are associated with maternal and infant health. More complex and more sophisticated techniques requiring special equipment, for example, bioelectrical impedence, may not be as well validated and as useful as simple anthropometry done carefully. Biochemical measurement of plasma proteins such as albumin is not recommended for assessment of overall nutritional status because of low sensitivity and specificity; in particular, many of these plasma proteins are affected by acute phase responses to infection. In addition, albumin levels naturally decrease during pregnancy owing to pregnancy-related hemodilution.

Iron

Iron deficiency is one of the most common nutrient deficiencies in the world, and the single most common cause of nutritional anemia. Pregnant women are at highest risk; anemia from iron and/or folate deficiency is the most frequent health and nutritional complication related to pregnancy. Severe anemia (hemoglobin (Hb) <70 g/L), to which iron deficiency is a major, but not the only contributor *(13)*, can adversely effect the mother and the fetus and result in prematurity, spontaneous abortions, low birth weight, and fetal death *(14)*. Malaria during pregnancy aggravates the risk of anemia and of low birth weight *(15)*.

Assessing iron status is notoriously difficult, especially in pregnancy as changes in maternal physiology (increase in plasma volume and erythropoiesis) significantly affect the iron-related hematological and biochemical parameters. Iron assessment methods can be grouped into those directed toward red blood cells and those that are not. The simplest and most common methods used in blood are hemoglobin (Hb) and hematocrit. Both lack sensitivity, but are simple and cheap to perform and thus widely used. Furthermore, these measure anemia and there is little evidence that less severe iron deficiency without anemia is associated with adverse effects on health *(14)*. Therefore, assessment of anemia alone is sufficient for many applications.

Circulating Hb level falls early in the first trimester, reaches its lowest point at the end of the second trimester, and gradually rises again during the third. A Hb level of 110 g/L in the late first and third trimester, and of 105 g/L in the second trimester, are suggested as lower limits for Hb concentration *(16)*. The cyanmethemoglobin spectrophotometric method is the gold standard method for assessing Hb *(17)*. Other methods are more useful for rapid testing in the field, for example, the HemoCue™ hemoglobinometer (Angelholm, Sweden). This transportable instrument uses disposable cuvets that draw blood by capillary action. The cuvets are placed into the instrument where the Hb is read after several seconds. The HemoCue™ can be used by nonclinical personnel after training. However, the test cuvets are often considered too expensive for routine use in clinics or primary health care centres in many countries.

The most frequently used nonred blood cell measure of iron status is serum ferritin. It is the most sensitive measure of iron status because it reflects iron stores rather than heme synthesis, is easy and relatively cheap to measure, and uses very small amounts of serum. A low serum ferritin is diagnostic of iron deficiency. However, a normal or high serum ferritin cannot be so unambiguously interpreted, because ferritin is an acute phase protein and plasma levels increase dramatically after infection (even subclinical infection) or trauma. In the third trimester of pregnancy, a high ferritin level is a marker of maternal infection and is associated with preterm delivery (18). Ferritin is usually measured by immunoassay, which requires a reasonable degree of laboratory sophistication. Commercial kits are available, or cheaper in-house assays using commercially available reagents (for example, Dako, Cambridge, UK) can be set up by a more experienced technician (19).

Measurement of serum transferrin receptors (TfR) is an alternative technique for assessing iron status. TfR reflects cell receptor levels that rise as cells sense an increased need or decreased availability of iron. The technique requires very small amounts of serum and is a sensitive measure of iron status. Unlike serum ferritin, TfR levels are unaffected by most types of acute or chronic inflammation, although there is conflicting evidence concerning TfR changes during malaria (19). TfR was unaffected by undernutrition and pregnancy in a study of Zairean women (20), but other studies have shown variation in TfR throughout normal pregnancy, which would complicate the use of TfR to assess iron status (21). Results for TfR concentrations can vary considerably depending on the commercial kit used. A reliable kit is available from Ramco Laboratories Inc (Ati-Atlas Ltd; Chichester, UK). Different anticoagulants in the sample collection tubes can also affect results—ethylene diamine tetraacetic acid (EDTA) tubes should not be used—as can time delay between sample collection and centrifugation (22). TfR levels can be measured in blood spots collected on filter paper (6).

Retinol (Vitamin A)

Retinol is important for immune function, visual processes, and reproduction. Vitamin A is important for resistance to infection, although most of the data come from studies involving young children (23). A recent study among Nepali women found the risk of death related to pregnancy (during and postpartum) was 40% lower among women supplemented weekly with vitamin A (24).

Vitamin A requirements increase slightly during pregnancy, but almost double during lactation. Healthy term infants are born with very low stores of vitamin A in their livers, and need to accumulate adequate stores during lactation. Unlike many other micronutrients, where breast milk levels remain adequate despite maternal undernutrition, retinol in breast milk varies with maternal status (25).

Maternal history of night blindness during a recent pregnancy is an indicator of the vitamin A status of a population (23). Night blindness can be assessed easily in epidemiological surveys and a prevalence of greater than 5% indicates a vitamin A deficiency problem of public health importance. The existence of a well-recognized local term for night blindness can also suggests that vitamin A deficiency is common in the population. Where night blindness is prevalent, less severe vitamin A deficiency is also likely to be common and it may not be necessary to assess individual plasma retinol before intervening to improve vitamin A status.

Plasma retinol concentrations are homeostatically regulated and reflect vitamin A stores only at the extremes of deficiency or toxicity. During the acute-phase response to infection or trauma, plasma retinol levels decrease; thus it is not a suitable indicator of vitamin A status during infection. During lactation, the concentration in breast milk (expressed per volume or per gram of the fat content) is an alternative index to plasma levels (26). Breast milk retinol content varies with stage of lactation and its interpretation can be complex. Although plasma retinol circulates bound to retinol binding protein (RBP), in milk, retinol is mainly in the form of retinyl esters associated with fat globules. Consequently, laboratory techniques for measuring breast milk retinol are more difficult than those for plasma retinol (27) and the cheap internal standard, retinyl acetate, that is commonly used for plasma cannot be used.

Pregnancy hemodilution appears to decrease plasma retinol levels, although a formal allowance for this effect on retinol has not been made as it has been for Hb. Table 2 shows plasma retinol during the third trimester of pregnancy, compared with levels 6 wk postpartum in Zambian women (unpublished). High-performance liquid chromatography (HPLC) is considered to be the only laboratory technique sufficiently reliable for routine determination of plasma or breast milk retinol (27).

The relative dose response (RDR) and modified relative dose response (MRDR) tests are designed to estimate liver retinol stores and are more sensitive to deficiency than is plasma retinol (26,28). The tests measure a change in plasma retinol or didehydroretinol several hours after ingestion of a small test dose. Although useful in research or in a subsample of a larger survey, these tests require both greater subject compliance and more sophisticated or precise HPLC techniques than for plasma retinol.

Table 2
Plasma Retinol and α-Tocopherol Levels
(mean [SD]) in Zambian Women During Pregnancy and Postpartum

	35 wk gestation	6 wk postpartum
	$n = 276$	$n = 194$
Retinol (μmol/L)	1.09 (0.39)	1.50 (0.51)
α-tocopherol (μmol/L)	26.1 (6.41)	21.3 (5.44)

Source: Kasonka, Makasa, Chisenga, Newens. (2002) Personal communication.

Measurement of plasma RBP has been suggested as an alternative to plasma retinol to which it is highly correlated. Plasma levels of RBP are decreased by the presence of an acute-phase response, protein-energy malnutrition, and in acutely stressful situations (for example, just before parturition) (29). RBP can be measured by radial immunodiffusion (for example, The Binding Site, Inc., San Diego, CA) or enzyme-linked immunoabsorbent assay (ELISA), techniques that are less expensive and require less sensitive equipment than the HPLC method for plasma retinol. Field methods allowing immediate analysis, as well as dried blood spot methods for retinol and RBP, are being developed. Currently, the major problem with the use of RBP for vitamin A assessment is the lack of international standards and agreed cut-offs for deficiency, but these problems are potentially solvable (30).

α-Tocopherol (Vitamin E)

The main function of vitamin E is its role as an antioxidant, required for the protection of polyunsaturated fatty acids, mainly in membranes. Antioxidants such as vitamin E are particularly important for cells of the immune system that are exposed to high concentrations of free-radical products as a result of immune activation. Studies in dairy animals indicate that oxidative stress and immune dysfunction are associated with mastitis, and that vitamin E supplementation reduces the incidence of mastitis in cows (31). Evidence of a similar reduction of subclinical mastitis after micronutrient supplementation also exists for women (11,32).

Plasma α-tocopherol can be measured by HPLC using techniques similar to that for plasma retinol. The two vitamins can be measured simultaneously if the HPLC system has a variable wavelength detector. α-Tocopherol is subject to oxidation, which can be enhanced by light or heat exposure. Samples should be handled out of direct light, and stored at −70°C, with minimal freeze-thawing.

In contrast to plasma retinol, plasma levels of α-tocopherol increased during pregnancy in Zambian women (see Table 2), in parallel with an increase in total lipids *(33)*. Plasma α-tocopherol levels should be expressed relative to fat, that is, cholesterol or triglyceride levels.

Iodine

Iodine deficiency during pregnancy increases the risk of stillbirth, abortion, and low birth weight *(34)*. The decreased availability of iodine to the fetus leads to decreased synthesis of thyroid hormones, preventing normal development of the brain and body. Methods for assessing iodine status in a wide range of laboratory settings are published *(35)*. Manual assessment of the prevalence of goiter at the population level is cheap and relatively simple, but indicates only deficiency that is sufficiently severe and prolonged to result in clinical symptoms. More sensitive techniques of detecting iodine deficiency measure plasma concentrations of the thyroid hormones, thyroxine (T4) and triiodothyronine (T3), or of the related proteins, thyroglobulin and thyroid stimulating hormone. Commercial radioimmunoassays and immunochemiluminometric assays for the above are widely available and the compounds can be reliably measured in dried blood spots from both maternal and cord whole blood samples. Total T3 and T4 increase during pregnancy, but the unbound or free hormone concentrations generally remain in the normal range for nonpregnant women.

Measurement of iodine in urine is easy, inexpensive, rapid, sensitive, and specific to iodine status *(35)*. Several hundred samples can be run by a technician in a day, with the method's greatest application probably being in smaller laboratories where equipment is limited. Other than pipets, the only instruments needed are a spectrophotometer and a heating block or water bath. However, the use of urinary iodine to estimate iodine sufficiency during pregnancy can be misleading because pregnancy causes increased iodine excretion, resulting in a relative increase in urinary iodine concentration, giving a false sense of adequacy of iodine nutrition *(36)*.

Vitamin D

The importance of vitamin D for immune function and resistance to infection, as well as the high prevalence of vitamin D deficiency even in sunny climates, is being increasingly recognized. Pregnancy and lactation may impose an increased requirement for vitamin D *(37)*. The recommended indicator of vitamin D status is plasma concentration of 25-hydroxyvitamin D3 [25(OH)D$_3$]. Plasma levels of 25(OH)D$_3$ remain relatively constant during pregnancy. Commercial radioimmunoassay kits (for example Nichols Institute Diagnostics, San Juan Capistrano, CA) are a good method for measuring 25(OH)D$_3$ in most laboratories, although the use of radioisotopes requires a laboratory licensed for their safe use and disposal.

Zinc

Zinc is an important trace element for immune function. About 80% of pregnant women worldwide may be zinc deficient *(38)*, but this is speculative because of the great difficulty in assessing zinc status. During pregnancy, maternal zinc status may directly affect fetal growth and birth weight, and influence neonatal growth and morbidity. Moderate zinc deficiency has been related to complications during labor and delivery, but trials of zinc supplementation during pregnancy have not convincingly improved outcome *(39)*. However, the majority of these trials have been performed in developed countries where zinc deficiency was probably not severe.

An established functional or enzymatic marker of zinc status is not available. Serum or plasma levels are considered a useful indicator of population status, but are unreliable for assessment of individual status. Plasma zinc levels vary throughout the day by 15–20%, and are affected by infection and pregnancy *(39)*. During pregnancy, plasma zinc concentrations fall from the 10th week of gestation onward, partly because of hemodilution. Serum and plasma levels may not be an adequate measure of marginal zinc status because they appear to adapt in populations where the dietary zinc intake is low. Serum and plasma zinc levels can be measured by atomic absorption spectroscopy. Great care must be taken to avoid sample contamination with environmental zinc *(40)*. Even slight hemolysis of blood samples, resulting from rough handling of samples or prolonged time between sample collection and centrifugation, can release enough zinc from red blood cells to invalidate the measurement of plasma zinc.

Evaluation of Immune Function or Infection

Overall tests of immune function, such as total or differential blood leukocyte count, antibody responses to vaccines, and delayed type hypersensivity, can be used, but lack sensitivity. Commonly used vaccines have been selected for high immunogenicity, and responses may be normal in women with modest immunodeficiency. The assays provide limited mechanistic information. Antibody and delayed hypersensitivity responses involve numerous cell types and soluble factors, and it is unclear which is responsible when a defective overall response is seen. Therefore, there is interest in assays for specific components of the immune response to obtain more sensitive or mechanistic information.

Cytokines

Cytokines are a heterogeneous group of glycoproteins that are key regulators of immune functions. Cytokines are synthesized by numerous cell types including leukocytes that are normally considered part of the immune system and also by, for example, epithelial cells at the mucosal surface. The capacity for and the profile of cytokine production reflects immunologic status.

The maternal immune system is modulated during pregnancy to avoid rejecting the fetus. A few studies in humans have suggested that a bias toward T-helper type-2 (Th2) anti-inflammatory responses exists in normal pregnancy, and a T-helper type-1 (Th1) bias in women with high-risk pregnancies. Infection during pregnancy (systemic or of the genital tract) can negatively affect outcome, for example, preterm birth and infant development, partly through changes in cytokine balance *(41–43)*. These changes fall into two broad categories: excessive production of inflammatory cytokines such as interleukins (IL) 1 and 6 and tumor necrosis factor (TNF)-α, and an increase in Th1 cytokines such as interferon (IFN)-γ relative to Th2 cytokines such as IL-4 and IL-10.

Abnormal activation of the immune system, interacting with nutritional status, plays a role in the etiology of preeclampsia. Antioxidant micronutrients (vitamin C or E) have been implicated in cell-mediated immunity, affecting both inflammatory cytokine levels and tissue damage. Damage from oxidative stress and lipid peroxidation has been etiologically involved in a variety of physiological, pathological, and clinical conditions including pregnancy and its complications, mainly preeclampsia *(44)*. Supplementation with vitamins C and E has proved beneficial in the prevention of preeclampsia in women at increased risk of the disease *(45)*. Micronutrient deficiencies in pregnancy may also increase the risk of vertical transmission of HIV from mother to infant *(46)*, via impairment of systemic immune function, weakening of epithelial integrity of the placenta and genital tract, and increased viral shedding in breast milk from inflamed breast tissue.

ELISA assays, both commercial and homemade, and higher-tech Flow cytometry and microarray techniques can be used to measure cytokine-producing cells, circulating cytokines, or cytokines produced in vitro. Various assays for mRNA such as Northern blot, RNAse protection assay, semiquantitative reverse transcription polymerase chain reaction, and *in situ* hybridization can be used to measure cytokine production at the cellular level. However, interpretation of the results obtained can be more difficult than performing the assay. mRNA levels may not correlate well with actual protein level due to variations in posttranscriptional modifications, cytokines produced can be bound to cells, or to binding proteins that can either promote or downregulate their function. Bound cytokine is often not measurable by immunoassays unless the assay is specifically designed to measure total, rather than free, cytokine. In vitro culture of blood cells can provide information on constitutive and stimulated cytokine production. Separation of total blood leukocytes or a particular subpopulation and normalizing the cell number in samples from different subjects can reduce the variability between subjects and permit determination of key cell populations involved. However, these same procedures may distort the system so far from what it was in vivo that the results cannot easily be extrapolated back to the whole individual. Culture of whole blood has the opposite problem in that it may better reflect the in vivo situation, but at some loss of understanding of mechanisms. Whole blood cultures have an advantage in field situations: sterile tubes with necessary immunologic stimuli or other reagents can be prepared in a central laboratory and samples can be simply added to tubes in the field with no further manipulation. Finally, many key immunological responses involved in resistance to infection in vivo take place at mucosae and mucosal immune functions are largely distinct from those in circulating leukocytes. However, the problems of measuring and interpreting cytokines, even in readily available mucosal fluids such as breast milk, are even greater than for plasma or cell culture because of the complex matrix of milk.

Proxy Markers of Cytokine Production

In view of the difficulties of measuring cytokines and interpreting the results, several proxy markers, for example, neopterin and acute phase proteins, are used to assess immunocompetence. Research is ongoing to determine how well their measurement in pregnancy can be used to monitor women at risk of obstetric complications. Because many of the indicators of micronutrient status are affected by the acute phase response, and may not reflect micronutrient status during infection, assessing for concurrent clinical and subclinical infections by monitoring the acute phase response can improve interpretation of micronutrient results. The latter can be done on fresh blood samples, using the older assay for erythrocyte sedimentation rate, or easily and cheaply on stored plasma samples by measuring acute phase protein concentrations.

Neopterin

Neopterin is a product of IFN-γ-activated macrophages, and is closely associated with activation of the cellular immune system. Serum and urine levels are increased in a variety of infections, chronic inflammatory states, autoimmune disorders, and malignancies, and levels correlate with disease severity. Neopterin increases early with infection and may precede the clinical manifestation, especially in viral infections, or the increase in antibody titer. Neopterin has recently been quantified in pregnancy and the postpartum period, and has been suggested as a marker of high risk of complications such as intraamniotic fluid infections and severe preeclampsia *(47,48)*.

In comparison with the direct measurement of IFN-γ, the determination of neopterin level presents important advantages. IFN-γ is subject to fast degradation and can be bound to soluble or cell bound receptors and the biologically effective concentration can differ greatly from the obtained free concentration. These problems do not occur with neopterin, which is not modified or bound chemically in vivo, but is excreted quantitatively by the kidney. Neopterin can be assayed in serum, plasma, or urine using commercially available immunoassay kits (for example, BRAHMS Diagnostica, Berlin).

Acute Phase Proteins

Plasma acute phase proteins such as C-reactive protein (CRP), α1-antichymotrypsin (ACT) and α1-acid glycoprotein (AGP) are well-established markers for monitoring clinical and subclinical inflammation. Easier to assay than the inflammatory cytokines that induce them, with longer plasma half-lives, they play a major role in the assessment of the acute phase response to infection, injury, or other inflammatory stimuli (49). Acute phase proteins are synthesized mainly by hepatocytes and secreted into the plasma. CRP plasma concentrations increase within 10 h of the onset of acute inflammation; the protein has a short plasma half-life and thus concentrations normalize rapidly (49). Plasma ACT concentrations also increase early, but remain elevated for a longer time than CRP concentrations (49). Plasma AGP concentrations only begin to rise more than 24 h after the onset of inflammation, but remain elevated even weeks into convalescence (49). Women who delivered prematurely had higher plasma CRP levels early in the second trimester than those with term deliveries (50). In healthy women, there is a major acute phase response during parturition, with CRP levels peaking at 24 h after vaginal delivery or at 48 h after caesarean section, declining during the days following the birth (51,52).

Commercial assays for CRP by ELISA are widely available. The newer assays with lower detection limits are recommended over the older assays with detection limits around 5 mg/L because it is now apparent that even plasma levels lower than this can be associated with negative outcomes in nonpregnant adults. CRP is also easily measured by a sensitive homemade sandwich ELISA using commercial reagents (for example, Dako, Cambridge, UK; Behring Diagnostics Milton Keynes, UK) (19).

Commercial assays for acute phase proteins other than CRP are less widely available, but homemade assays can be readily developed. Turbidimetric methods work well for ACT and AGP but require equipment such as autoanalyzers (for example, COBAS centrifugal analysers), which may not be widely available. AGP and ACT can also be measured by ELISA using commercially available antibody and other reagents (Dako, Cambridge, UK) (19).

Subclinical Mastitis

Subclinical mastitis can be used to determine maternal morbidity in the postpartum period, which is also a time of increased vulnerability. Subclinical mastitis is defined as raised breast milk sodium accompanied by raised milk inflammatory cytokines in the absence of symptoms of mastitis, and has been shown to be common in several populations (11,53). Subclinical mastitis results from several causes and represents a nonspecific marker of poor maternal health. The causes include poor lactation practice, maternal infection, or deficiencies of micronutrients, particularly the antioxidants (11,32). Subclinical mastitis is associated with poor infant growth and with increased milk HIV viral load, a risk factor for mother-to-child HIV transmission (53,54). Therefore, screening for and the prevention and treatment of subclinical mastitis are potentially very important. A raised Na/K ratio can tentatively be used as a nonspecific marker of mother–infant dyads at risk.

Breast milk sodium concentration is controlled at around 5–6 mmol/L by tight junctions between alveolar cells of the breast tissue. During clinical or subclinical mastitis, inflammation leads to opening of the tight junctions, allowing plasma to enter the milk and increasing milk sodium levels. Milk sodium can be expressed as a ratio to potassium, which is fairly constant in mature milk (12–16 mmol/L), in order to ignore the variable proportion of milk fat in spot milk samples. Normal Na/K ratios are less than about 0.6. Ratios greater than 1.0 (about 16 mmol/L sodium) indicate breastfeeding problems severe enough to impair infant weight gain. Milk Na/K measurement is useful for its simplicity but, like neopterin and acute phase proteins, it lacks specificity for particular conditions. Breast milk sodium and potassium levels can be cheaply and easily determined by flame photometry or by ion-specific electrode. The inflammation itself can be detected by measurement of inflammatory cytokines such as IL-8 (11).

Conclusions

Techniques to measure nutritional status of pregnant and lactating women are fairly well established because of longstanding appreciation of the importance of nutrition to maternal and infant health. Both high and low technology methods of assessing nutritional status are available and, in many cases, have been compared and standardized with each other and across laboratories. Measures of immune function are generally less advanced in terms of such standardization and of how different measures correlate with clinically important outcomes. Sophisticated immunological assays are available, but research is needed on their use in populations where infections are common and as important determinants of maternal and infant health, especially in low-income countries.

Acknowledgments

We are grateful to L. Kasonka, M. Makasa, M. Chisenga, and K. Newens for the Zambian vitamin A and E data. Specific commercial reagents mentioned are those used successfully in the authors' laboratory and do not necessarily preclude the use of similar reagents from other sources.

References

1. Costello, A. and Osrin, D. (2003) Micronutrient status during pregnancy and outcomes for newborn infants in developing countries. *J. Nutr.* **133**, 1757S–1764S.
2. Konje, J.C. and Ladipo, O.A. (2000) Nutrition and obstructed labor. *Am. J. Clin. Nutr.* **72**, 291S–297S.
3. Steketee, R.W., Nahlen, B.L., Parise, M.E., and Menendez, C. (2001) The burden of malaria in pregnancy in malaria-endemic areas. *Am. J. Trop. Med. Hyg.* **64**, 28–35.
4. Li, X.F., Fortney, J.A., Kotelchuck, M., and Glover, L.H. (1996) The postpartum period: the key to maternal mortality. *Int J. Gynecol. Obstet.* **54**, 1–10.
5. Thurnham, D.I., McCabe, G.P., Northrop-Clewes, C.A., and Nestel, P. (2003) Effects of sub-clinical infection on plasma retinol concentrations and assessment of the prevalence of vitamin A deficiency. *Lancet* **362**, 2050–2058.
6. McDade, T.W. and Shell-Duncan, B. (2002) Whole blood collected on filter paper provides a minimally invasive method for assessing human transferrin receptor level. *J. Nutr.* **132**, 3760–3763.
7. Rondo, P.H. and Tomkins, A.M. (2002) Folate and intrauterine growth retardation. *Ann. Trop. Paediat.* **20**, 253–258.
8. Rogerson, S.J., Mkundika, P., and Kanjala, M.K. (2003) Diagnosis of Plasmodium Falciparum malaria at delivery: comparison of blood film preparation methods and of blood films with histology. *J. Clin. Microbiol.* **41**, 1370–1374.
9. Neville, M.C., Keller, R.P., Seacat, J., Casey, C.E., Allen, J.C., and Archer, P. (1984) Studies on human lactation. I. Within-feed and between-breast variation in selected components of human milk. *Am. J. Clin. Nutr.* **40**, 635–646.
10. Lucas, A., Gibbs, J.A., Lyster, R.L., and Baum, J.D. (1978) Creamatocrit: simple clinical technique for estimating fat concentration and energy value of human milk. *Br. Med. J.* **1**, 1018–1020.
11. Filteau, S.M., Lietz, G., Mulokozi, G., Bilotta, S., Henry, C.J., and Tomkins, A.M. (1999) Milk cytokines and subclinical breast inflammation in Tanzanian women: effects of dietary red palm oil or sunflower oil supplementation. *Immunol.* **97**, 595–600.
12. World Health Organization. The use and interpretation of anthropometry; report of the WHO expert committee on physical status. Geneva: WHO, 1995. (WHO Tech. Rep. Ser., 854).
13. United Nations's Children's Fund, United Nations Univ., World Health Organization. (2001) Iron deficiency anemia: assessment, prevention, and control. A guide for program managers. WHO, Geneva: (WHO/NHD/01.3)

14. Stoltzfus, R.J. (2001) Iron-deficiency anemia: reexamining the nature and magnitude of the public health problem. Summary: implications for research and programs. *J. Nutr.* **131**, 697S–700S.
15. Steketee, R.W. (2003) Pregnancy, nutrition, and parasitic diseases. *J. Nutr.* **133**, 1661S–1667S.
16. Centers for Disease Control and Prevention. (1989) Criteria for anemia in children and childbearing-aged women. *Morb. Mortal. Wkly. Rep.* **38**, 400–404.
17. National Committee for Clinical Laboratory Standards. (2000) Procedure for the quantitative determination of haemoglobin in blood; Approved standard. 3rd ed. Pennsylvania, USA: NCCLS document **20**, H15–A3.
18. Scholl, T.O. (1998) High third-trimester ferritin concentration: associations with very preterm delivery, infection, and maternal nutritional status. *Obstet. Gynecol.* **92**, 161–166.
19. Beesley, R., Filteau, S.M., Tomkins, A.M., et al. (2000) Impact of acute malaria on plasma concentrations of transferrin receptors. *Trans. R. Soc. Trop. Med. Hyg.* **94**, 295–298.
20. Kuvibidila, S., Warrier, R.P., Ode, D., and Yu, L. (1996) Serum transferrin receptor concentrations in women with mild malnutrition. *Am. J. Clin. Nutr.* **63**, 596–601.
21. Choi, J.W., Im, M.W., and Pai, S.H. (2000) Serum transferrin receptor concentrations during normal pregnancy. *Clin. Chem.* **46**, 725–727.
22. De Jongh, R., Vranken, J., Vundelinckx, G., Bosmans, E., Maes, M., and Heylen, R. (1997) The effects of anticoagulation and processing on assays of IL-6, sIL- 6R, sIL-2R and soluble transferrin receptor. *Cytokine* **9**, 696–701.
23. Sommer, A. and Davidson, F.R. (2002) Assessment and control of vitamin A deficiency: The Annecy Accords. *J. Nutr.* **132**, 2845S–2850S.
24. West, K.P., Jr., Katz, J., Khatry, S.K., et al. (1999) Double blind, cluster randomised trial of low dose supplementation with vitamin A or beta-carotene on mortality related to pregnancy in Nepal. *Brit. Med. J.* **318**, 570–575.
25. Miller, M., Humphrey, J., Johnson, E., Marinda, E., Brookmeyer, R., and Katz, J. (2002) Why do children become vitamin a deficient? *J. Nutr.* **132**, 2867S–2880S.
26. Rice, A.L., Stoltzfus, R.J., De Francisco, A., and Kjolhede, C.L. (2000) Evaluation of serum retinol, the modified-relative-dose-response ratio, and breast-milk vitamin A as indicators of response to postpartum maternal vitamin A supplementation. *Am. J. Clin. Nutr.* **71**, 799–806.
27. Tanumihardjo, S.A. and Penniston, K.L. (2002) Simplified methodology to determine breast milk retinol concentrations. *J. Lipid. Res.* **43**, 350–355.
28. Tanumihardjo, S.A. (1994) The relative dose-response assay in *A Brief Guide to Assessing Vitamin A Status*, (Underwood, B.A. and Olson, J.A., eds.) Washington, DC: Nutrition Foundation, Inc., pp. 12–13.
29. Gamble, M.V., Ramakrishnan, R., Palafox, N.A., Briand, K., Berglund, L., and Blaner, W.S. (2001) Retinol binding protein as a surrogate measure for serum retinol: studies in vitamin A-deficient children from the Republic of the Marshall Islands. *Am. J. Clin. Nutr.* **73**, 594.

30. De Pee, S. and Dary, O. (2002) Biochemical indicators of vitamin A deficiency: serum retinol and serum retinol binding protein. *J. Nutr.* **132**, 2895S–2901S.
31. Hogan, J.S., Weiss, W.P., and Smith, K.L. (1993) Role of vitamin E and selenium in host defense against mastitis. *J. Dairy Sci.* **76**, 2795–2803.
32. Gomo, E., Filteau, S.M., Tomkins, A.M., Ndhlovu, P., Fleischer Michaelsen, K., and Friis, H. (2003) Subclinical mastitis among HIV-infected and uninfected Zimbabwean women participating in a multimicronutrient supplementation trial. *Trans. R. Soc. Trop. Med. Hyg.* **97**, 212–216.
33. Horwitt, M.K., Harvey, C.C., Dahm, C.H., Jr., and Searcy, M.T. (1972) Relationship between tocopherol and serum lipid levels for determination of nutritional adequacy. *Ann. NY Acad. Sci.* **203**, 223–236.
34. Lamberg, B.A. (1991) Endemic goitre—iodine deficiency disorders. *Ann. Med.* **23**, 367–372.
35. Dunn, J.T., Crutchfield, H.E., Gutekunst, R., and Dunn, A.D. (1993) Methods for measuring iodine in urine. Wageningen: ICCIDD/UNICEF/WHO.
36. Soldin, O.P. (2002) Controversies in urinary iodine determinations. *Clin. Biochem.* **35**, 575–579.
37. Specker, B.L. (1994) Do North American women need supplemental vitamin D during pregnancy or lactation? *Am. J. Clin. Nutr.* **59**, 484S–490S.
38. Caulfield, L.E., Zavaleta, N., Shankar, A.H., and Merialdi, M. (1998) Potential contribution of maternal zinc supplementation during pregnancy to maternal and child survival. *Am. J. Clin. Nutr.* **68**, 499S–508S.
39. Osendarp, S.J.M., West, C.E., and Black, R.E. (2003) The need for maternal zinc supplementation in developing countries: an unresolved issue. *J. Nutr.* **133**, 817S–827S.
40. Lakomaa, E.L., Mussalo-Rauhamaa, H., and Salmela, S. (1998) Avoidance of contamination in element analysis of serum samples. *J. Trace Elem. Electrolytes Health Dis.* **2**, 37–41.
41. Gomez, R., Ghezzi, F., Romero, R., et al. (1995) Premature labor and intra-amniotic infection. Clinical aspects and role of the cytokines in diagnosis and pathophysiology. *Clin. Perinatol.* **22**, 281–342.
42. Dammann, O. and Leviton, A. (1997) Maternal intrauterine infection, cytokines, and brain damage in the preterm newborn. *Pediatr. Res.* **42**, 1–8.
43. Fried, M., Muga, R.O., Misore, A.O., and Duffy, P.E. (1998) Malaria elicits type 1 cytokines in the human placenta: IFN-gamma and TNF-alpha associated with pregnancy outcomes. *J. Immunol.* **160**, 2523–2530.
44. Sagol, S., Ozkinay, E., and Ozsener, S. (1999) Impaired antioxidant activity in women with pre-eclampsia. *Int. J. Gynaecol. Obstet.* **64**, 121–127.
45. Chappell, L.C., Seed, P.T., Briley, A.L., et al. (1999) Effect of antioxidants on the occurrence of pre-eclampsia in women at increased risk: a randomised trial. *Lancet* **354**, 810–816.
46. Dreyfuss, M.L. and Fawzi, W.W. (2002) Micronutrients and vertical transmission of HIV-1. *Am. J. Clin. Nutr.* **75**, 959–970.

47. Burns, D.N., Nourjah, P., Wright, D.J., et al. (1999) Changes in immune activation markers during pregnancy and postpartum. *J. Reprod. Immunol.* **42**, 147–165.
48. Radunovic, N., Kuczynski, E., Rebarber, A., Nastic, D., and Lockwood, C.J. (1999) Neopterin concentrations in fetal and maternal blood: a marker of cell-mediated immune activation. *Am. J. Obstet. Gynecol.* **181**, 170–173.
49. Thompson, D., Milford-Ward, A., and Whicher, J.T. (1992) The value of acute phase protein measurements in clinical practice. *Ann. Clin. Biochem.* **29**, 123–131.
50. Hvilsom, G.B., Thorsen, P., Jeune, B., and Bakketeig, L.S. (2002) C-reactive protein: a serological marker for preterm delivery? *Acta Obstet. Gynecol. Scand.* **81**, 424–429.
51. de Villiers, W.J., Louw, J.P., Strachan, A.F., et al. (1990) C-reactive protein and serum amyloid A protein in pregnancy and labour. *Br. J. Obstet. Gynaecol.* **97**, 725–730.
52. Staven, P., Suonio, S., Saarikoski, S., and Kauhanen, O. (1989) C-reactive protein (CRP) levels after normal and complicated caesarean section. *Ann. Chir. Gynaecol.* **78**, 142–145.
53. Willumsen, J.F., Filteau, S.M., Coutsoudis, A., et al. (2003) Breastmilk RNA viral load in HIV-infected South African women: effects of subclinical mastitis and infant feeding. *AIDS* **17**, 407–414.
54. Semba, R.D. (2000) Mastitis and transmission of human immunodeficiency virus through breast milk. *Ann. NY Acad. Sci.* **918**, 156–162.
55. Tietz, N.W. (1995) *Clinical Guide to Laboratory Tests.* 3rd ed. WB Saunders, Philadelphia.

4 Severe Undernutrition and Immunity

ALAN A. JACKSON AND PHILIP C. CALDER

CONTENTS

KEY POINTS

- Severely undernourished children are severely immunocompromised.
- Severely undernourished children are highly susceptible to infection, and the interaction leads to a vicious negative cycle.
- Ongoing infection leads to specific nutrient deficiencies.
- Severe undernutrition is associated with very high morbidity and mortality that is directly related to the lack of immunocompetence.
- Infection is often silent because the reductive adaptation of severe undernutrition impairs the immune responses.
- Nonspecific defenses and cell-mediated immunity are most severely affected.
- The proliferative responses of T-lymphocytes are decreased.
- The acute phase response is less active in undernutrition.
- Antioxidant defenses are impaired.
- An increase in free iron promotes prooxidant cellular damage.

From: *Handbook of Nutrition and Immunity*
Edited by: M. E. Gershwin, P. Nestel, and C. L. Keen © Humana Press, Totowa, NJ

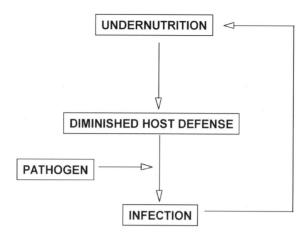

Fig. 1. Bidirectional interaction between nutrition, immune function, and infection. Undernutrition impairs immune defenses and lowers resistance to invading pathogens. In turn, infection alters nutrient status (*see* Fig. 2) and contributes to the undernourished state.

- Successful treatment requires a staged approach, in which cellular function is restored before any attempt is made to restore the weight deficit.
- Cellular function is restored by treating infections, correcting specific nutrient deficiencies, and not giving supplemental iron or an excessive intake of energy, protein, or sodium.

Introduction

Undernutrition is a strong determinant of morbidity and mortality from infection, especially in young children. Globally, it is estimated that 10.4 million children under the age of 5 die each year. Infections are the underlying cause of death for the majority: acute respiratory infections, 24%; diarrhea, 19%; malaria, 7%; measles, 6%. However, undernutrition is the main underlying or associated cause in 49% of all deaths *(1)*. The severity of undernutrition determines the severity of an infection and risk of death *(2–7)*. Undernutrition and infection interact in a vicious negative cycle (*see* Fig. 1). Poor nutrition weakens the body's defenses and increases the likelihood of an infection taking place, although infection itself leads to loss of appetite and increased losses of nutrients from the body and, therefore, a poorer nutritional status (*see* Fig. 2). In many situations, infection is the major precursor for the onset of undernutrition *(8)*. The nutrition-infection problem is most common among children from households that have least assurance of a secure supply of food and have limited resources. Ineffective breast feeding, poor feeding practices, lack of water, fail-

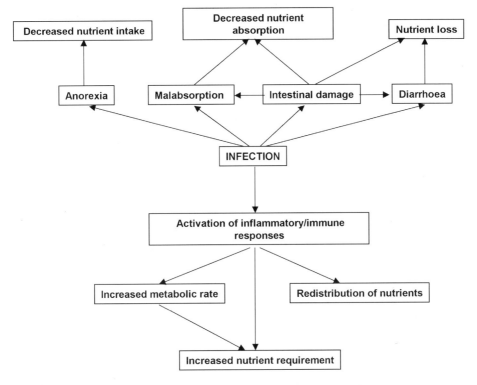

Fig. 2. Mechanisms by which infection can affect nutrient status.

ure of simple hygienic measures, and failure to dispose of solid and other waste adequately contribute substantially to the persistence of the problem. However, a failure to understand the nature of the interaction between poor nutrition and infection and to institute appropriate treatment contributes to the ongoing high mortality. The case mortality rate for severe undernutrition remains unacceptably high—over 30–40% in many health centers around the world *(9)*. Even in resource-poor settings, mortality is expected to be less than 5–10% *(10)*; and inappropriate clinical care makes an unacceptably high contribution to this mortality *(11)*.

This chapter outlines the changes in immune function that occur with severe undernutrition, and which are associated with increased susceptibility to infection, and clarifies some of the important aspects that underlie effective approaches to treatment. Various terms have been and some continue to be used to describe the wide range of different clinical presentations of severe undernutrition. These terms are either descriptive or carry implications about the underlying dietary cause of the disorder and the pathological changes that take place. The terms marasmus, kwashiorkor, wasting, oedematous malnutrition, protein deficiency, and protein-energy deficiency have all been used. Each term emphasizes a particular aspect of a complex condition that has been useful in screening and diagnosis, but often unhelpful in treatment. This is partly because the terms fail to emphasize sufficiently the extent to which infection is present, and the effect of infection on the nutritional state of the individual. Protein-energy malnutrition has been used to describe a condition in which there is significant weight loss. This weight loss has been ascribed to an inadequate intake of food, or an inadequate diet that lacks energy and/or protein in terms of quantity or quality. However, weight loss may not be simply caused by an inadequate intake of macronutrients, as more complex changes are almost invariably taking place owing to a range of nutrient insufficiencies and imbalances. Thus, the terms marasmus, kwashiorkor, and marasmic kwashiorkor have been replaced by the more general terms undernutrition, severe undernutrition, and edematous malnutrition, which do not make any *a priori* judgment about the specific etiology or pathophysiology *(12)*. It can be assumed that most, if not all, severely undernourished children are infected, and making this assumption is one of the key elements in any successful treatment regimen *(10,13)*.

Humankind is continuously exposed to a range of infectious organisms, and an individual's ability to resist these is determined by their capacity to respond appropriately. The response may vary in general or in detail for specific infecting organisms but, at all ages, the flexibility to respond appropriately is fundamental to survival. Young children are particularly vulnerable because the ability to respond most effectively develops with age, and this capability becomes more refined with growth and development and with maturation of the immune response. Therefore, the extent to which an individual is particularly vulnerable is mainly dependent on the interaction of two factors: the extent to which adequate nutrition provides the body with the capability to maintain its function and to protect itself, and the hostility of the environment with which the body has to cope.

Food supply and availability are often uncertain and the body copes by adapting, that is, by bringing mechanisms into play that enable it to maintain function *(14–16)*. However, the extent to which these processes can cope is limited, and they can fail if the degree of undernutrition is sufficiently severe. These processes operate at the cellular, tissue, and whole body levels, and involve the systems that are activated by infection and usually provide adequate protection against infection. As undernutrition becomes progressively more severe, this ability to cope is increasingly eroded and, in the more extreme situations, may be lost completely. Infection induces changes in the body, including a loss of appetite, and frequently leads to a deterioration of nutritional state and a decreased ability to cope. Unless broken at an early stage, this vicious cycle of infection and deteriorating nutrition leads to a progressively worsening state, which can only be treated effectively if due consideration is given to the effect that each has on the other. In this section, the pathophysiological changes that take place in the interaction between nutrition and infection have been used as the starting point for describing the effective management of severe undernutrition. Critically important to a successful outcome is the order in which the different elements of care are brought into play *(10)*.

Nature of Severe Undernutrition

Severe undernutrition is the consequence of two interacting and often concurrent processes, one quantitative change and the other qualitative. The quantitative change is a reduction in total food intake, so that the energy provided by the food is inadequate to meet the needs of the body. The qualitative change is deficiencies of specific nutrients, with the pattern and extent of these deficiencies being variable. Deficiencies are often associated with a poor diet, but importantly are often brought about or made worse by increased losses of specific nutrients during periods of stress such as infection (*see* Fig. 2). The clinical presentation of severe undernutrition usually depends on the extent to which energy intake is inadequate and the particular pattern of specific nutrient deficiencies. This pattern can be very variable and accounts for the widely different clinical presentation from one location to another and, indeed, gave rise to the wide range of descriptive terminology mentioned earlier. This terminology has contributed partly to the persisting high rates of mortality, because it has been presumed that the clinical presentation is an indication of a particular underlying nutritional etiology that has not been corrected. Nevertheless, an inadequate intake of food leads to an unbalanced loss of body tissue, which can be detected clinically as wasting, and on screening as a low body weight-for-age and a low body weight-for-height. Specific nutritional deficiencies (water- and fat-soluble vitamins; trace elements such as zinc, copper, selenium; and minerals such as potassium and magnesium) and their immunologic effect are described in other chapters. They are very common in severe undernutrition, but the pattern of individual nutrient deficiencies and the severity of the deficiency can vary extensively from location to location. Each will have an effect on the body's resistance to infection and will contribute to the variability in clinical presentation in terms of the extent of edematous swelling, skin changes, fatty enlargement of the liver, heart failure, renal impairment, and brain function.

Reductive Adaptation

Reductive adaptation refers to the changes that take place in the body to accommodate a situation where energy intake is insufficient to meet the requirements for maintaining the normal structure and function of cells and tissues *(13–16)*.

The activity of all cells depends upon a continuous supply of energy in a useable form. For most situations, the ability to generate adequate ATP is critical, and for the whole body this is associated with the availability of oxygen and a substrate ultimately derived from carbohydrate, lipid, or amino acids (proteins). This substrate is derived from the body's resources and is replaced on an intermittent basis by the substrate in food consumed. If dietary intake is insufficient to meet the rate at which energy is used by the body, tissues become progressively lost and body weight decreases. The loss of tissue to supply the substrate required to generate energy are not shared evenly among all tissues in the body. The losses are relatively greater for muscle and subcutaneous adipose tissue than other tissues, and there is relative preservation of the brain and the visceral tissues including the kidneys, liver, heart and lungs, leading to a change in the proportions of tissues within the body. The lymphoreticular system is affected by the loss of tissue mass, and undernourished children have a reduced size thymus and spleen and small local lymph nodes (see later).

As dietary energy intake fails to meet the needs of the body, the level of work (energy expenditure) being carried out cannot be maintained. The amount of work performed can be reduced by a decrease in external work, for example, physical activity, or a decrease in internal work, namely, tissue mass. The functions and processes that contribute to the overall internal work of the cells of the system also slow down. The two most obvious processes that place a high demand on the available energy are the pumps in the plasma membrane, which maintain the intra- and extracellular environments in an appropriate state for cell function to occur, and the rate at which proteins are synthesized. Normally, there is a high concentration of potassium within the cell and a high concentration of sodium in the extracellular space that bathes the cells. Achieving and maintaining this difference in the distribution of potassium and sodium is critical for normal cellular function, and this largely occurs through the activity of a pump, the Na/K ATPase, which sits in the plasma membrane. Energy is used to pump sodium from inside the cell to the extracellular fluid, and potassium into the cell from the extracellular fluid. When the availability of energy is limited, this pump slows down, which allows the level of potassium within the cell to fall and the level of sodium to rise, thereby changing the microenvironment within which cellular processes have to take place. Protein synthesis from amino acids uses a substantial proportion of the body's energy requirements. These proteins fulfill a wide range of functions as structural elements, as enzymes to catalyze the chemical processes within the body, as nutrient and hormone transporters, and as hormones or other signaling molecules that integrate the complex range of functions carried out by the body.

Normally, the range and extent of the proteins synthesized are substantially greater than are likely to be needed on a minute-by-minute basis. However, this excess provides an important reserve of function should an unusual situation arise. Thus, the ability of the body to cope immediately with an unusual or extreme situation is dependent upon this "reserve capacity." When the available energy is reduced, it is not possible to maintain this reserve capacity in all cells and tissues at the same level, and the ability to respond to sudden or unusual changes that stress metabolism is impaired. How this impaired ability is expressed or manifested will vary from situation to situation, depending upon the nature and severity of the stressor, and the degree of reductive adaptation in the host.

Effect of Undernutrition on the Immune Response

An important characteristic of life is the body's ability to protect itself from the range of adverse environmental insults to which it is exposed daily. These insults include infection with bacteria and other organisms, and protection is provided by a complex multilayered system of defenses that may be general or highly specific. The first layer of defense, the physical and chemical barrier provided by the skin and mucous membranes, is highly dependent on cellular replication, mucin secretion, and the secretion of protective molecules, such as gastric acid, lysozyme, and secretory immunoglobulins. Once these barriers are breached, increasing reliance is placed on the ability of the body to mount an effective cellular immune response.

In clinical practice, the presence of an infection is indicated by the host's response to that infection. The changes that indicate infection may be a part of a general response, such as the presence of fever, increased pulse, increased respiratory rate, feeling unwell, or the loss of appetite. The site of the infection is localized by the activation of an immune response and the presence of an inflammatory infiltrate. In severe undernutrition, both the generalized and localized responses are often diminished and may be completely absent; these individuals are severely immunocompromised (14,17). Therefore, as in any other immunocompromised state, the presence of an ongoing infection must be highly suspected. Multiple foci of bacterial infection often exist and frequently involve the surface barriers of the skin, respiratory, urinary, and gastrointestinal tracts, but more invasive infection also takes place and can occur with organisms that are not usually considered pathogenic (18–20).

A large number of animal studies have demonstrated the adverse effects of a low-protein diet on immunity (21,22) and these effects have been confirmed in human settings involving protein-energy malnutrition (23–28). Both wasting and stunting are associated with impaired immune function and increase the risk of infectious morbidity and mortality. In severely undernourished children, there may be multiple foci of infection *(18–20,29)*. Not unexpectedly, an inadequate or low-protein diet diminishes the immune responses and increases susceptibility to infection because immune defenses are dependent on cell replication and the production of proteins with biological activities, for example, immunoglobulins, cytokines, and acute phase proteins. It is, however, important to note that low-protein diets are often characterized as being inadequate in micronutrients and low in energy and macronutrients. Nutritional status is further impaired in the presence of infection, which leads to loss of appetite and reduced food intake, as well as an increase in the losses of micronutrients from the body *(see* Fig. 2). Therefore, the exact nature and extent of the immune impairments observed will reflect the nature and extent of the nutrient deficiencies present.

Practically all forms of immunity can be affected by severe undernutrition, but nonspecific defenses and cell-mediated immunity appear to be more severely affected than humoural (antibody) responses *(see* Table 1) *(21,22, 30,31)*. Severe undernutrition causes atrophy of the lymphoid organs (thymus, spleen, lymph nodes, tonsils) in laboratory animals and humans. The corticomedullary regions of lymphoid organs are affected to a greater extent than the epithelium, although the latter is also altered. There is also loss of bone marrow reserves of leukocytes *(32,33)*. The circulating white blood cell count can be increased owing to increased numbers of neutrophils *(34)*; the absolute and relative numbers of monocytes, T-lymphocytes, $CD4^+$ cells, and $CD8^+$ cells are decreased, as is the CD4 to CD8 ratio *(25,35,36)*. The extent of decline in lymphocyte numbers is proportional to the extent of undernutrition *(28)* *(see* Fig. 3). The proliferative responses of T lymphocytes to mitogens and antigens are decreased by undernutrition *(34,35,37)*, as is the synthesis of interleukin (IL)-2 and interferon (IFN). The effect on IFN-γ appears greater than that on IL-2 *(38)*. Animal studies indicate that the production of the Th2 cytokines IL-4, IL-5, and IL-10 may be unaffected by protein deficiency even when production of the Th1 cytokine IFN-γ is markedly depressed *(39,40)*. Likewise, antigen processing and presentation capacity of macrophages may remain intact in undernutrition *(41)*. Natural killer cell activity is decreased in undernutrition *(42,43)*, as is the production of tumour necrosis factor (TNF)-α, IL-1, and IL-6, by stimulated monocytes *(39,44–47)*. The delayed-type hypersensitivity response to antigens is decreased by undernutrition *(48–51)* and the extent of the decrease is related to the degree of undernutrition *(28)* *(see* Fig. 3). Bactericidal activity and respiratory burst of neutrophils are decreased by undernutrition, but the phagocytic capacity of neutrophils and monocytes appears to be unaffected *(32,52)*. The concentration of the complement factor C3 is decreased in severe undernutrition *(48,53,54)*. B-cell numbers and circulating immunoglobulin levels are not affected or may even be increased by undernu-

Table 1
Summary of the Effects
of Protein-Energy Malnutrition on Various Aspects of Immune Function

Component or function	Effect of protein-energy malnutrition
Mucus production	⇓
Mucus structure	Altered
Integrity of the intestinal mucosa	⇓
Weight of thymus, spleen, tonsils, and lymph nodes	⇓
White blood cell counts	⇔ or ⇑
Number of T-lymphocytes in the bloodstream	⇓
Number of CD4 and CD8 cells in the bloodstream	⇓
Ratio of CD4 to CD8 cells in the bloodstream	⇓
Proliferation of T lymphocytes	⇓
Production of Th1-type cytokines (IL-2, IFN-γ)	⇓
Production of Th2-type cytokines (IL-4, IL-5, IL-10)	? ⇔
Delayed-type hypersensitivity	⇓
Number of B-lymphocytes in the bloodstream	⇔
Concentration of immunoglobulins in the bloodstream	⇔ or ⇑
Antibody response to immunization	⇔ or ⇓ depending upon the response involved
Concentration of sIgA in tears, saliva, and so on	⇓
Concentration of C3 in the bloodstream	⇓
Natural killer cell activity	⇓
Phagocytosis by neutrophils	⇔
Respiratory burst by neutrophils	⇓
Phagocytosis by monocytes/macrophages	⇔
Bacterial killing by neutrophils	⇓
Antigen presentation by monocytes	⇔
Production of TNF, IL-1, and IL-6 by monocytes/macrophages	⇓
Concentration of acute phase proteins in the bloodstream	⇓

trition (34,35,48,49,55). The elevated levels may be the result of concurrent infection. Antibody responses to diphtheria, tetanus toxoids, and pneumococcal polysaccharides appear unaffected by undernutrition (48,49). However, the antibody responses to immunization with viral vaccines, which are T-cell-dependent antigens, are diminished (23). Although the level of secretory IgA in tears, saliva, and intestinal washings is decreased by undernutrition (56–58), this may relate to decreased expression of the polymeric Ig receptor that is responsible for transepithelial transport of IgA, rather than to reduced IgA synthesis (58,60).

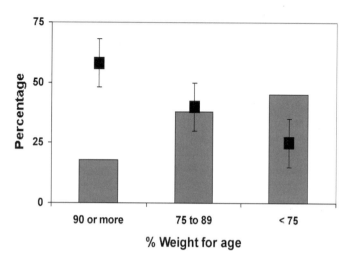

Fig. 3. Relationship between extent of protein-energy malnutrition in children and immune function. Weight-for-age among undernourished children is an indicator of the malnutrition-induced body wasting. T-lymphocytes as a percentage of total blood lymphocytes (black squares) and the percentage of children showing a negative response to tuberculin (shaded bars) are associated with body wasting. Data are taken from ref. *28*.

Low Birth Weight

The fetus accumulates several nutrients such as zinc, copper, iron, and vitamin A during the last trimester of pregnancy, especially during the last 6–8 wk. Thus, premature babies, whether they are small-for-gestational age or appropriate-for-gestational-age, are born with lower nutrient reserves than term infants *(61,62)*. IgG is transferred from the mother to fetus beyond 32 wk of gestation and babies delivered before this time have low serum concentrations, which is thought to contribute to the high frequency of respiratory infections and sepsis in low-birth-weight (LBW) babies. In addition to immaturity of the respiratory system and the gastrointestinal tract, the LBW infants are born with an immature immune system and a reduction in the size of lymphoid organs. LBW babies have decreased numbers of circulating lymphocytes, T-lymphocytes, and CD4+ cells, a decreased CD4 to CD8 ratio, a diminished lymphocyte proliferative response, and a decreased ability of neutrophils to kill bacteria *(63–66)*. LBW babies have lower circulating immunoglobulin concentrations, apart from IgE that is elevated, and normal numbers of B-cells. Some of the immune abnormalities persist beyond 12 mo of age *(64,66)*. LBW increases susceptibility to diarrhea and pneumonia, and increases risk of death from diarrhea, pneumonia, and measles *(67)*.

Barrier Function

Anatomic barriers (skin, mucous membranes) and secretory substances (lysozyme, stomach acid, mucus, secretory IgA) form part of innate host defense. Alterations of anatomic barriers such as skin lesions favor the penetration of infectious microorganisms. Changes in the surface of the gastrointestinal tract can favor pathogen colonization *(68)*, and bacterial translocation *(17)*. Undernutrition alters the quantity of mucus maintained on epithelial surfaces and can also affect its structure *(69,72)*. The intestinal mucosa too may atrophy *(68)*. Decreased secretory IgA has been observed in undernutrition (see above). Salivary flow was reduced and the chemical composition of saliva altered in undernourished children *(73)* and rats *(74)*. Gastric acid secretion is significantly reduced increasing the likelihood of significant numbers of bacteria reaching the small intestine. This, together with a slowing in intestinal transit, contributes to the increased risk of bacterial overgrowth in the small intestine and further impairs the ability to digest and absorb food normally *(17)*.

Acute Phase Response

The acute phase response is attenuated in advanced human protein-energy malnutrition and in protein-deficient rodents. This conclusion is based on measurements of acute phase proteins in serum of children following natural infection *(75)* or vaccination *(76)*, and in weanling rats following a sterile inflammatory stimulus *(77)*. Synthesis of TNF-α, IL-1, and IL-6 is suppressed by stimulated monocytes from children with wasting protein-energy malnutrition *(46,47)*, as is IL-6 by macrophages in wasting protein-deficient young adult rats *(39)*. Thus, the decreased hepatic production of acute phase proteins may reflect, in part, a decreased production of the promoters of their synthesis *(78)*.

Effect of Acute Phase Response on Nutrition

The metabolic response to a severe infection leads to an increase in energy expenditure, increased whole body protein turnover, loss of weight, and negative nitrogen balance *(79–81)*. These responses are muted in severe undernutrition as a direct consequence of the process of reductive adaptation *(17,45,78)*, and are the underlying cause of the significantly increased morbidity and mortality. Clinical signs of infection indicate a more fundamental change in the reordering of the body's metabolic behavior as an integral part of the immune response. Nutrients are repartitioned between tissues and the losses from the body increased, with the magnitude of these losses being greater than might be expected from the degree of negative nitrogen balance. Loss of minerals such as potassium, trace elements such as zinc and copper, and vitamins such as retinol, folate, and B_{12} is increased *(14,17)*. One important consequence of these increased losses is that a marginally adequate diet prevents effective recovery, and deficiencies of specific micronutrients will further impair the ability of cells in general and the cells of the immune system in particular to function adequately and effectively *(16)*. An important exception to this increase in micronutrient losses is iron. Erythrocyte production is reduced in severe undernutrition and infection, and the available iron that is not used for erythrocyte formation increases. There are no mechanisms through which iron can be excreted from the body. Free iron is highly chemically reactive and potentially toxic and is usually transported in blood or stored in a nontoxic form, bound to transferrin or ferritin *(82,83)*. In severe undernutrition, either because of excess iron availability or a limit to the amount that can be stored as ferritin, the amount of free iron in liver and bone marrow increases *(84–87)*. Free iron increases the risk of free radical generation and prooxidant damage to cells *(88)*.

An important aspect of being able to clear an infection is the leukocyte respiratory burst that is impaired in undernutrition. Under normal circumstances, the respiratory burst leads to an increased generation of potentially toxic oxidant damage caused by unbalanced generation of free radicals *(89)*. Usually, the integrity of the system is maintained by the balance being maintained by cellular antioxidant systems and processes. One of the more important changes in cellular function that limits the ability of undernourished children to cope with infection is impaired antioxidant defenses *(90,91)*, Many micronutrient-based components are an integral part of this system, but central to this is the ability to maintain the cellular concentration of the tripeptide antioxidant glutathione (GSH) *(91–93)*. Although energetically expensive, the formation and maintenance of cellular levels of GSH is fundamental. The significant difference in edematous malnutrition is a failure to maintain GSH, which leads directly to excess peroxidative damage of cellular lipids and impaired function *(94–96)*. The repair of cellular GSH status requires sufficient nonessential amino acids such as glycine and cysteine *(97,98)* that are, in turn, dependent on adequate folate, B_2, B_6, B_{12}, zinc, and copper status.

The integration within the body of these complex changes at the cellular and tissue levels depends on an appropriate pattern of hormonal signals and cytokine responses. These responses are modulated by the availability of nutrients, and central to this modulation is the changes that take place in liver function. A large proportion of the proteins synthesized are made in the liver and secreted into the circulation *(14)*. These proteins fulfill a range of functions, among which the transport and delivery of nutrients to other tissues is significant. Examples of transport proteins include albumin, apolipoproteins, transferrin, retinol binding protein, and transthyretin *(99–101)*. The amount and rate at which each of the different proteins is synthesized and secreted varies and, to an extent, is sensitive to the nutrient intake. This property has been used as a biochemical measure of nutritional status *(102,103)*. However, the rate at which these proteins are synthesized and secreted is also modified profoundly during an infection. During an acute phase response, the synthesis of nutrient transport proteins is substantially reduced in favor of the synthesis of acute phase proteins *(78,99–101)*. This shift in the pattern of proteins secreted by the liver exerts a substantial effect on nutrient delivery to all other tissues in the body. In the past, the fall in the plasma albumin concentration was the focus of great attention and taken as a marker for dietary intake. In practice, the significant fall in albumin concentration in undernutrition is more likely to be caused by the acute phase response than to a simple dietary deficiency *(16,83,99,104)*. Indeed, the changes in plasma concentration taking place, as a consequence of alterations in the synthesis of albumin, reflect the changed pattern of synthesis and secretion of the other nutrient transport proteins *(99–101)*. With effective treatment of infection and specific nutrient deficiencies, substantial clinical improvement can take place well in advance of significant improvement in the synthesis rate or plasma concentration of the nutrient transport proteins *(99–101)*. Importantly, transferrin synthesis is reduced as is its concentration in serum, which is another factor that contributes to a general difficulty in handling available iron safely and effectively *(83,84)*. With appropriate treatment the synthesis of transferrin returns to normal *(100)*.

Nature of the Problem to be Managed in Treating a Child With Severe Undernutrition and Infection

The most common infections are acute diarrheal diseases and respiratory tract infections. Standard hygiene practices, including handwashing and effective disposal of contaminated materials, is the basis of limitation and control. However, the weakened immune defenses of undernourished individuals are often incapable of coping with the usual dangers of a modestly contaminated environment. The constant challenge to the immune system allows ongoing nutrient losses. The mainstay of effective treatment requires an integrated approach that has been presented as a 10-step process by the World Health Organization, and which essentially consists of four major elements for the treatment of the acute stages *(10)* (*see* Table 2).

Step 1. Undernutrition As a Medical Emergency

Severely undernourished children often present as a medical emergency with the combination of infection, hypothermia, and hypoglycemia. In addition to general supportive therapy, "silent" infections must be seriously suspected and

Table 2
Principles of Effective Staged Treatment of Severe Undernutrition

---

1. Infection, hypothermia, and hypoglycemia are linked and have to be
   treated aggressively and together as a matter of urgency
2. Normal homeostasis can only be achieved when cells have been repaired
   and can function competently. This requires that all infections are
   under effective control and specific nutrient deficiencies have been
   corrected
3. Growth can only be achieved by cells that can function competently.
   Therefore, an excess of energy or protein, which drives growth, before
   cellular repair has been completed is more likely to increase morbidity
   than lead to an improvement
4. Iron, which cannot be used effectively by metabolic processes, is potentially toxic. Undernourished children tend to have an excess of iron in
   their body, and further supplements increase mortality

---

treated aggressively with suitable wide spectrum antibiotics. Body temperature is maintained by decreasing heat loss, by effectively covering the child,
and providing an external source of warmth, which may simply be the warmth
of the mother's body. As nighttime temperatures can fall to low levels, the
child has to be protected from hypothermia in the early hours of the morning.
Treating infections and maintaining body temperature in themselves help to
maintain blood glucose, but during the early stages, intravenous glucose or
drinks of sucrose or glucose are often necessary while waiting to establish a
regular feeding regimen.

Step 2. Repair Cellular Machinery

The wasting process and loss of specific nutrients impairs the normal function of the cell. An overgrowth of organisms is common and recognizing and
effectively treating small bowel overgrowth may be critical to reducing the
continuing loss of nutrients through the gastrointestinal tract. Potassium deficiency is an important cause of edema and impaired cellular function, and gen-
erous supplements of potassium are central to restoring cellular function and
competence. Because excess sodium is always present in cells and tissues, limiting the intake of sodium ensures that further sodium retention does not make
case management even more difficult. All other specific nutrient deficiencies
need to be corrected progressively. By ensuring an adequate intake of antioxidant nutrients (a vitamin and mineral mixture) it is possible to limit free-radical-mediated oxidative damage. These interventions are of specific importance
for competent cells of the immune system, but are also of general importance
in restoring the function of all cells.

Step 3. Limit Energy and Protein

Screening for undernutrition is based on weight and height; thus drawing attention to the loss of tissue rather than an underlying disturbance of cellular function. If the problem is identified as tissue loss, the natural response is to attempt to replace the lost tissue as quickly and effectively as possible. However, this is potentially dangerous because the damaged cells do not have the ability to grow and replicate. Therefore, the first priority is to repair the machinery required for normal cellular function. This involves correction of micronutrient status that will, in turn, provide the ability to handle macronutrients that will be deposited effectively as new tissue. Excessive energy intake, even as little as 10% of the maintenance requirement, will promote a drive to net tissue deposition. The drive for tissue growth represents a competitive demand for available nutrients and, if excessive, leads to recovery syndrome and possible death. Therefore, energy intake should be limited to cover the needs for maintaining weight (90 kcal/kg/d) and avoid a drive to tissue deposition. Similarly, excessive protein can have an adverse effect if the cellular machinery is not sufficiently repaired to effectively detoxify an excess of amino acids. Those amino acids that cannot be deposited as tissue have to be excreted, and if the excretory systems are impaired, the residues are very toxic. Higher protein diets during this period have been associated with excess mortality. In general, it is not necessary to provide more than 1 g protein/kg/d *(16,105)*.

Step 4. Do Not Give Iron Supplements During the Acute Stage of Treatment

Additional iron is not usually given during the acute and early stages of treatment, because excess iron is associated with greatly increased mortality. If there is direct evidence of specific iron deficiency, clinical judgement is required, but under this circumstance, great caution should be exercised in the administration of iron.

The above regimen effectively treats infection and restores the body's ability to control metabolic balance. Depending upon the severity of the condition, this period may take a few days to a week to complete successfully. The rate at which the immune capability responds is similar to that of other tissues, and cell-mediated immune function may be improved over a period of days to weeks. A failure to improve may reflect a failure to correct an undefined specific nutrient deficiency, for example, the need for adequate zinc repletion *(13,50)*.

The treatment regimen may need to be adapted to manage specific infections most effectively. For example, particular considerations may exist for treating tuberculosis, HIV, malaria, or other parasites. Patients with tuberculosis may not have obvious symptoms when undernourished, but they develop significant symptomatology during treatment once the ability to mount an effective immune response is restored. The increase in symptoms as nutritional status improves may be mistaken for a deterioration in the condition and a worsening of the underlying infection. Severe iron deficiency may be present in individuals with malaria, and caution is required in correcting the iron deficiency at an appropriate rate without stressing the patient. Increasingly, children presenting with undernutrition are likely to have HIV/AIDS *(106)*. The general principles of treatment do not differ from those that apply to any other infected-undernourished individual and, if anything, even greater care is required in the nutritional support needed to improve metabolic control. Certainly, more effective management of any infected undernourished person is likely to lead to a better response to standard pharmaceutical interventions.

Conclusion

A great deal remains to be learned about the nature of the complex interaction between a host's immune response and infection, and how this interaction affects nutritional status. However, there is sufficient understanding of the principles of these interactions to significantly improve the care that is offered to undernourished individuals and to reduce the morbidity and mortality, even under the most resource-poor conditions.

References

1. World Health Organization. (2000) Nutrition for health and development: a global agenda for combating malnutrition. WHO, Geneva: (WHO/NHD/00.6).
2. Kielmann, A.A. and McCord, C. (1978) Weight-for-age as an index of risk of death in children. *Lancet* i, 1247–1250.
3. Alam, N., Wojtymiak, B., and Rahaman, M.M. (1989) Anthropometric indicators and risk of death. *Am. J. Clin. Nutr.* **49**, 884–888.
4. Lutter, C.K., Mora, J.O., Habicht, J.P., et al. (1989) Nutritional supplementation: effects on child stunting because of diarrhea. *Am. J. Clin. Nutr.* **50**, 1–8.
5. Victoria, C.G., Barros, F.C., Kirkwood, B.R., and Vaughan, J.P. (1990) Pneumonia, diarrhea, and growth in the first 4 years of life: a longitudinal study of 5914 urban Brazilian children. *Am. J. Clin. Nutr.* **52**, 391–396.
6. Pelletier, D.L. and Frongillo, E.A. (2003) Changes in child survival are strongly associated with changes in malnutrition in developing countries. *J. Nutr.* **133**, 107–119.
7. Pelletier, D.L., Frongillo, E.A., Schroeder, D.G., and Habicht, J.P. (1995) The effects of malnutrition on child mortality in developing countries. *Bull. WHO* **73**, 443–448.
8. Scrimshaw, N.S., Taylor, C.E., and Gordon, J.E. (1968) *Interactions of Nutrition and Infection*. Geneva, Switzerland: WHO.

9. Schofield, C. and Ashworth, A. (1996) Why have mortality rates for severe malnutrition remained so high? *Bull. World Hlth. Organiz.* **74**, 223–229.

10. Management of severe malnutrition: a manual for physicians and senior health workers. Geneva, Switzerland: WHO, 1999.

11. Chopra, M. and Wilkinson, D. (1995) Treatment of severe malnutrition. *Lancet* **345**, 788–789.

12. Physical status: the use and interpretation of anthropometry. (1995) Report of a WHO Expert Committee. WHO Technical Report Series 854. Geneva, Switzerland: WHO.

13. Jackson, A.A. and Golden, M.H.N. (1987) Severe malnutrition in *Oxford Textbook of Medicine*. (Weatherall, D.J., Ledingham, J.G.G., Warrell, D.A., eds.) Oxford Medical Publications, Oxford, England, pp. 12–28.

14. Waterlow, J.C. (1992) *Protein-Energy Malnutrition*. Edward Arnold, London, England.

15. Waterlow, J.C. (1968) Observations on the mechanism of adaptation to low protein intakes. *Lancet* **ii**, 1091–1097.

16. Jackson, A.A. (1990) The aetiology of kwashiorkor, in *Diet and Disease in Traditional and Developing Societies*. (Harrison, G.A. and Waterlow, J.C., eds.) Cambridge, England: Cambridge University Press, pp. 76–113.

17. Alleyne, G.A.O., Hay, R.W., Picou, D.I., Stanfield, J.P., and Whitehead, R.G. (1997) *Protein-energy malnutrition*. Edward Arnold, London, England.

18. Christie, C.D.C., Heikens, G.T., and Black, F.L. (1990) Acute respiratory infections in ambulatory malnourished children: a serological study. *Trans. Roy. Soc. Trop. Med. Hyg.* **84**, 160–161.

19. Christie, C.D.C., Heikens, G.T., and McFarlane, D.E. (1998) Nosocomial and community acquired infections in malnourished children. *J. Trop. Med. Hyg.* **91**, 173–180.

20. Christie, C.D.C., Heikens, G.T., and Golden, M.H.N. (1992) Coagulase negative staphylococcal bacteraemia in severely malnourished Jamaican children. *Ped. Infect. Dis. J.* **11**, 1030–1036.

21. Gross, R.L. and Newberne, P.M. (1980) Role of nutrition in immunologic function. *Physiol. Rev.* **60**, 188–302.

22. Woodward, B. (2001) The effect of protein-energy malnutrition on immune competence in *Nutrition, Immunity and Infectious Diseases in Infants and Children*. (Tontisirin, K. and Suskind, R., eds.) Basel, Switzerland: Karger, pp. 89–120.

23. Chandra, R.K. (1975) Reduced secretory antibody response to live attenuated measles and poliovirus vaccines in malnourished children. *Brit. Med. J.* **2**, 583–585.

24. Chandra, R.K. (1979) Serum thymic hormone activity in protein-energy malnutrition. *Clin. Exp. Immunol.* **38**, 228–230.

25. Chandra, R.K. (1983) Numerical and functional deficiency in T helper cells in protein-energy malnutrition. *Clin. Exp. Immunol.* **51**, 126–132.

26. Chandra, R.K., Gupta, S., and Singh, H. (1982) Inducer and suppressor T cell subsets in protein-energy malnutrition. *Nutr. Res.* **2**, 21–26.

27. Chandra, R.K., Chandra, S., and Gupta, S. (1984) Antibody affinity and immune complexes after immunization with tetanus toxoid in protein-energy malnutrition. *Am. J. Clin. Nutr.* **40**, 131–134.

28. Rivera, J., Habicht, J.-P., Torres, N., et al. (1986) Decreased cellular immune response in wasted but not in stunted children. *Nutr. Res.* **6**, 1161–1170.

29. Freidland, I.R. Bacteraemia in severely malnourished children. (1992) *Ann. Trop. Paediatr.* **12**, 433–440.

30. Kuvibidila, S., Yu, L., Ode, D., and Warrier, R.P. (1993) The immune response in protein-energy malnutrition and single nutrient deficiencies in *Nutrition and Immunology*. (Klurfield, D.M., ed.) Plenum, London, England, pp. 121–155.

31. Woodward, B. (1998) Protein, calories and immune defences. *Nutr. Rev.* **56**, S84–S92.

32. Edelman, P., Kulapongs, P., Suskind, R.M., and Olson, R.E. (1977) Leukocyte mobilization in Thai children with kwashiorkor in *Malnutrition and the Immune Response*. (Suskind, R.M., ed.) Raven, New York, pp. 265–269.

33. Borelli, P., Mariano, M., and Borojevic, R. (1995) Protein malnutrition: effect on myeloid cell production and mobilzation into inflammatory reactions in mice. *Nutr. Res.* **15**, 1477–1485.

34. Chandra, R.K. (1972) Immunocompetence in undernutrition. *J. Ped.* **81**, 1184–1200.

35. Kulapongs, P., Suskind, R.M., Vithayasai, V., and Olson, E.D. (1977) In vitro cell-mediated immune response in Thai children with protein-calorie malnutrition in *Malnutrition and the Immune Response*. (Suskind, R.M., ed.) Raven, New York, pp. 99–104.

36. Salimonu, L.S., Johnson, A.O.K., Williams, A.I.O., Iyabo-Adeleye, G., and Osunkoya, B.O. (1982a) Lymphocyte populations and antibody levels in immunized malnourished children. *Brit. J. Nutr.* **48**, 7–14.

37. Sellmeyer, E., Bhettay, E., Truswell, A.S., Meyers, O.L., Hansen, J.D.L. (1972) Lymphocyte transformation in maslnourished children. *Arch. Dis. Child.* **47**, 429–435.

38. Mengheri, E., Nobili, F., Crocchioni, G., and Lewis, J.A. (1992) Protein starvation impairs the ability of activated lymphocytes to produce interferon-γ. *J. Interferon Res.* **12**, 17–21.

39. Hill, A.D.K., Naama, H., Shou, J., Calvano, S.E., and Daly, J.M. (1995) Antimicrobial effects of granulocyte-macrophage colony-stimulating factor in protein-energy malnutrition. *Arch. Surg.* **130**, 1273–1278.

40. Shi, H.N., Scott, M.E., Stevenson, M.M., and Koski, K.G. (1998) Energy restriction and zinc deficiency impair functions of murine T cells and antigen-presenting cells during gastrointestinal nematode infection. *J. Nutr.* **128**, 20–27.

41. Redmond, H.P., Gallagher, H.J., Shou, J., and Daly, J.M. (1995) Antigen presentation in protein-energy malnutrition. *Cell Immunol.* **163**, 80–87.

42. Salimonu, L.S., Ojo-Amaize, E., Williams, A.I., et al. (1982) Depressed natural killer cell activity in children with protein-calorie malnutrition. *Clin. Immunol. Immunopathol.* **24**, 1–7.

43. Ingram, K.G., Croy, B.A., and Woodward, B.D. (1995) Splenic natural killer cell activity in wasted, protein-energy malnourished weanling mice. *Nutr. Res.* **15**, 231–243.
44. Bhaskaram, P., Madhusudham, J., Radhakrishna, K.V., and Reddy, V. (1986) Immune response in malnourished children with measles. *J. Trop. Ped.* **32**, 123–126.
45. Kauffman, C.A., Jones, P.G., and Klorges, M.J. (1982) Fever and malnutrition: endogenous pyrogen/interleukin-1 in malnourished patients. *Am. J. Clin. Nutr.* **44**, 449–452.
46. Doherty, J.F., Golden, M.H.N., Remick, D.G., and Griffin, G.E. (1994) Production of interleukin-6 and tumor necrosis factor-α in vitro is reduced in whole blood of severely malnourished children. *Clin. Sci.* **86**, 347–351.
47. Munoz, C., Arevalo, M.T., Lopez, M., and Schlesinger, L. (1994) Impaired interleukin-1 and tumor necrosis factor production in protein-calorie malnutrition. *Nutr. Res.* **14**, 347–352.
48. Kielmann, A.A., Uberoi, I.V., Chandra, R.K., and Vehra, V.L. (1976) The nutritional status on immune capacity and immune responses in preschool children in a rural community in India. *Bull. World Hlth. Organiz.* **54**, 477–483.
49. Neumann, C.G., Lawlor, G.I., Stiehm, E.R., et al. (1975) Immunologic responses in malnourished children. *Am. J. Clin. Nutr.* **28**, 89–104.
50. Golden, M.H.N., Golden, B.E., Harland, P.S.E.G., and Jackson, A.A. (1978) Zinc and immunocompetence in protein-energy malnutrition. *Lancet* **i**, 1226–1228.
51. Shell-Duncan, B. (1997) Evaluation of infection and nutritional status as determinants of cellular immunosuppression. *Am. J. Hum. Biol.* **9**, 381–390.
52. Seth, V. and Chandra, R.K. (1972) Opsonic activity, phagocytosis and bactericidal capacity of polymorphs in undernutrition. *Arch. Dis. Child.* **47**, 282–284.
53. Chandra, R.K. (1977) Serum complement components in malnourished Indian children in *Malnutrition and the Immune Response*. (Suskind, R.M., ed.) Raven, New York, pp. 329–332.
54. McMurray, D.N., Loomis, S.A., Casazza, L.J., Rey, H., and Miranda, R. (1981) Development of impaired cell-mediated immunity in mild and moderate malnutrition. *Am J Clin Nutr* **34**, 68–77.
55. Ha, C-L., Paulino-Racine, L.E., and Woodward, B.D. (1996) Expansion of the humoral effector cell compartment of both systemic and mucosal immune systems in a weanling murine model which duplicates critical features of human protein-energy malnutrition. *Brit. J. Nutr.* **75**, 445–460.
56. McMurray, D.N., Rey, H., Casazza, L.J., and Watson, R.R. (1977) Effects of moderate malnutrition on concentration of immunoglobulins and enzymes in tears and saliva of young Colombian children. *Am. J. Clin. Nutr.* **30**, 1944–1948.
57. Watson, R.R., McMurray, D.N., Martin, P., and Reyes, M.A. (1985) Effect of age, malnutrition and renutrition on free secretory component and IgA in secretions. *Am. J. Clin. Nutr.* **42**, 281–288.
58. Sullivan, D.A., Vaerman, J-P., and Soo, C. (1993) Influences of severe protein malnutrition on rat lacrimal, salivary, and gastrointestinal immune expression during development, adulthood and aging. *Immunol.* **78**, 308–317.

59. Ha, C-L. and Woodward, B.D. (1997) Reduction in the quantity of the polymeric immunoglobulin receptor is sufficient to account for the low concentration of intestinal secretory immunoglobulin A in a weanling mouse model of wasting protein-energy malnutrition. *J. Nutr.* **127**, 427–435.

60. Ha, C-L. and Woodward, B.D. (1998) Depression in the quantity of intestinal secretory IgA and in the expression of the polymeric immunoglobulin receptor in caloric deficiency of the weanling mouse. *Lab. Invest.* **78**, 1255–1266.

61. Farrell, P.M., Zachman, R.D., and Gutcher, G.R. (1985) Fat soluble vitamins A, E and K in the premature infant in *Vitamin and Mineral Requirements in Preterm Infants.* (Vtsang, R.C., ed.) Marcel Dekker, New York, pp. 63–98.

62. Powers, H.J. (1993) Micronutrient deficiencies in the preterm neonate. *Proc. Nutr. Soc.* **52**, 285–291.

63. Ferguson, A.G., Lawlor, G.J., Neumann, C.G., Oli, W., and Stiehm, E.R. (1974) Decreased rosette-forming lymphocytes in malnutrition and intrauterine growth retardation. *J. Ped.* **85**, 717–723.

64. Chandra, R.K. (1975) Fetal malnutrition and postnatal immunocompetence. *Am. J. Dis. Child.* **129**, 450–454.

65. Chandra, R.K., Ali, S.K., and Chandra, S. (1977) Thymus-dependent lymphocytes and delayed hypersensitivity in low birthweight infants. *Biol. Neonate* **31**, 15–18.

66. Neumann, C.G., Stiehm, E.R., Zahradnick, J., et al. (1984) Immune function in intrauterine growth retardation. *Nutr. Res.* **4**, 399–419.

67. Ashworth, A. (2001) Low birth weight infants, infection and immunity in *Nutrition, Immunity and Infectious Diseases in Infants and Children.* (Totinsirin, K. and Suskind R., eds.) Karger, Basel, pp. 121–136.

68. Deitch, E.A., Ma, W-J., Ma, L., Berg, R.D., and Specian, R.D. (1990) Protein malnutrition predisposes to inflammatory-induced gut-origin septic states. *Ann. Surg.* **211**, 560–567.

69. Alleyne, G.A.O., Hay, R.W., Picou, D.I., Stanfield, J.P., and Whitehead, R.G. (1977) *Protein-energy malnutrition.* Edward Arnold, London.

70. Sherman, P., Forstner, J., Roomi, N., Khatri, L., and Forstner, G. (1985) Mucin depletion in the intestine of malnourished rats. *Am. J. Physiol.* **248**, G418–G423.

71. Enwonwu, C.O. (1995) Interface of malnutrition and peridontal diseases. *Am. J. Clin. Nutr.* **61**, 430S–436S.

72. Redmond, H.P., Shou, J., Kelley, C.J., et al. (1991) Immunosuppressive mechanisms in protein-calorie malnutrition. *Surgery* **110**, 311–317.

73. Johansson, I., Saellstrom, A-K., Rajan, B.P., and Parameswaran, A. (1992) Salivary flow and dental caries in Indian children suffering from chronic malnutrition. *Caries. Res.* **26**, 38–43.

74. Johansson, I. and Ericson, T. (1987) Biosynthesis of salivary bacteria-agglutinating glycoprotein in the rat during protein deficiency. *Caries. Res.* **21**, 7–14.

75. Duran-Chavez, C., Sanchez-Herrera, G., Canedo-Solares, I., and Perez-Ortiz, B. (1994) C-reactive protein in severely malnourished children. *Nutr. Res.* **14**, 967–975.

76. Doherty, J.F., Golden, M.N.H., Raynes, J.G., Griffin, R.E., and McAdam, K.P.W.J. (1993) Acute-phase protein response is impaired in severely malnourished children. *Clin. Sci.* **84**, 169–175.
77. Jennings, G., Bourgeois, C., and Elia, M. (1992) The magnitude of the acute phase protein response is attenuated by protein deficiency in rats. *J. Nutr.* **122**, 1325–1331.
78. Reid, M., Badaloo, A., Forrester, T., Morlese, J.F., Heird, W.C., and Jahoor, F. (2002) The acute-phase protein response to infection in edematous and nonedematous protein-energy malnutrition. *Am. J. Clin. Nutr.* **76**, 1409–1415.
79. Tomkins, A.M., Garlick, P.J., Schofield, W.N., and Waterlow, J.C. (1983) The combined effects of infection and malnutrition on protein metabolism in children. *Clin. Sci.* **65**, 313–324.
80. Manary, M.J., Broadhead, R.L., and Yarasheski, K.E. (1998) Whole-body protein kinetics in marasmus and kwashiorkor during acute infection. *Am. J. Clin. Nutr.* **67**, 1205–1209.
81. Reid, M., Badaloo, A., Forrester, T., Heird, W.C., and Jahoor, F. (2002) Response of splanchnic and whole body leucine kinetics to treatment of children with edematous and noedematous protein-energy malnutrition accompanied by infection. *Am. J. Clin. Nutr.* **76**, 633–640.
82. McFarlane, H., Reddy, S., Adcock, K.J., Adeshina, H., Cooke, A.R., and Akene, J. (1970) Immunity, transferrin, and survival in kwashiorkor. *Br. Med. J.* **2**, 268–270.
83. Reeds, P.J. and Laditan, A.A.O. (1976) Serum albumin and transferrin in protein energy malnutrition. *Br. J. Nutr.* **36**, 255–263.
84. Waterlow, J.C. (1948) Fatty liver disease in infant in the British West Indies. MRC Special Report Series No. 263, HMSO, London.
85. Dempster, W.S., Sive, A.A., Rosseau, S., Malan, H., and Heese, H.V. (1995) Misplaced iron in kwashiorkor. *Eur. J. Clin. Nutr.* **49**, 208–210.
86. Sive, A.A., Dempster, W.S., Rosseau, S., Kelly, M., Malan, H., and Heese, H.D. (1996) Bone marrow and chelatable iron in patients with protein energy malnutrition. *S. Afr. Med. J.* **86**, 1410–1413.
87. Sive, A.A., Dempster, W.S., Malan, H., Rousseau, S., Heese, H.D. (1997) Plasma free iron: a possible cause of oedema in kwashiorkor. *Arch. Dis. Child.* **76**, 54–56.
88. Ramdath, D. and Golden, M.H.N. (1989) Non-haematological aspects of iron nutrition. *Nutr. Res. Rev.* **2**, 29–49.
89. Golden, M.H. and Ramdath, D. (1987) Free radicals in the pathogenesis of kwashiorkor. *Proc. Nutr. Soc.* **46**, 53–68.
90. Sive, A.A., Subotzky, E.F., Malan, H., Dempster, W.S., and Heese, H.D. (1993) Red blood cell antioxidant enzyme concentrations in kwashiorkor and marasmus. *Ann. Trop. Paediatr.* **13**, 33–38.
91. Jackson, A.A. (1986) Blood glutathione in severe malnutrition in childhood. *Trans. R. Soc. Trop. Med. Hyg.* **80**, 911–913.
92. Reid, M., Badaloo, A., Forrester, T., et al. (2000) In vivo rates of erythrocyte glutathione synthesis in children with severe protein-energy malnutrition. *Am. J. Physiol.* **278**, E405–E412.

93. Ramdath, D.D. and Golden, M.H. (1993) Elevated glutathione S-transferase activity in erythrocytes from malnourished children. *Eur. J. Clin. Nutr.* **47**, 658–665.

94. Mayatepek, E., Becker, K., Gana, L., Hoffman, G.F., Leichsenring, M. (1993) Leukotrienes in the pathophysiology of kwashiorkor. *Lancet* **342**, 958–960.

95. Lenhartz, H., Ndasi, R., Anninos, A., et al. (1998) The clinical manifestations of the kwashiorkor syndrome is related to increased lipid peroxidation. *J. Pediatr.* **132**, 879–881.

96. Manary, M.J., Leeuwenberg, C., and Heinecke, J.W. (2001) Increased oxidative stress in kwashiorkor. *J. Pediatr.* **137**, 421–424.

97. Persaud, C., Forrester, T., and Jackson, A.A. (1996) Urinary 5-L-oxoproline (pyrogluamic acid) is increased during recovery from severe childhood malnutrition and responds to supplemental glycine. *J. Nutr.* **126**, 2823–2830.

98. Badaloo, A., Reid, M., Forrester, T., Heird, W.C., and Jahoor, F. (2002) Cysteine supplementation improves the erythrocyte glutathione synthesis rate in children with severe edematous malnutrition. *Am. J. Clin. Nutr.* **76**, 646–652.

99. Morlese, J.F., Forrester, T., Badaloo, A., del Rosario, M., and Frazer, M. (1996) Albumin kinetics in edematous and nonedematous protein-energy malnourished children. *Am. J. Clin. Nutr.* **64**, 952–959.

100. Morlese, J.F., Forrester, T., del Rosario, M., Frazer, M., and Jahoor, F. (1997) Transferrin kinetics are altered in children with severe protein-energy malnutrition. *J. Nutr.* **127**, 1469–1474.

101. Morlese, J.F., Forrester, T., del Rosario, M., Frazer, M., and Jahoor, F. (1998) Repletion of the plasma pool of nutrient transport protein occurs at different rates during nutritional rehabilitation of severely malnourished children. *J. Nutr.* **128**, 214–219.

102. Shetty, P., Watrasiewicz, K., Jung, R., and James, W. (1979) Rapid turnover proteins: an index of subclinical protein-energy malnutrition. *Lancet* **ii**, 230–232.

103. Golden, M.H.N. (1982) Transport proteins as indices of protein status. *Am. J. Clin. Nutr.* **35**, 1159–1165.

104. James, W.P.T. and Hay, A.M. (1968) Albumin metabolism: effect of the nutritional state and the dietary protein intake. *J. Clin. Invest.* **47**, 1958–1972.

105. Collins, S., Myatt, M., and Golden, B. (1998) Dietary treatment of severe malnutrition in adults. *Am. J. Clin. Nutr.* **68**, 193–199.

106. Mgone, C.S., Mhalu, F.S., Shao, J.F., et al. (1991) Prevalence of HIV-1 infection and symptomatology of AIDS in severely malnourished children in Dar Es Salaam, Tanzania. *J. AIDS* **4**, 910–913.

5 Infection, Immunity, and Vitamins

USHA RAMAKRISHNAN, AMY L. WEBB, AND KAREN OLOGOUDOU

CONTENTS

KEY POINTS

- Vitamin deficiencies, especially A and the B-complex, are widespread in many developing countries and impair both innate and adaptive immunity.
- Vitamin A is the most widely studied micronutrient and deficiency results in:
  - decreased barrier function
  - decreased natural killer activity
  - decreased T- and B-lymphocytes and abnormal cytokine function.
- Vitamin A supplementation:
  - decreases child mortality
  - decreases measles related morbidity and mortality
  - decreases the severity and duration of diarrhea
  - has no effect on acute lower respiratory infection and vertical transmission of HIV.
- Vitamin E and C have antioxidant properties and supplementation and
  - increase immune function in elderly
  - may decrease HIV progression.
- The B vitamins and vitamins D and K are less studied, especially in humans.

From: *Handbook of Nutrition and Immunity*
Edited by: M. E. Gershwin, P. Nestel, and C. L. Keen © Humana Press, Totowa, NJ

- Multiple micronutrient supplements offer promise as a cost-effective strategy to increase immune function in the elderly and HIV/AIDS patients, but more studies are needed in developing countries.

Introduction

Inadequate food intake and poor dietary quality result in micronutrient deficiencies and affects a large number of people in developing countries, as well as subgroups such as the elderly and HIV infected individuals in developed countries. The most extensively studied vitamin deficiency is that for vitamin A, which affects up to 254 million young children worldwide (1). Women of reproductive age are also at high risk of vitamin A deficiency (VAD) in many developing countries. Vitamin A supplementation improves breast milk quality alleviates anemia, and may reduce maternal mortality (2). Other common vitamin deficiencies include the B vitamins, especially folic acid, B_6, B_{12}, thiamin (B_1), riboflavin (B_2), as well as vitamin C, although reliable data on the magnitude of these deficiencies are limited (3). Deficiencies of the other fat-soluble vitamins, namely D, E, and K are less common, and subgroups may be at risk.

The synergistic association between nutrition and infections has been well known for several decades. Scrimshaw (4) demonstrated protein-energy malnutrition in young children increased their susceptibility to common childhood illness such as diarrhea and acute respiratory infections which, in turn, increased their risk of being undernourished as a result of reduced food intake and increased losses from poor absorption and metabolism. Over the last 30 yr, considerable progress has been made in understanding the mechanisms by which undernutrition—and more recently specific micronutrient deficiencies—can affect the immune system and thus the response to infections (5,6). This chapter summarizes the role of vitamins in immune function and response to infections. The role of vitamins in common childhood illnesses including diarrhea, measles, and respiratory infections as well as malaria and HIV/AIDS is discussed.

Single Vitamins and Immune Infection

Vitamin A

The role of vitamin A in immune function was first recognized at the beginning of the 20th century, when it was dubbed the "antiinfective" vitamin (7). Since then, both its role in modulating disease-specific immunity and the mechanisms through which it may exert its antiinfective effects have been elucidated (8). Vitamin A supplementation can reduce all-cause child mortality by almost one-third in areas where VAD is common (9). For measles and diarrhea, this decreased the severity and duration of illness rather than the incidence of the disease *(2,10)*. Ongoing research related to vitamin A supplementation in malaria and HIV/AIDS will provide additional understanding of how vitamin A functions in immunity.

Mechanisms

INNATE IMMUNITY

Vitamin A is essential for maintaining normal epithelial tissue integrity and is critical to barrier function. Deficiency is associated with hyperkeratosis of the skin, squamous metaplasia of respiratory epithelium, and decreased numbers of goblet cells and mucus secretions in the epithelial lining of the gut *(8,11)*. Vitamin A supplementation improved gut epithelial integrity and the gut's regenerative ability in children in India and the Gambia *(12)*. VAD has been associated with reduced numbers and activity of natural killer cells and eosinophils and diminished phagocytic and oxidative burst capabilities of macrophages and neutrophils *(8,13)*. Increased production of interleukin (IL)-12 and tumor necrosis factor (TNF)-α in the vitamin A deficient state, and a subsequent increase in activated but inefficient macrophages, may promote an excessive inflammatory response and its accompanying pathologies *(8)*. Repletion and supplementation reverse these cellular abnormalities *(11,13)*. In summary, vitamin A is essential to a competent innate response; deficiency suppresses innate immunity, hindering the formation of a rapid response in the event of infections and insults. β-carotene, the nontoxic precursor of vitamin A, may also have similar effects but data are limited and more research is needed to elucidate the role of β-carotene in the immune response and in specific diseases.

ADAPTIVE RESPONSE

Vitamin A appears to maintain the normal antibody-mediated (or T-helper type-2 [Th2]) response by suppressing IL-12 and TNF-α production *(6,8)*. Deficiency results in abnormal production of these cytokines and subsequent suppression of the Th2 response, and individuals with VAD have an impaired ability to defend against extracellular pathogens (*see* Table 1). Additionally, VAD is associated with a decrease in the number of antigen specific plasma cells, a diminished immunoglobulin (Ig) A response to cholera toxin and influenza, diminished IgG1 and IgE response to *Schistosoma mansoni* and *Trichinella spiralis (6,8)*. The diminished antibody response and suppression of Th2 cytokine production have been shown to be reversible with supplementation *(6,8,11)*.

Morbidity

The role of vitamin A and its deficiency in specific diseases, especially childhood diseases, has been a subject of interest for decades. Some of the key findings for several common causes of child mortality are described below.

MEASLES

Vitamin A has long been associated with morbidity and mortality outcomes from measles. Serum retinol concentrations are inversely related to increased severity of measles, and community-based and clinical trials have shown that large dose vitamin A supplementation (200,000 IU) decreased measles-specific mortality by more than 50% *(14)*. These findings led the World Health Organization (WHO) to recommend that all children receive a large-dose vitamin A supplementation of 200,000 IU (100,000 for children under the age of 1 yr) at the onset of measles. In areas where VAD is a public health concern, WHO and UNICEF recommend two doses. Recent studies have also shown that large dose vitamin A supplementation reduces the incidence and duration of infections secondary to measles *(see* Table 2). A systematic review *(21)* that included six randomized controlled trials found that vitamin A supplementation significantly reduced the incidence of croup and otitis media and the duration of diarrhea, pneumonia, hospital stay, and fever.

DIARRHEA

Studies reporting a role for vitamin A in alleviating and/or preventing diarrhea are mixed *(see* Table 3). Several randomized controlled trials failed to detect any reduction in the incidence of diarrhea and it is now accepted that the primary role of vitamin A in reducing diarrhea-associated mortality is by reducing the severity and duration of a diarrheal episode *(2,10)*. Some studies found the beneficial effects of vitamin A supplementation appeared to be modulated by the individual's nutritional status and/or the infectious agent. Work in Bangladesh, the Congo, and Tanzania illustrate the emerging dichotomy of how vitamin A affects those with diarrhea. Supplementing Bangledeshi children ameliorated diarrhea caused by shigellosis, but had no effect on diarrhea of rotavirus or *Escherichia coli* origin *(24,32)*. The suppression of the Th2 response during VAD may provide insight into this discrepancy. A hospital study on Congolese children found decreased risk of diarrhea among those with protein-energy malnutrition who received vitamin A supplementation and an increased risk of diarrhea among those without protein-energy malnutrition who received vitamin A supplementation *(33)*. In Tanzania, the benefits of supplementation were more evident in stunted children *(39)*. It is hypothesized that in well-nourished children, large doses of vitamin A may escalate a normal inflammatory response whereas, in children with suboptimal status, large doses of vitamin A may normalize the Th1 response and restore an optimal Th2 response in addition to improving gut integrity *(8,13)*.

RESPIRATORY INFECTIONS

In contrast to measles and diarrhea, vitamin A does not diminish the incidence, severity, or duration of respiratory infections that are not secondary to measles. In fact, some studies have indicated that vitamin A supplementation, especially in well-nourished individuals, may exacerbate respiratory infections *(10,39)*. Studies in Guatemala, Brazil, and Tanzania found no effect of vitamin A supplementation on reducing respiratory-related mortality; duration of hospital stay; or fever, tachynpea, or hypoxia in hospitalized children, whereas a study in Peru found significant increases in persistence of retractions on day 3 after supplementation with 300,000 IU vitamin A *(39)*. Only one study (in Vietnam) found that a 400,000 IU vitamin A supplement was associated with decreased hospital stay in undernourished children hospitalized for respiratory infections. Community-based trials corroborate the findings of a lack of effect. Studies in India and Australia found vitamin A supplementation did not alter the incidence of acute lower respiratory tract infection (ALRI), whereas studies in Indonesia and Ecuador found that the effect was dependent on nutritional status *(31,34)*. In Indonesia *(31)*, vitamin A supplementation was associated with increased incidence of ALRI among nonstunted children; no effects were observed among stunted children. The Ecuador study *(34)* found a significantly decreased incidence of respiratory infections among underweight children, but increased incidence among supplemented children with normal nutritional status, and no effect among stunted children. It has been hypothesized that in normally nourished children, vitamin A supplementation may increase the inflammatory response, thus exacerbating damage to the respiratory tract *(8)*.

MALARIA

Animal studies have long provided support for a role of vitamin A in malaria morbidity and malaria resistance *(40)*. A study in Papua New Guinea found significantly reduced malarial episodes, and nonsignificantly diminished parasite load and decreased spleenomegaly among preschool children supplemented with vitamin A. Other studies in humans, however, were confounded or biased and their results must be interpreted with caution *(40)*. Based on animal and human studies, it appears that VAD potentiates malaria morbidities. The exact of role of supplementation in alleviating malaria illness, however, has not been fully studied. Controlled intervention trials in adults and children and in individuals of varying stages of nutritional deficit are

Table 1
Role of Vitamins in Immune Function

Vitamin	INNATE IMMUNITY	Adaptive immunity				
		T cells	B cells	Cytokines	Th1	Th2
A	• Decreased Barrier Integrity • Squamous metaplasia of epithelial linings • Hyperkeratosis • Decreased mucus secretion • Increased gut permeability • Increased number of circulating neutrophils and natural killer (NK) cells • Decreased killing ability of NK cells, macrophages, and neutophils • Increased number of activated macrophages	• Decreased number of antigen specific plasma cells	• Decreased IgG1, IGE, and IgA response	• Abnormal cytokine pattern • Increased production of IL-12 and IFN-γ	Increased	Decreased
Folic Acid	• Decreased NK cell activity	• Decreased DTH response			Decreased	?
B$_6$	• Decreased lymphocyte proliferation • Decreased NK cell activity	• Decreased T-helper cells		• Decreased IL-2	Decreased	?

B$_{12}$	• Increased lymphocyte activity and NK activity with supplementation	• Decreased DTH response		?	Decreased?
C	• Decreased phagocytosis and microbial activity			?	?
D$_3$	• Inhibits NK in dose-dependent manner	• Inhibits T-lymphoctyte proliferation			
E	• Decreased phagocytosis in conjunction with vitamin C • Decreased NK cytoxicity	• Increased lymphocyte proliferation in response to mitogen • Impaired DTH skin response	• Decreased IL-2 formation in response to specific mitogen • Increased IL-4	Decreased	

Table 2
Effect of Vitamin A Supplementation on Measles

Country (Yr)	Study Sample	Intervention	Results
Tanzania, 1987 (15)	180 children admitted to hospital for measles	• 200,000 IU vitamin A on days 1 and 2 of hospital stay • 1 mo follow up	• No effect on mortality from measles or pneumonia
South Africa, 1990 (16)	189 children <13 yr admitted to hospital	• 200,000 IU vitamin A on days 1 and 2 of hospital stay • Follow up for length of hospital stay	• Decreased hospital deaths • Decreased duration of measles-associated pneumonia, diarrhea, and hospital confinement • Decreased incidence of croup
South Africa, 1991 (17)	60 children 4–24 mo	• 200,000 IU vitamin A on days 1, 2, and 8 of hospital stay • Follow up for length of hospital stay	• No effect on mortality • Decreased duration of clinical measles and measles-associated pneumonia

Study	Population	Intervention	Results
Kenya, 1993 (18)	294 children <5 yr	• 200,000 IU vitamin A in single dose • Followed up for length of hospital stay	• No effect on hospital death • No effect on incidence of measles-specific pneumonia • No effect on incidence of measles-specific diarrhea • Decreased incidence of otitis media
Zambia, 1996 (19)	200 children <5 yr	• 380,000 IU vitamin A in single dose • 1 mo follow up	• No effect on mortality • No effect on incidence of pneumonia
Zambia, 2002 (20)	200 acute measles patients (5 mo–17 yr) stratified by vitamin A deficiency	• 200,000 IU vitamin A in single dose • 1 mo follow up	• Decreased incidence of measles-associated pneumonia in VAD children receiving supplement-placebo and VA sufficient • Increased incidence of measles-associated pneumonia in VA sufficient receiving supplementation compared to placebo

Table 3
Effect of Vitamin A Supplementation on Diarrhea

Country (Yr)	Study Sample	Intervention	Results
Indonesia, 1991 (22)	28,861 children 1–5 yr	200,000 IU vitamin A every 6 mo for 1 yr	• No effects on prevalence of diarrhea
India, 1991 (23)	15,419 children 6–60 mo	~8000 IU vitamin A/wk for 1 yr	• Increased incidence of chronic diarrhea among stunted children
Bangladesh, 1992 (24)	83 children 1–5 yr	200,000 single dose vitamin A	• No effect on diarrhea (predominantly due to *E. coli* and rotavirus)
Haiti, 1993 (25)	11,124 children 6–83 mo	200,000 IU vitamin A 4x/mo	• Increased prevalence of diarrhea
China, 1993 (26)	172 children 6–36 mo	200,000 IU vitamin A every 6 mo	• Decreased incidence of diarrhea
Brazil, 1994 (27)	1240 children 6–48 mo	200,000 IU vitamin A (100,000 in <1 yr) every 4 mo for 1 yr	• Decreased incidence of diarrhea • Decreased incidence of severe diarrhea
India, 1994 (28)	900 children 12–60 mo with acute diarrhea	200,000 IU vitamin A	• No effect on incidence
India, 1995 (29)	216 children 6–60 mo	200,000 IU vitamin A	• No effect on duration • Decreased incidence of severe episodes
India, 1995 (30)	583 children 6–36 mo	200,000 IU vitamin A (100,000 <1 yr) every 4 mo for 1 yr	• No effect on incidence • Decreased duration of diarrhea episode
Indonesia, 1996 (31)	1407 children 6–47 mo	200,000 IU vitamin A (100,000 <1 yr) every 4 mo for 1 yr	• No effect on incidence of diarrhea
Bangladesh, 1998 (32)	83 children 1–7 yr with shigellosis	200,000 single dose vitamin A	• Reduced duration

102

Study (location, year, ref)	Subjects	Intervention	Results
...(33)	300 children 0–72 mo	200,000 single dose vs daily low dose (5000 IU) 40 wk	• Decreased incidence of severe diarrhea in PEM children receiving daily supplements • Increased risk of diarrhea in non-PEM children receiving single high dose
Ecuador, 1999 (34)	400 children 6–36 mo	10,000 IU vitamin A/wk for 40 wk	• Decreased risk of severe diarrhea in children 18–23 mo • Reduced risk of severe diarrhea
Tanzania 2000 (35)	687 children hospitalized with pneumonia 6–60 mo	200,000 IU vitamin A on d 1, d 2, mo 4 and 8	• Decreased risk of acute diarrhea in wasted children • Increased risk of acute diarrhea in children with normal nutritional status
Bangladesh, 2001 (36)	96 moderately malnourished children with persistent diarrhea 6–24 mo	4 intervention groups Zn: 20 mg and multivitamin daily VA: 26,666 IU vitamin A/d + multivitamin daily Zn + vitamin A: 26,666 IU vitamin A + 20 mg Zn + multivitamin daily Placebo 7-d study	• Zn and not vitamin A decreased stool output, prevented weight loss, and promoted earlier recovery
Bangladesh, 2001 (37)	800 children 12–35 mo	Four intervention groups Zn: 20 mg/daily for 14 d Vitamin A: 200,000 IU on d 14 Zn +VA Placebo 6 mo follow up	• Both vitamin A and Zn decreased the prevalence and incidence of diarrhea, separately and in combination • Decreased prevalence of dysentery for vitamin A + Zn only
Tanzania, 2002 (38)	687 children 6–60 mo hospitalized with pneumonia	200,000 IU vitamin A on day 1, d 2, mo 4, and 8	• Increased growth patterns observed among those who had suffered severe diarrhea

needed. Furthermore, the ability of vitamin A to alleviate anemia *(41)*, while concurrently alleviating malaria-related illness, offers hope in improving the health outcomes of pregnant women, who suffer from the compounded effects of malaria induced anemia.

HIV

The two primary areas of research on vitamin A and HIV relate to maternal-to-child transmission (MTCT) of HIV and HIV pathogenesis and progression. With respect to MTCT, VAD is associated with increased risk of viral shedding via genital secretions, epithelial cornification of the lower genital tract, diminished placental integrity in rats, and increased viral shedding in human breast milk. Observational studies in Malawi, Rwanda, and the United States have also shown that low serum retinol levels were associated with increased risk of vertical transmission of HIV *(42)*. However, supplementation trials of pregnant HIV$^+$ women in Malawi, Tanzania, and South Africa, failed to demonstrate any benefits.

With respect to HIV/AIDS pathogenesis and progression VAD, but not supplementation *per se*, appears to be the primary modulator. In adults, low serum vitamin A has been associated with increased mortality and disease progression *(43,44)*. However, some studies found vitamin A supplementation had a U-shaped relationship with disease progression and death *(45)*. Supplementation had no effects on viral load in HIV$^+$ intravenous drug users *(42)*, or in improving T-cell counts in HIV$^+$ Tanzanian women *(46)*. Thus, vitamin A supplementation in adults may be important in HIV/AIDS only in the context of remedying deficiency. In contrast, several studies have demonstrated that vitamin A supplementation, provided three or four times a year to children under the age of 5 yr, reduced AIDS-related morbidities, particularly diarrhea, and death *(47)*. Additionally, vitamin A supplementation in HIV-infected children has not been associated with the adverse effects observed in some studies involving uninfected children *(42)*.

Vitamin B Complex

Understanding of the role of the B vitamins in immunity is difficult because of the lack of well-designed human studies. The knowledge base is limited to what can be gleaned from intervention trials that use multiple micronutrient or vitamin supplements, animal studies, and a limited number of human trials most involving the elderly or those with HIV/AIDS. The better understood B vitamins include folate, B_{12}, and B_6, which are implicated in cell proliferation and erythrocyte production. Deficiencies of these three micronutrients result in anemia: microcytic anemia in B_6 deficiency and megaloblastic anemia in folate and/or B_{12} deficiency, rendering it difficult to determine whether the immunocompromised state is a result of the specific nutrient deficiency or to the general, anemic state.

Mechanisms

Folate, B_{12}, and B_6 appear to aid in the maintenance of both the innate and the adaptive response. Folate and B_6 deficiencies are associated with thymic atrophy. Rat offspring of B_6 deficient dams were noted as having significantly smaller spleens and thymus glands *(48,49)*, indicating a role for these vitamins in the maintenance of immune organs (*see* Table 1).

Vitamins

VITAMIN B_6

Numerous animal studies have demonstrated that vitamin B_6 deficiency is associated with reductions in antibody producing cells, reduced delayed type hypersensitivity (DTH) response, decreased proliferation of lymphocytes, and diminished cytotoxicity of T-cells *(49)*. Human studies investigating B_6 mediated immunity in the elderly observed an association between B_6 deficiency and decreased antibody production and Th cell populations *(50)*. Additionally, decreased IL-2 production, T-lymphocyte numbers, and T-lymphocyte proliferation were observed in individuals undergoing B_6 depletion studies *(6)*. Reduced lymphocyte proliferation and diminished natural killer cell activity were observed in B_6-deficient patients with HIV/AIDS *(45)*. Repletion studies showed B_6 supplementation restored proper immune function, and supplementation studies in the elderly and those with HIV/AIDS improved immune response *(5)*. Taken together, researchers hypothesize that B_6 deficiency may suppress Th1 activity while repletion enables a proper Th2 response *(6)*.

FOLATE

Folate is required for thymidine production and the normal cycle of cell division and proliferation and, therefore, affects the proliferative response of immune cells. Animal and human studies in folate deficient subjects have demonstrated reduced lymphocyte numbers *(48)* and proliferation in response to mitogens, as well as diminished DTH response and natural killer cell activity *(6)*. With respect to specific morbidities, folate-deficient animals developed increased susceptibility to infections with various pathogens including shigella, salmonella, murine rotavirus, *trypanasoma flexniri*, *plasmodium yoelli*, and the Newcastle virus *(48)*. Depletion studies in humans have demonstrated that single deficiencies of either folate or B_{12} result in diarrhea *(51)*. Folic acid deficiency and megaloblastic anemia may increase malaria-associated morbidities and susceptibility to malarial infection *(41)*. Researchers hypothesize that folate deficiency may act mechanistically by inducing suppression of the Th1 response *(6)*, but few have examined the benefits of improving folate status in reducing morbidity.

VITAMIN B$_{12}$

Vitamin B$_{12}$ is also important in erythrocyte production and cellular proliferation. Deficiency leads to megaloblastic anemia and, with respect to immune cells, impaired neutrophil function. Deficiency is also associated with declining CD4 counts and increased disease progression among men with HIV/AIDS *(43)*. B$_{12}$ supplementation has been shown to improve antibody function and lymphocyte production. In B$_{12}$-deficient AIDS patients, supplementation improved lymphocyte counts, CD8^{+} counts, and natural killer cell activity *(43)*. Its role in the Th2/Th1 response has not been elucidated, although researchers speculate that B$_{12}$ deficiency may suppress the Th2 response *(6)*.

RIBOFLAVIN

Riboflavin has been relatively well studied in the context of malaria and deficiency appears to protect against malaria infection and malaria-related morbidities. It is hypothesized that the malaria parasite requires riboflavin and is deprived in the deficient state *(52)*. However, more recent research involving high-dose riboflavin supplementation has demonstrated that riboflavin can suppress parasite growth, although the mechanisms have not been elucidated *(53)*.

OTHER B VITAMINS

Few studies have examined the roles of the remaining B vitamins (thiamin, pantothenic acid, niacin, and biotin) in immune function and those in humans have been carried out in the context of multivitamin supplements. Thus, their individual effects are difficult to determine. Preliminary research in rats hints at an increased requirement for biotin by lymphocytes during the proliferative response *(54)*, although studies in biotin deficiency have found that immune markers are not altered in the deficient state compared with a normal state of nutriture *(55)*.

Vitamin C

Mechanism

Vitamin C is found in high concentration in leukocytes and is readily mobilized during infection. Human and animal studies have shown it to be a strong modulator of immunity. Vitamin C deficiency in animals has been associated with decreased phagocytosis and antimicrobial activity of macrophages. In contrast, high levels of vitamin C have been associated with increased mitogen-induced production of antibodies by the peripheral blood lymphocytes, increased DTH response, and decreased T-cell death, as well as enhanced neutrophil function *(6,13)*.

Morbidity

ACUTE RESPIRATORY INFECTIONS

Although it is commonly accepted that vitamin C can 'boost' immunity, few studies have looked at the effect of ascorbate on specific morbidities. One study suggests potential benefits: elderly patients admitted for acute respiratory infection and supplemented with 200 mg vitamin C/d for 4 wk reportedly fared much better than the unsupplemented ones *(56)*.

HIV/AIDS

More recently, vitamin C has been implicated in the progression of HIV to AIDS. In a randomized clinical trial of HIV$^+$ subjects, daily supplementation for 3 mo with both vitamin C and vitamin E (1000 mg ascorbic acid and 800 IU dl-α-tocopherol) decreased lipid peroxidation and indicated a trend toward a reduced viral load *(57)*. In vitro experiments using HIV-infected human cell lines demonstrated that exposure to high doses of vitamin C decreased proliferation and survival of the infected cells and reduced viral production *(58)*. These findings appear to confirm a role for vitamin C independent of vitamin E, although more research is needed.

Vitamin D

Mechanism

In its active form, 1,24-dihydroxyvitamin D_3, vitamin D has been shown to act as a powerful immunoregulator that is capable of suppressing Th1 response. It has been shown to inhibit T-lymphocyte proliferation and immunoglobulin production, decrease natural killer cell toxicity, and decrease the production of IL-2, IL-12, and IFN-γ. In contrast, 1,25-dihydroxyvitamin D_3 increases synthesis of IL-4, IL-5, and IL-12, as well as IgA, and it is thought this vitamin may act to promote a Th2 response *(6)*.

Morbidity

How the above findings translate into morbidity remains unclear as few studies have looked at the role of vitamin D in specific disease states. Several observational studies suggest a role of vitamin D deficiency in various respiratory infections including tuberculosis and, to a lesser extent, pneumonia *(59)*.

Vitamin E

Mechanism

Vitamin E is the primary lipid-soluble antioxidant in the body and is essential for protecting the cell membranes against lipid peroxidation, a damaging process that is immunosuppressive. For this reason, vitamin E is thought to be essential in optimizing and even enhancing immune function. Long and short term supplementation with vitamin E in healthy elderly subjects increased IL-2 levels and its associated lymphocyte proliferation in response to specific mitogens, increased helper-T activity, and improved the DTH skin response that is a marker of cell-mediated immunity *(60,61)*. Vitamin E also increases natural killer cell toxicity and, when given with vitamin C, promotes phagocytosis *(62)* (*see* Table 1).

Morbidity

Few large-scale studies have looked at the effect of vitamin E supplementation on specific infections and disease state. Evidence from cross-sectional data shows an inverse association between blood vitamin E levels and overall incidence of infectious diseases in the preceding three years in noninstitutionalized, healthy, elderly subjects *(63)*.

HIV/AIDS

Serum vitamin E levels have been negativity associated with viral load and disease progression in HIV-infected populations. In a 9-yr follow-up study of HIV⁺ men in Baltimore, US, investigators found a significant 35% reduction in the risk of progression to AIDS when comparing the highest and lowest quartiles of serum vitamin E. Median AIDS-free survival time was 1.5 yr longer in the highest serum vitamin E quartile compared with the lowest one *(43)*. Although not statistically significant, the results suggest vitamin E may protect against HIV progression in infected subjects.

MALARIA

Despite the overall benefits of good vitamin E nutriture to protect against infection, observational evidence suggests that low serum levels may be protective against malarial infection *(64)*. It is hypothesized that vitamin E suppresses the parasite-damaging oxidative stress reaction generated by the immune system, thus increasing survival of the *Plasmodium falciparum* parasite.

Vitamin K

One of the least studied vitamins is vitamin K, a fat-soluble vitamin that is widely available in plants and animal foods as phylloquinone (vitamin K_1). An analog, menaquinone (vitamin K_2) can be synthesized endogenously in the liver of most mammalians organisms and by bacteria found in the human gut.

The importance of vitamin K in proper coagulation of the blood has long been known and vitamin K-dependent proteins and factors have been identified. In recent years, vitamin K has also been found to play a role in bone calcification.

Vitamin K deficiency is rare in healthy adults. Because they are born with low vitamin K stores, a sterile gut, and because breastmilk is low in vitamin K, newborn infants are especially vulnerable to vitamin K deficiency in the first few days of life. Prophylactic vitamin K supplementation in newborns with the purpose of preventing hemorrhagic disease of the newborn is a common practice, especially in premature infants. Other than this routine supplementation, little is known about a potential role of vitamin K in the prevention of other disease states or the association between vitamin K and the immune function.

Multiple Micronutrient Supplementation

Micronutrients do not act in isolation; they probably exert a synergestic effect within the body to promote optimal health. Likewise, micronutrient deficiencies rarely occur in isolation. Subclinical deficiencies of multiple micronutrients, rather than single micronutrient deficiencies, are likely to be highly prevalent in developing countries where access to high-quality food is limited and the majority of household income is spent on a few simple staples (65). Interventions such as multiple micronutrient supplementation or fortification of commonly consumed foods, such as wheat flour with several micronutrients, are attractive because they have potential to alleviate simultaneously multiple subclinical deficiencies in a cost-effective manner compared with single micronutrient interventions. Although multiple micronutrient and vitamin supplements are widely consumed in some developed countries, and are being promoted in developing countries, little is known about their benefits for health and disease.

A few studies have examined the role of multiple micronutrient supplements in the immune system and on morbidity outcomes, primarily among the elderly in more developed countries and in HIV/AIDS patients. Regardless of their lessened generalizability to the developing world, elderly populations in developed countries are at increased risk of nutritional deficiencies for a variety of reasons and may represent an adequate, although not ideal, model for comparison. Additionally, in the absence of undernutrition, aging is associated with diminished cellular immunity (66). Patients with HIV/AIDS are also at increased risk of micronutrient deficiencies; thus results from these studies may also be applicable to developing countries. Several randomized controlled trials in elderly patients found that supplementation with multiple micronutrients improved cellular immune markers, specifically improved natural killer activity, enhanced DTH response, and/or cytokine production by lymphocytes. Intervention studies in the elderly have also observed improved immune responses, improved mirconutrient status, reduced frequency of illness, and improved self-perceived quality of life *(67)*. One study found these benefits to be most pronounced among those with type II diabetes and those with subclinical deficiencies in multiple nutrients *(67)*. Multiple micronutrient supplementation has been associated with improved immune function and delayed disease progression in HIV/AIDS patients, and more rigorous studies are needed *(68)*.

A few intervention trials using multiple micronutrient supplementation have been carried out among young children and pregnant women in developing countries. The main outcome in most of these trials was young child growth and the results have not been encouraging. Only one study, in Tanzania *(46)*, involved HIV$^+$ pregnant women and examined the effects of supplementation on immune function or morbidity. The results from the Tanzanian trial are promising and need to be replicated. Women who received daily prenatal multiple vitamins had significantly higher CD3$^+$, CD4$^+$, and CD8$^+$ counts, as well as improved infant outcomes compared with the control group who received iron-folate supplements that is the standard of care *(46)*. Studies of selected combinations of one or more vitamins along with minerals such as iron and zinc may help understand the mechanisms. More research is needed to determine which nutrients need to be included in a multiple micronutrient supplement, as well as the dose and method of delivery that will be most effective in developing country settings. Issues such as micronutrient interactions, safety, cost, accessibility, and quality also need to be addressed.

Conclusion

Vitamins are important immunomodulaters and play a key role in alleviating the burden of disease globally. Vitamin A is important for preventing adverse outcomes from common childhood diseases such as measles and diarrhea. Although less is known about the benefits of other vitamins, including C, D, and E, they play an important role in maintaining normal immunity and deficiencies are associated with impaired responses and immune function. The challenge is to find ways to reduce the prevalence of vitamin deficiencies in a cost-effective way and to better understand the interaction between vitamins and other risk factors of common illnesses that affect many people—especially young children—living in impoverished settings. Priority needs to be given to determining the efficacy of both multiple micronutrient supplements and the fortification of common foods with different micronutrients. More research is also needed on understanding the role of vitamins in emerging infections as well as infections, such as malaria, tuberculosis, and HIV/AIDS.

References

1. West, K.P., Jr. (2002) Extent of vitamin A deficiency among preschool children and women of reproductive age. *J. Nutr.* **132**, 2857S–2866S.
2. West, K.P. and Darnton-Hill, I. (2001) Vitamin A deficiency, in *Nutrition and Health in Developing Countries*. (Semba, R.D. and Bloem, M.W., eds.), Humana, Totowa, pp. 267–306.
3. Ramakrishnan, U. (2002) Prevalence of micronutrient malnutrition worldwide. *Nutr. Rev.* **60**, S46–S52.
4. Scrimshaw, N.S., Taylor, D.I., and Gordon, J.E. (1968) *Interaction of nutrition and infection.* WHO, Geneva.
5. Chandra, R.K. (2002) Nutrition and the immune system from birth to old age. *Eur. J. Clin. Nutr.* **56**, S73–S76.
6. Long, K.Z. and Santos, J.I. (1999) Vitamins and the regulation of the immune response. *Ped. Infect. Dis. J.* 283–290.
7. Greene, H.N. and Mellanby, E. (1928) Vitamin A as an anti-infective agent. *Br. Med. J.* **2**, 691696.
8. Stephenson, C.B. (2001) Vitamin A, infection, and immune function. *Annu. Rev. Nutr.* **21**, 167–192.
9. Beaton, G.H., Martorell, R., Aronson, K.J., et al. (1993) Effectiveness of vitamin A supplementation in the control of young child mortality in developing countries. Nutrition policy discussion paper No. 13. ACC/SCN, Geneva.
10. Ramakrishnan, U. and Martorell, R. (1998) The role of vitamin A in reducing child mortality and morbidity and improving growth. *Salud Publica Mex* **40**, 189–198.
11. Bhaskaram, P. (2002) Micronutrient malnutrition, infection, and immunity: An overview. *Nutr. Rev.* **60**, S40–S45.
12. Thurnham, D.I., Northrop-Clewes, C.A., McCullough, F.S.W., Das, B.S., and Lunn, P.G. (2000) Innate immunity, gut integrity, and vitamin A in Gambian and Indian infants. *J. Infec. Dis.* **182**, S23–S28.
13. Erickson, K.L., Medina, E.A., and Hubbard, N.E. (2000) Micronutrients and innate immunity. *J. Infect. Dis.* **182**, 5–10.
14. Sommer, A. (1997) Vitamin A prophylaxis. *Arch. Dis. Child.* **77**, 191–200.
15. Barclay, A.F.G., Foster, A., and Sommer, A. (1987) Vitamin A supplements and mortality related to measles: A randomized clinical trial. *Br. Med. J.* **294**, 294–296.
16. Hussey, G.D. and Klein, M. (1990) A randomized, controlled trial of vitamin A in children with severe measles. *N. Engl. J. Med.* **323**, 160–164.
17. Coutsoudis, A., Broughton, M., and Coovadia, H.M. (1991) Vitamin A supplementation reduces measles morbidity in young African children: A randomized, placebo-controlled, double-blind trial. *Am. J. Clin. Nutr.* **54**, 890–895.
18. Ogaro, F., Orinda, V., Onyango, F., and Black, R. (1993) Effect of Vitamin A on diarrhoeal and respiratory complications of measles. *Trop. Geograph. Med.* **45**, 283–286.
19. Rosales, F., Kjolhede, C., and Goodman, S. (1996) Efficacy of a single oral dose of 200,000 IU of oil-soluble vitamin A in measles-associated morbidity. *Am. J. Epidemiol.* **143**, 413–422.

20. Rosales, F.J. (2002) Vitamin A supplementation of vitamin A deficient measles patients lowers the risk of measles-related pneumonia in Zambian children. *J. Nutr.* **132**, 3700–3703.

21. D'Souza, R.M. and D'Souza, R.D. (2002) Vitamin A for preventing secondary infections in children with measles—a systematic review. *J. Trop. Pediatr.* **48**, 72–77.

22. Abdeljaber, M.H., Monto, A.S., Tilden, R.L., Schork, A., and Tarwotjo, I. (1991) The impact of vitamin A supplementation on morbidity: A randomized community intervention trial. *Am. J. Publ. Health* **81**, 1654–1656.

23. Rahamathullah, L., Underwood, B.A., Thulasiraj, R.D., and Milton, R.C. (1991) Diarrhea, respiratory infections and growth are not affected by a weekly low-dose vitamin A supplement: A masked controlled field trial in children of southern India. *Am. J. Clin. Nutr.* **54**, 568–577.

24. Henning, B., Stewart, K., Zaman, K., Alam, A.N., Brown, K.H., and Black, R.E. (1992) Lack of therapeutic efficacy of vitamin A for non-cholera watery diarrhoea in Bangladeshi children. *Eur. J. Clin. Nutr.* **46**, 437–443.

25. Stansfield, S.K., Pierre-Louis, M., Lerebours, G., and Augustin, A. (1993) Vitamin A supplementation and increased prevalence of childhood diarrhea and acute respiratory infections. Lancet **341**, 578–582.

26. Lie, C., Ying, C., En-Lin, W., Brun, T., and Geissler, C. (1993) Impact of large dose vitamin A supplementaion on childhood diarrhea, respiratory disease and growth. *Eur. J. Clin. Nutr.* **47**, 88–96.

27. Barreto, M.L., Santos, L.M.P., Assis, A.M.O., et al. (1994) Effect of vitamin A supplementation on diarrhoea and acute lower respiratory tract infection sin young children in Brazil. *Lancet* **344**, 228–231.

28. Bhandari, N., Bhan, M., and Sazawal, S. (1994) Impact of massive dose of vitamin A given to preschool children with acute diarrhoea on subsequent respiratory and diarrhoeal morbidity. *Br. Med. J.* **309**, 1404–1407.

29. Dewan, V., Patwari, A.K., Jain, M., and Dewan, N. (1995) A randomized controlled trial of vitamin A supplementation in acute diarrhea. *Ind. Pediatr.* **32**, 21–25.

30. Ramakrishnan, U., Latham, M.C., Abel, R., and Frongillo, J.E.A. (1995) Vitamin A supplementation and morbidity among preschool children in south India. *Am. J. Clin. Nutr.* **61**, 1295–1303.

31. Dibley, M.J., Sadjimin, T., Kjolhede, C.L., and Moulton, L.H. (1996) Vitamin A supplementation fails to reduce the incidence of acute respiratory illness and diarrhea in preschool-age Indonesian children. *J. Nutr.* **126**, 434–442.

32. Hossain, S., Biswas, R., Kabir, I., et al. (1998) Single dose vitamin A treatment in acute shigellosis in Bangladeshi children: A randomized double blind controlled trial. *Br. Med. J.* **316**, 422–426.

33. Donen, P., Dramaix, M., Brasseur, D., et al. (1998) Randomized placebo-controlled clinical trial of the effect of a single high dose or daily low doses of vitamin A on morbidity of hospitalized malnourished children. *Am. J. Clin. Nutr.* **62**, 1254–1260.

34. Sempertegui, F., Estrella, B., Camaniero, V., et al. (1999) The beneficial effects of weekly low-dose vitamin A supplementation on acute lower respiratory infections and diarrhea in Ecuadorian children. *Pediatr.* **104**, E1.
35. Fawzi, W.W., Mbise, R., Speigelman, D., Fataki, M., Hertzmark, E., and Ndossi, G. (2000) Vitamin A supplements and diarrheal and respiratory tract infections among children in Dar es Salaam, Tanzania. *J. Pediatr.* **137**, 660–667.
36. Khatun, U.H.F., Malek, M.A., Black, R.E., Sarkar, N.R., Wahed, M.A., and Roy, S.K. (2001) A randomized controlled clinical trial of zinc, vitamin A or both in undernourished children with persistent diarrhea in Bangladesh. *Acta. Pediatric.* **90**, 376–380.
37. Rahman, M.M., Vermund, S.H., Wahed, M.A., Fuchs, G.J., Baqui, A.H., and Alvarez, J.O. (2001) Simultaneous zinc and vitamin A supplementation in Bangladeshi children: A randomized double blind controlled trial. *Br. Med. J.* **323**, 314–318.
38. Villamor, E., Mbise, R., Spiegelman, D., et al. (2002) Vitamin A supplements ameliorate the adverse effect of HIV-1, malaria, and diarrheal infections on child growth. *Pediatr.* **109**, e6.
39. Villamor, E. and Fawzi, W.W. (2000) Vitamin A supplementation: Implications for morbidity and mortality in children. *J. Infect. Dis.* S122–S133.
40. Shankar, A.H. (2001) Malaria, in *Nutrition and health in developing countries.* (Semba, R.D. and Bloem, M.W., eds.) Humana, Totowa, pp. 177–208.
41. Allen, L.H. and Casterline-Sabel, J. (2001) Prevalence and causes of nutritional anemias, in *Nutritional anemias.* (Ramakrishnan U, ed.) CRC, Boca Raton, FL, pp. 7–21.
42. Semba, R.D. and Gray, G.E. (2001) Human immunodeficiency virus infection, in *Nutrition and health in developing countries.* (Semba RD, Bloem MW, eds.) Humana, Totowa, pp. 237–266.
43. Patrick. (2000) Nutrients and HIV: Part two vitamins A and E, zinc, B-vitamins, and magnesium. *Altern. Med. Rev.* **5**, 39–51.
44. Tang, A.M., Graham, N.M.H., Semba, R.D., and Saah, A.J. (1997) Association between serum vitamin A and E levels and HIV disease progression. *AIDS* **11**, 613–620.
45. Fawzi, W. (2000) Nutritional factors and vertical transmission of HIV-1: Epidemiology and potential mechanisms. *Ann. NY Acad. Sci.* **918**, 99–114.
46. Fawzi, W.W., Msamanga, G.I., Spiegelman, D., et al. (1998) Randomized trial of effects of vitamin supplements on pregnancy outcomes and T cell counts in HIV-1-infected women in Tanzania. *Lancet* **351**, 1477–1482.
47. Fawzi, W.W., Msmanga, G.I., Wei, R., et al. (2003) Effect of providing vitamin supplements to human immunodeficiency virus-infected, lactating mothers on the child's morbidity and CD4+ cell counts. *HIV/AIDS* **36**, 1053–1062.
48. Dhur, A., Galan, P., and Hercberg, S. (1991) Folate status and the immune system. *Prog. Food Nutr. Sci.* **15**, 43–60.
49. Chandra, R.K. and Sudharkan, L. (1991) Regulation of the immune response by vitamin B6. *Ann. NY Acad. Sci.* **585**, 404–423.

50. Rall, L.C. and Meydani, S.N. (1993) Vitamin B6 and immune competence. *Nutr. Rev.* **51**, 217–225.

51. Beard, J.L. (2001) Functional consequences of nutritional anemia in adults, in *Nutritional anemias*. (Ramakrishnan U, ed.) CRC, Boca Raton, FL, pp. 111–128.

52. Shankar, A.H. (2000) Nutritional modulation of malaria morbidity and mortality. *J. Infect. Dis.* **182**, S37–S53.

53. Akompong, T., Ghori, N., and Haldar, K. (2000) In vitro activity of riboflavin against the human malaria parasite Plasmodium falciparum. *Antimicrob. Agents Chemother.* **44**, 88–96.

54. Zempleni, J. and Mock, D.M. (2000) Utilization of biotin in proliferating human lymphocytes. *J. Nutr.* **130**, 335S–337S.

55. Helm, R.M., Mock, N.I., Simpson, P., and Mock, D.M. (2001) Certain immune markers are not good indicators of mild to moderate biotin deficiency in rats. *J. Nutr.* **132**, 3231–3236.

56. Hunt, C., Chakravorty, N.K., Annan, G., Habibzadeh, N., and Schorah, C.J. (1994) The clinical effects of vitamin C supplementation in elderly hospitalised patients with acute respiratory infections. *Int. J. Vit. Nutr. Res.* **64**, 212–219.

57. Allard, J.P., Aghdassi, E., Chau, J., et al. (1998) Effects of vitamin E and C supplementation on oxidative stress and viral load in HIV-infected subjects. *AIDS* **12**, 1653–1659.

58. Rivas, C.I., Vera, J.C., Guaiquil, V.H., et al. (1997) Increased uptake and accumulation of vitamin C in human immunodeficiency virus 1-infected hematopoietic cell lines. *J. Biol.* **272**, 5814–5820.

59. Sasidharan, P.K., Rajeev, E., and Vijayakumari, V. (2002) Tuberculosis and vitamin D deficiency. *J. Ass. Phys. India* **50**, 554–558.

60. Meydani, S.N., Barklund, M.P., Liu, S., et al. (1990) Vitamin E supplementation enhances cell-mediated immunity in healthy elderly subjects. *Am. J. Clin. Nutr.* **52**, 557–563.

61. Meydani, S.N., Meydan, M., Blumberg, J.B., et al. Vitamin E supplementation and in vivo immune response in healthy elderly subjects. *J. Am. Med. Assoc.* **277**, 1380–1386.

62. de la Fuente, M., Ferrandez, M.D., Burgos, M.S., Soler, A., Prieto, A., and Miquel, J. (1998) Immune function in aged women is improved by ingestion of vitamins C and E. *Can. J. Physiol. Pharmacol.* **76**, 373–380.

63. Chavance, M., Herbert, B., Fournier, C., Janot, C., and Vernhes, G. (1989) Vitamin status, immunity and infections in an elderly population. *Eur. J. Clin. Nutr.* **43**, 827–835.

64. Levander, O.A., Ager, A.L., Jr. (1993) Malarial parasites and antioxidant nutrients. *Parasitol* **107**, S95–S106.

65. Ramakrishnan, U. and Huffman, S. (2001) Multiple micronutrient malnutrition: What can be done? in *Nutrition and Health in Developing Countries*. (Semba, R.D. and Bloem, M.W., eds.) Humana, Totowa, pp. 365–391.

66. High, K.P. (1999) Micronutrient supplementation and immune function in the elderly. *Clin. Inf. Dis.* **28**, 717–722.

67. Barringer, T.A., Kirk, J.K., Santaniello, A.C., Foley, K.L., and Michielutte, R. (2003) Effect of a multivitamin and mineral supplement on infection and quality of life. *Ann. Intern. Med.* **138**, 365–371.

68. Buys, H., Hendricks, M., Eley, B., and Hussey, G. (2002) The role of nutrition and micronutrients in paediatric HIV infection. *S. Afr. Dis. J.* **57**, 454–456.

6 Trace Elements/Minerals and Immunity

CARL L. KEEN, JANET Y. URIU-ADAMS, JODI L. ENSUNSA,
AND M. ERIC GERSHWIN

CONTENTS

KEY POINTS

- Mineral deficiencies:
  - Arise through a variety of mechanisms.
  - Occur frequently in both developed and developing countries.
  - Can influence all components of the immune system.
- Mineral deficiency-induced abnormalities in the immune system are particularly profound when they occur during early development.
- Copper deficiency inhibits interleukin (IL)-2 production by affecting gene transcription; IL-2 is a cytokine involved in normal T-cell metabolism.
- The effect of iodine deficiency on the immune system has not been well characterized.
- Iron deficiency can be a risk factor for an impaired immune system. However, supplementation may enhance the virulence of some agents.
- While severe magnesium deficiency is thought to be rare in humans, low plasma magnesium concentrations are a common clinical finding. The thymus is vulnerable to magnesium deficiency-induced oxidative damage.

From: *Handbook of Nutrition and Immunity*
Edited by: M. E. Gershwin, P. Nestel, and C. L. Keen © Humana Press, Totowa, NJ

- Manganese deficiency is rare in humans. Manganese plays a role in neu-trophil adhesion and degranulation, and reduces superoxide-mediated inflammatory and autoimmune responses via manganese superoxide dismutase.
- Selenium intakes are very low in some populations. An individual's risk for infection from some viruses is influenced by their selenium and over-all antioxidant status.
- Zinc influences multiple components of the immune system, and the risk for infectious disease is increased with zinc deficiency.

Introduction

A large number of trace elements are found in human tissues, but few have been shown to be essential for survival (1,2). A prolonged dietary deficit in any essential trace element in the adult organism results in morbidity and poten-tially death. Deficiency during prenatal or early postnatal development can result in profound disturbances in development, including prenatal and early postnatal death, congenital abnormalities, low birth weight, and functional dis-turbances of systems including the neurological, cardiac, pulmonary, and immune systems. In experimental animals, many of these disturbances can per-sist after correcting the nutrient deficiency.

The essential trace elements include cobalt, copper, iodine, iron, manga-nese, molybdenum, selenium, and zinc (2). However, because little is known about the effects of cobalt and molybdenum deficiencies in humans, these trace elements are not included in this chapter. Many countries (3) have dietary rec-ommendations for fluoride (1) (for its benefits on dental health) and chromium (2) (for its putative ability to increase insulin action in certain individuals) and both influence immunity in experimental animal models (4,5), but neither ele-ment meets the classical definition of essentiality; thus they too are not included in this chapter. Arsenic, boron, nickel, and vanadium may be essential trace elements for some species (2). Nevertheless, because of the lack of consensus concerning their essentiality in humans, they are not discussed here. For macrominerals, only magnesium is included in this chapter as deficits of cal-cium, phosphorus, and potassium are not thought to induce abnormalities in the immune system (1). Because of space constraints, in many places review articles rather than primary references are cited.

Mechanisms Underlying the Develpment of Essential Trace Elements and Mineral Deficiencies

Before discussing the immune defects associated with deficiencies of spe-cific essential trace elements and minerals, it is important to recognize the multiple pathways by which their deficiencies may arise (see Table 1). A pri-mary deficiency and potentially the death of the individual can occur as a con-

Table 1
Causative Factors in Mineral Deficiencies

Primary deficiency: low dietary intake of a micronutrient

Secondary (conditioned) deficiency
- Genetic factors
  - Mutant genes (e.g., acrodermatitis enteropathica and Menkes disease)
  - Polymorphisms (e.g., mutations in the methylenetetrahydrofolate reductase gene)
  - Multiple gene defects
- Nutritional interactions
  - Dietary binding factors (e.g., fiber and phytate)
  - Micronutrient-micronutrient interactions (e.g., zinc–copper, iron–manganese, cadmium–zinc, and zinc–vitamin A interactions)
- Physiological stressors
  - Disease-associated changes in micronutrient metabolism (e.g., diabetes and hypertension-induced changes in mineral metabolism)
- Drugs or other chemicals and toxicants
  - Antimetabolites (e.g., dicumarol)
  - Metal chelation (e.g., decreased absorption and increased excretion)
  - Decreased gut absorption and/or increased kidney loss (secondary to tissue damage)
- Toxicant-induced changes in tissue pools (secondary to inflammatory or acute phase response)

sequence of a prolonged inadequate dietary intake of an element. In principle, an individual's risk of a primary deficiency of any essential element can be determined from an analysis of their dietary intake. The prevalence of primary trace element and mineral deficiencies in most developed countries is thought to be low (1,2), but the opposite is true for developing countries. The exceptions are iron and zinc deficiencies that are widespread throughout the world (2). However, a primary deficiency of an essential nutrient rarely occurs in isolation, and in most cases multiple deficiencies coexist. This makes it difficult to extrapolate the results from experimental animal studies, in which single nutrient deficiencies are typically studied, to humans.

A secondary or conditioned deficiency can occur where the dietary intake would otherwise be adequate (6). Conditioned deficiencies can arise through different mechanisms. First, genetic factors can create a higher than normal requirement for a nutrient. For example, individuals with acrodermatitis enteropathica require a higher than normal intake of zinc owing to a genetic defect in zinc absorption, whereas those with Menkes disease require additional copper because of defects in copper absorption and transport. In addition to single gene defects, multiple gene polymorphisms can contribute to the development of essential mineral deficiencies. For example, the frequency of enzootic ataxia (a cluster of developmental defects observed in newborn lambs from ewes that had been on copper deficient diets during pregnancy) varies considerably among different breeds of sheep, even when grazed on the same pasture. Similar "strain" differences in the response to diets low in essential trace elements (copper, iron, manganese, zinc) have also been reported for the rat, mouse, chicken, and dog *(7)*. The extent to which multiple gene abnormalities contribute to altered mineral metabolism in humans is unknown but, given the widespread occurrence of these abnormalities in other species, it is reasonable to speculate that they may occur with relatively high frequency.

Second, different nutritional interactions can produce conditioned deficiencies. Dietary binding factors, such as fiber and phytate (myoinositol hexaphosphate) form complexes with divalent essential minerals in the gut and limit their absorption. This inhibition of absorption can be profound, resulting in marked increases in dietary zinc requirements in populations characterized by high phytate diets. Mineral–mineral interactions can also result in conditioned deficiencies through multiple mechanisms, including:

- where one mineral is involved in the metabolism of another, a deficit of one can influence the metabolism of the other. Examples are the altered iron and selenium metabolism often observed with copper deficiency *(8,9)*;
- when two metals share a common transport site or ligand, ions that have similar physiochemical properties (for example, similar orbitals, size, and coordination numbers) can be predicted to be antagonistic to each other in biological systems. Chemical determinants of some potential mineral–mineral interactions are shown in Table 2. Examples of nutritionally relevant mineral–mineral interactions, that is where high intakes of one metal are thought to interfere with the absorption of the other, include zinc–copper, cadmium–zinc, iron–zinc, iron–manganese, and calcium–magnesium. Although these interactions can result in the "induction" of a deficiency of an essential trace element or mineral, the same type of interaction can result in an excessive tissue accumulation of a nonessential metal. For example, lead and cadmium uptake from the diet can increase with zinc deficiency *(3)*. The extent to which an excess concentration of nonessential minerals contributes to the immune system abnormalities observed in individuals with a deficiency of an essential mineral is unknown;
- when the deficiency of one mineral is severe enough to cause tissue injury. When this occurs in the gastrointestinal tract, a general malabsorption syndrome can result and affect the uptake of several essential minerals.

Table 2
Chemical Determinants of Potential Mineral–Mineral Interactions

Ion	Orbital	Coordination number	Group
Cu^+	d^{10}	4	Ib
Cu^{2+}	d^9	4	Ib
Zn^{2+}	d^{10}	4	IIb
Fe^{2+}	d^6	6	VIII
Fe^{3+}	d^5	6	VIII
Mn^{2+}	d^5	6	VIIa
Cd^{2+}	d^{10}	4	IIb

Third, drugs or other chemicals can affect the metabolism of the mineral. Drug/chemical–mineral interactions can be separated into two categories.

- Drugs that act by chelating the metal. For example, copper and zinc by D-penicillamine and ethylenediaminetetraacetate (EDTA), respectively (7).
- Drugs that indirectly influence the normal metabolism of the mineral. Mineral uptake from the gastrointestinal tract can be reduced following drug-induced intestinal cell damage, as well as by drug-induced reductions in gastrointestinal transit time (7). Similarly, diuretics can markedly increase the excretion of some minerals; magnesium deficiency secondary to the use of diuretics is a frequent finding (10). Finally, drugs and chemicals can alter the metabolism of numerous minerals through the acute phase response. Although the acute phase response may provide immediate benefits, if it persists, it can result in profound changes in zinc, copper, iron, and selenium metabolism (6). The extent to which acute phase response-induced changes in the metabolism in the above minerals attenuates or augments the disease process is unclear.

Fourth, stressor-induced physiological changes in mineral metabolism can occur. In some cases the stressor, often a disease or trauma, can result in an excessive loss of a mineral; for example, excessive losses of copper, zinc, and magnesium with chronic diarrhea and diabetes-associated polyuria (11,12). In other cases the stressor may influence the metabolism of minerals through the acute phase response; for example, the hypozincemia, hypoferremia, and hypercupremia associated with hypertension, diabetes, alcoholism, and AIDS (6,13).

Copper and Immune Function

Copper is essential for the immune system in humans and animals. In infants, neutropenia is a clinical sign of copper deficiency that responds to copper treatment *(14)*. In human adults, experimental copper deficiency induced by a low-copper diet (0.38 mg Cu/d) resulted in a decreased ability of peripheral blood mononuclear cells to proliferate when stimulated with mitogens *(15)*. The percentage of circulating B-cells (CD 19[1]) also increased, whereas other populations of immune cells (for example, leukocytes, lymphocytes, monocytes, neutrophils, and so on) were unaffected. When the above subjects were fed a diet adequate in copper, indices of copper status normalized but the alterations in immune function persisted.

Severe copper deficiency in animals results in anemia, thymic hypoplasia, and splenomegaly *(14)*. Lower lymphocyte stimulation indices for phytohemagglutinin and concanavalin A, and lower immunoglobulin (Ig)M concentrations have also been noted. Copper-deficiency has been shown to suppress the maturation and function of splenic T-helper cells and the bactericidal activity of promonocytic cells and macrophages. When diets are marginal in copper, neutropenia can occur and the ability of neutrophils and macrophages to generate superoxide anion is reduced leading to decreased bactericidal activity. The maturation of copper-deficient neutrophils also appears to be arrested *(14)*. Importantly, copper supplementation to copper-deficient mice can reverse impaired immune function. For example, mice fed copper-deficient diets over lactation and weaning exhibited impaired antibody response to sheep erythrocytes, which was reversed with copper supplementation *(16)*. Copper supplementation also reversed the copper deficiency-induced decrease in total T-cells and CD4[+] (helper) cells *(14,17)*.

The reduction in T-cell proliferation and differentiation may be attributed to copper deficiency-induced reduction in IL-2, a cytokine essential for normal T-cell metabolism *(14)*. Indeed, the addition of IL-2 to copper-deficient splenocytes in culture restores their proliferative capacity. Similar reversibility of effects was noted in vivo in copper-deficient animals that were repleted with dietary copper. The copper deficiency-induced decrease in IL-2 mRNA was owing to inhibition of transcription of the IL-2 gene *(18)*.

A secondary copper deficiency can be induced by administration of molybdenum. Superoxide anion and hydrogen peroxide formation after stimulation with phorbal myristate acetate (PMA) and opsonized zymosan (OpZ) were decreased in copper-deficient bovine macrophages *(19)*. A marked increase in monocytes and a decrease in B-lymphocytes were also noted. In cattle, copper deficiency has also been noted to decrease antibody production, and reduce production of interferon and tumor necrosis factor by mononuclear cells *(20)*. The compromised immune function can lead to an increased susceptibility to microbial infections and endotoxin.

Genetic abnormalities in copper metabolism can precipitate copper deficiencies. In a murine model for Menkes syndrome, a human genetic copper disorder, the macular mutant mouse exhibited lymphoid tissue atrophy unless treated with copper *(21)*. These mice had a decreased T-cell dependent response, for example, decreased antibody production against sheep red blood cells in vivo and in vitro, compared with normal mice.

Although severe copper deficiency is uncommon, marginal copper deficiency may be prevalent in humans *(1)*. Environmental or physiological conditions that perturb copper metabolism can trigger a subclinical copper deficiency. For example, exercise, infection, inflammation, diabetes and hypertension, and the consumption of zinc supplements and diets high in fructose can alter copper metabolism. High levels of zinc intake (100–300 mg/d) can induce copper deficiency resulting in neutropenia, anemia, and impaired immune function *(1)*. Failla et al. *(22)* investigated the contributory effects of starch versus fructose on copper deficiency-induced impairment in immune function. Rats fed starch-based copper-deficient diets exhibit reduced antibody titers after primary immunization with sheep erythrocytes, and decreased copper concentrations in thymus and spleen. These effects were even more pronounced when fructose was substituted for the starch. Again, repletion of copper rapidly restored immunocompetence and stimulated thymic growth indicating an immunomodulatory role for copper.

With regard to excess copper, mice exposed to high concentrations of copper in drinking water showed a reduced proliferative response to concanavalin A *(23)*. Elevated serum copper and ceruloplasmin can also reduce the in vitro response of lymphocytes to mitogens, indicating that copper may be immunosuppressive in high amounts *(24)*.

Indicators of Copper Status

Indicators of copper status include serum, plasma, and urinary copper concentrations, plasma ceruloplasmin activity, erythrocyte copper, zinc superoxide dismutase (CuZnSOD) activity, and leukocyte or platelet cytochrome-*c* oxidase activity *(1)*. Physiological stressors such as inflammation, infection, and disease can result in an acute phase response with subsequent production of ceruloplasmin. Thus, ceruloplasmin and plasma copper levels may not accurately reflect copper status and the use of more than one copper status indicator has been suggested.

Iodine and Immune Function

Iodine deficiency disorders (goiter, mental retardation, hypothyroidism, cretinism, and various growth and developmental abnormalities) are one of the world's major public health problems, with over one billion individuals living in areas where the soil and, therefore, food is deficient in iodine *(2)*.

Iodine is an essential component of the two thyroid hormones, thyroxine (T4) and triiodothyronine (T3), and this hormonal activity is its only confirmed physiological function. However, in vitro, iodine has been reported to work

with myeloperoxidase from white cells to inactivate bacteria. Iodine can stimulate IgG synthesis in human lymphocytes in vitro *(25)*. Deficiency has been
reported to be a risk factor for gastric cancer, and iodine is thought to protect
the stomach through antioxidant mechanisms *(26)*. Whereas iodine deficiency
has been reported to be a risk factor for the development of immune deficiencies *(27)*, the mechanisms underlying these putative deficiencies have not been
identified. Iodine supplementation in areas characterized by a high incidence
of severe iodine deficiency is associated with reductions in infant mortality
(28), although it is thought that this is primarily as a result of the prevention of
hypothyroidism rather than a result of improvements in immune defense. In
China, populations characterized by low iodine intakes are often also characterized by low selenium and copper intakes *(9)*; thus, observed immune abnormalities in these populations can have multiple origins.

Excessive iodine intakes can result in hypothyroidism, as well as acute
hyperthyroidism, which can be characterized by impaired natural killer cell
activity *(29)*. Excessive dietary iodine has been linked with an increase in the
risk for autoimmune thyroiditis. Iodine may induce stereochemical changes in
the conformation of thyroglobulin that increase its antigenicity *(30)*. Although
serum concentrations of thyroid antibodies have been reported in some studies
to be lower in individuals with mild iodine deficiency than in individuals with
moderate deficiencies *(31)*, this is not a consistent finding *(32)*.

Indicators of Iodine Status

Urinary iodine is the standard method for assessing iodine status and
adequacy of intake. Levels below 20 µg/L indicate severe deficiency, 20–49
µg/L moderate deficiency, and 50–99 µg/L mild deficiency. Values between
100 and 200 µg/L are considered satisfactory. Thyroid function tests should be
conducted when urine iodine concentrations are low.

Iron and Immune Function

Iron deficiency is the most common known mineral deficiency in the world.
It is most prevalent among young children and pregnant women *(2)*, groups
characterized by a high risk for infections and morbidity. The most recognized
consequences of iron deficiency include anemia, impaired work performance,
impaired child development, and, when severe, mortality *(33)*. A reduction in
plasma iron concentration is an important component of the acute phase
response and can limit the growth of some pathogens. However, prolonged
iron deficiency can result in multiple immunological abnormalities. Characteristic changes include reduced inflammatory responses such as the delayed-type
hypersensitivity reaction; impairments in neutrophil and macrophage cytotoxic
activity; reductions in lymphocyte proliferation, T-cell numbers, cytokine

release, and antibody production; and lymphoid tissue atrophy *(2)*. Although reduced resistance to infection is commonly accepted to be an early effect of iron deficiency in experimental animals, as well as in humans, few papers have been published on this topic *(34)*. A recent review of 28 randomized controlled trials *(35)* concluded that there was no clear effect of iron supplementation on the overall incidence of infectious illness in young children, although there was an increased risk for developing diarrhea. De Silva et al. *(36)* found iron supplementation reduced morbidity from upper respiratory tract infection in Sri Lankan children. Iron supplementation trials for malarial disease have yielded conflicting results; malarial anemia is reduced with iron supplementation, but the risk for incidence or reactivation of disease may be increased *(37)*. The adverse effects of iron supplementation on malaria have been attributed to increased peripheral availability of young erythrocytes, increased iron reserves for parasite development, and the loss of the inhibitory effects of microcytosis on intraerythrocytic parasites *(37)*. Iron supplementation has been reported to be a potential risk factor for HIV progression and morbidity *(38,39)*, although others have argued that the potential risks and benefits of iron supplementation for HIV-infected individuals, particularly young children, have not been sufficiently studied *(40)*. The effects of iron deficiency on the immune system reflect the multiple roles of iron in mitochondrial energy production, the respiratory burst, and its function as a component of numerous enzymes including NO synthase, COX, lipoxygenase, and catalase.

Indicators of Iron Status

Iron status is typically assessed using multiple indicators. Plasma ferritin is a measure of iron stores, but it is an acute phase protein and can be elevated in inflammation. Plasma transferrin and plasma total iron binding capacity are elevated with storage iron-depletion before anemia develops. Plasma-soluble serum transferrin receptor (sTfR) concentration increases with functional deficits, and its use as an indicator of iron status is rapidly gaining acceptance in non malarial areas *(41,42)*.

Magnesium and Immune Function

Magnesium, an abundant intracellular divalent cation, is involved in numerous metabolic processes including the immune system. In experimental animals, chronic magnesium deficiency is associated with thymic atrophy, reduced cellular and humoral immune response, as well as induction of malignant T-cell lymphoma *(43)*. Rats and guinea pigs fed magnesium-deficient diets have been reported to be at an increased risk for anaphylactic shock *(44)*, perhaps because of increased levels of histamine. Degranulation of mast cells occurs during the first few weeks of magnesium deficiency resulting in high histamine levels in the blood. Histamine release by the mast cells is partly regulated by the actions of calcium and magnesium on cAMP formation; magnesium can act as a calcium antagonist in numerous situations and can affect calcium influx or mobilization in cells *(45)*.

Besides the classical symptoms of inflammation, including peripheral vasodilation and hyperemia of the ears, magnesium-deficient rats also exhibit an increase in circulating leukocytes, including neutrophils, eosinophils, basophils, and monocytes *(46)*. Macrophages from magnesium-deficient rats have a higher respiratory burst activity that control macrophages, both at basal conditions and after PMA stimulation *(46)*. The superoxide anion production of human leukocytes following PMA activation is increased when cultured in low magnesium conditions and decreased with high magnesium concentrations *(47)*. Magnesium-deficient rats challenged with live bacteria, bacterial endotoxin, or platelet-activating factor (PAF) as a model for anaphylaxis show increased mortality compared with controls *(46,48)*, indicating that magnesium-deficient animals have an abnormal reactivity to immune stress. In magnesium deficiency, the activated macrophages are primed to produce proinflammatory cytokines. Indeed, acute magnesium deficiency has been associated with elevated plasma concentrations of several inflammatory cytokines including IL-1, IL-6, and TNF-α *(49)* as well as nitric oxide *(50)*. The increase in a number of acute phase response proteins such as α2-macroglobulin, α1-acid glycoprotein, and fibrinogen may be a consequence of the magnesium deficiency-induced elevation of IL-6 *(46)*.

The inflammatory response induced by magnesium deficiency results in an increase in both reactive oxygen and reactive nitrogen species (ROS, RNS) *(51)*. Whereas ROS/RNS can play an important role in signal transduction, excessive or inappropriate activation of neutrophils and the concomitant increased production of ROS/RNS can lead to oxidative damage to biomolecules including protein, lipid, and DNA, as well as to tissue injury and cell death. The thymus appears to be particularly vulnerable to magnesium deficiency-induced oxidative damage. Petrault et al. *(52)* have shown that the expression of numerous genes that respond to oxidative stress (for example, CuZnSOD, HSP70 and HSP84, glutathione transferase, TNF receptor 1, IL-1 receptor type I, and growth arrest and DNA damage inducible protein 45 (GADD45) are upregulated after only 2 d of experimental magnesium deficiency *(52)*. Apoptosis seems to be one early mechanism underlying the accelerated thymus involution induced by magnesium deficiency *(43)*. Magnesium deficiency, which can increase intracellular calcium concentrations, may trigger the endonucleolytic processes leading to cell death *(43)*. Lowering the calcium/magnesium ratio by feeding a diet that is low in both magnesium and calcium significantly protects against the proinflammatory effect of magnesium deficiency (53).

In rats, gestational magnesium deficiency has been reported to result in thymic and splenic hypoplasia in the offspring, and a reduced plaque-forming response to sheep erythrocytes. Rat pups born to dams fed low magnesium diets during pregnancy were characterized by low numbers of T-helper and cytotoxic T-cells; these defects persisted until week 6 postnatal (54). In vitro Tc-cell-mediated lysis of target cells is proportional to magnesium concentrations, an effect that may be mediated through interactions with adhesion molecules. The adhesion of immune T-lymphocytes to specific antigen-bearing ascites tumor target cells also requires magnesium.

Whereas severe magnesium deficiency is rare in humans, low plasma magnesium concentrations are a common clinical finding. A number of studies suggest that most population groups including young children and pregnant women may not ingest adequate magnesium and, therefore, have compromised magnesium status (55,56). Magnesium intake has decreased over the years caused partly by increased consumption of refined and processed foods that generally have low magnesium content.

Some investigators have argued that marginal magnesium deficiency is common in specific population groups, including diabetics and alcoholics (1), although this is an area of considerable debate. A low magnesium intake and status may be involved in the development of asthma and chronic obstructive airway disease (57). The beneficial effects of dietary magnesium supplementation, or inhaled or intravenous magnesium administration, on improving asthma symptoms have been noted in some (58) but not all studies (59). Oxidative stress can lead to inflammation, bronchial hyperreactivity and bronchoconstriction, changes in mucus secretion, increased epithelial damage in airway vasculature, and ultimately lung pathology (60). Additional studies on the effects of magnesium deficiency on all aspects of the immune system are clearly warranted.

Excessive intakes of dietary magnesium have not been associated with the induction of immune system abnormalities in either experimental animals or humans.

Indicators of Magnesium Status

A variety of indicators are used to assess magnesium nutriture (1). Serum or plasma magnesium levels may not reflect overall magnesium status, but they are the most widely used measures in clinical practice. Some researchers consider the concentration of ionized magnesium levels in serum/plasma (measured by ion-selective electrodes) or free intracellular magnesium levels in erythrocytes (measured by nuclear magnetic resonance) to be better indicators than serum or plasma magnesium concentrations. Intravenous magnesium loading (magnesium tolerance test) also seems to be an accurate method to assess magnesium status in adults.

Manganese and Immune Function

There is a dearth of data on the effects of manganese on the immune system. In experimental animal models, developmental manganese deficiency is associated with the occurrence of congenital ataxia (secondary to the abnormal development of the otoliths), a high incidence of neonatal mortality, impaired postnatal growth, skeletal abnormalities, abnormal carbohydrate, lipid and protein metabolism, impaired insulin production, pancreatic damage, elevated evidence of tissue oxidative damage, and an increased risk of epilepsy (61). To a large extent, these abnormalities can be linked to roles manganese plays as a constituent of several enzymes including glycosyl transferase, arginase, pyruvate carboxylase, phosphoenolpyruvate carboxykinase, manganese superoxide dismutase (MnSOD), and glutamine synthetase. Immune system abnormalities are not considered to be a common sign of manganese deficiency in experimental animals.

Manganese deficiency is thought to be rare in human subjects, although low blood manganese has been reported to be associated with several diseases including osteoporosis and epilepsy (61). Healthy human adult males fed a low manganese diet for 39 d were characterized by low blood manganese concentrations and a high incidence of a fleeting dermatitis, Miliaria crystalline, that resolved upon correction of the deficiency (62). Although the frequency of severe manganese deficiency in humans is probably rare, conditions of marginal manganese deficiency may be common because of the use of iron supplements that can interfere with manganese absorption. Lymphocyte MnSOD activity was reported to be low in adult women who received a combined iron-manganese supplement for 124 d compared with values in women who received a manganese supplement alone (63). Similarly, high dietary iron intakes have been associated with low blood manganese concentrations and low lymphocyte MnSOD activities in healthy women (64). In vitro, manganese has been shown to induce macrophages to spread on glass surfaces, and to specifically induce the high-affinity conformation of the β_1- and β_2-integrins, proteins that allow neutrophils to adhere to distinct proteins of the extracellular matrix (61,65,66). Manganese in combination with PMA has also been shown to increase neutrophil degranulation (67). Additionally, manganese is a component of the T-cell mitogen concanavalin A (68).

Experimental animals fed a manganese-deficient diet have shown deficient antibody synthesis and/or secretion (69). After adding manganese to the diet, antibody production improved. However, when manganese is added in excessive amounts, inhibition in antibody production may occur. The mechanism(s) by which manganese affects antibody synthesis or release have not been clearly elucidated, although the negative effect of excess manganese is thought to involve the plasma membrane.

Manganese also plays a role in immune processes via its antioxidant activity in MnSOD. MnSOD given as gene therapy in a plasmid or adenoviral vector, or administration of a low molecular weight MnSOD mimetic (a compound with a redox-active metal center that dismutases superoxide and can easily traverse cell membranes and is nonimmunogenic), has been shown to affect immune and autoimmune processes in a variety of studies, including reducing tissue inflammation owing to irradiation, prolonging the time to rejection in pancreatic islet cell allografts, and inhibiting lung inflammation as a result of tobacco smoke (70,71). Gene therapy has also been used to induce MnSOD in mice given islet cell transplants by injection of an IL-10 containing adeno-associated viral vector (72). In these animals, IL-10 serum levels were positively associated with prolonged graft survival and induction of antioxidant enzymes, including MnSOD.

There are numerous reports of human manganese toxicity (2,61), and typical signs include severe neurological damage and behavioral abnormalities. Immune system abnormalities are not typically reported to be complications of manganese toxicosis in either humans or experimental animals. However, Srisuchart et al. (73) reported that mice injected with high amounts of manganese are characterized by an increase in mitogen and mixed lymphocyte responses, and a decrease in antibody production. Finally, at very high dietary manganese intakes a secondary iron deficiency can arise (61), creating the potential for iron deficiency-induced immune system abnormalities.

Indicators of Manganese Status

Plasma and whole blood manganese concentrations reflect dietary intake; whole blood manganese concentrations can reflect soft tissue concentrations. Lymphocyte MnSOD activity can also be reflective of manganese status. Magnetic resonance imaging is increasingly being used to assess manganese concentrations in the globus pallidus, a target tissue for manganese toxicity (61,74).

Selenium and Immune Function

Most of the selenium in tissue is found as selenomethionine or selenocysteine. Unlike selenocysteine, selenomethionine is not synthesized in tissues and must be obtained from the diet. Selenocysteine is the predominant form of selenium used in biological processes. Since the discovery of selenocysteine, often referred to as the 21st amino acid, the field of selenium biology has rapidly expanded. There are at least 20 mammalian selenoproteins identified to date, with the selenium-dependent glutathione peroxidases (GSHPX) being the largest family *(75,76)*. GSHPx reduces H_2O_2 and free hydroperoxides. GSHPx-1 is the most common and is present in most tissues. GSHPx-2 is located in the gastrointestinal tract, GSHPx-3 is in the plasma, and GSHPx-4 is primarily in the testes. GSHPx-4 also has the ability to reduce fatty acid hydroperoxides *(77)*. In addition to its antioxidant function, GSHPx may have a specific role in the enzymatic oxidation of arachadonic acid by modulating the cyclooxygenase and lipoxygenase pathways. The former give rise to prostaglandins and thromboxanes, which tend to be antiinflammatory, whereas the latter give rise to leukotrienes, which are proinflammatory *(78,79)*.

Besides the GSHPxs, selenoenzymes form three families of thioredoxin reductases and three families of iodothyronine deiodinases, thus important interactions can occur between selenium and iodine *(9)*. Copper also plays a role in the synthesis of some selenoproteins, although the mechanisms are not yet clarified; thus copper status is important in the production of certain selenium-containing enzymes *(9)*. Selenoproteins P and W also have antioxidant functions *(75,76)*. With respect to the immune system a 15-kDa selenoprotein has been identified in T-cells, but its function has not been agreed upon *(75,76)*. Given the above, it is evident that selenium can influence multiple biological systems through its involvement in oxidant defense systems, redox-regulation, and thyroid hormones.

Dietary selenium intake is very low in some populations. In certain regions of China, selenium deficiency is a major contributor to Keshan Disease, a syndrome characterized by myocardial necrosis. Selenium deficiency also affects the immune system. Beck et al. *(80)* have postulated that deficiency results in a condition of prooxidative stress that transforms a benign strain of coxsackievirus to a virulent strain. This suggests that an individual's risk of infection from a number of viruses is influenced by their overall selenium and antioxidant status. Consistent with this concept, marginal selenium deficiency was reported to be associated with an increase in the virulence of an influenza virus *(80)*.

Independent of the above, selenium is essential for both innate and acquired immunity *(9)*. Selenium deficiency is associated with impaired mitogen-induced lymphocyte proliferation, and selenium-deficient macrophages show impaired chemotaxis and altered redox status *(81)*. Serum IgG and IgM concentrations were reduced with selenium deficiency *(9)*. Neutrophils obtained from selenium-deficient individuals showed impaired killing activity that was attributed to their GSHPx activity *(9)*. Marginal selenium deficiency was reported to be a risk factor for autoimmiune thyroiditis, and selenium supplementation was associated with reduced thyroid peroxidase antibody concentrations in a prospective study *(82)*. Selenium deficiency was a risk factor for HIV-related mortality *(83)*. Selenium supplementation improved lymphocyte response in patients with gut failure on home parenteral nutrition, in chronic uremic patients on hemodialysis, and in elderly people in institutionalized settings *(84,85)*.

Selenium supplementation reduced the risk for tumorigenesis in experimental animals *(86)*. In humans, selenium supplements were associated with improved immune system function *(87)*, and a reduced risk of lung, colorectal, and prostate cancers *(88,89)*. Selenium metabolism can be influenced by the acute phase response, with serum concentrations dropping during the early phase *(90)*; the functional significance of this drop is unknown.

Indicators of Selenium Status

Selenium requirements for adults have recently been established based on the criterion of maximizing plasma GSHPx activity. Blood and plasma selenium concentrations can reflect marginal or severe selenium deficiency, they are of limited value in identifying selenium toxicity. Urine selenium concentrations are thought to reflect recent dietary intake of the element rather than body status *(91)*.

Zinc and Immune Function

Zinc is involved in a variety of cellular functions including membrane stabilization, free radical defense, signal transduction, transcription, and cell replication *(2)*. It is required for the activity of over 300 enzymes and is involved in the regulation of numerous genes. Zinc is a widely used structural component with zinc-finger structures being in a vast array of transcription factors, membrane receptors, and nuclear hormone receptors. Zinc is known to influence endocrine function *(92–94)*. Given the multiple biological roles of zinc, deficiency of this element has immunological consequences. Classical signs of zinc deficiency include diarrhea and dermatitis, signs that are consistent with disruptions in the barrier component of the innate immune system, and decreased host resistance to infectious disease, attributable to defects in cell-mediated immunity *(95–97)*.

In experimental animals, immunological consequences of zinc deficiency include low thymic weights and T-cell defects. Several T-cell abnormalities can occur with zinc deficiency including reductions in T-cell numbers and responsiveness to mitogenic stimulation, T-cell participation in antibody production, delayed-type hypersensitivity reactions, thymic hormone production, Tc-cell activity, and T-cell maturation. Zinc deprivation increases corticosteroid production and enlarges the adrenal glands, which may contribute to corticosteroid-induced T-cell apoptosis. In contrast to T-cells, B-cell functions are only marginally affected by zinc deficiency. Other immune parameters such as natural killer cell activity and cytokine production have shown mixed results. Zinc deficiency can result in an increased susceptibility to numerous pathogens. Significantly, most of the above signs can be rapidly reversed following the correction of the zinc deficiency (6,96,98,99). An important exception is that some of the immunological defects associated with zinc deficiency, such as low immunoglobin production, can persist long after the correction of the deficiency if the initial dietary insult occurs during early development (6,54).

Similar to the findings with experimental animals, zinc deficiency in humans is associated with numerous immunological abnormalities. Acrodermatitis enteropathica, a genetic disorder of zinc malabsorption, is characterized by thymic atrophy, reduced lymphocyte proliferative responses, and a high frequency of infections (95). These signs resolve with zinc supplementation. Subjects fed low zinc diets under experimental conditions show low serum thymulin activities and impaired T-cell and natural killer cell activities. The production of IL-2 and interferon is decreased in experimental zinc deficiency, whereas the production of IL-4, IL-6, and IL-10 is relatively unaffected (100–102). Hypozincemia is a component of the acute phase response. Although it is reasonable to suggest that the reduction in plasma zinc concentration represents a positive response to certain infectious agents in a manner similar to hypoferremia, this has yet to be clearly demonstrated. A persistent acute phase response-induced hypozincemia may represent a significant risk to the individual if it occurs during pregnancy (6).

Randomized controlled trials of zinc supplementation have yielded conflicting results. In several studies, maternal zinc supplementation has been associated with improvements in neonatal immune status, early neonatal morbidity, and infant infections (103). Several authors have reported improved cell-mediated immunity and reductions in childhood infectious disease morbidity and mortality (104,105).

An excess intake of zinc can adversely affect the immune system. In healthy adult subjects, high levels of zinc supplementation can result in impaired lymphocyte proliferative responses and reduced polymorphonuclear leukocyte chemotaxis and phagocytosis (102). The above may be caused in part by a zinc-induced secondary copper deficiency. Zinc supplement use was reported to increase the risk of HIV progression and mortality (106,107), possibly because the additional zinc favored HIV replication by increasing the availability of the metal for zinc-dependent viral proteins.

Indicators of Zinc Status

Despite intensive investigative efforts, reliable biomarkers for zinc status have yet to be identified (2). Low plasma zinc concentrations may be indicative of suboptimal zinc status, but they may also simply reflect an inflammatory state with an accompanying acute phase response. Hair zinc concentrations may be useful for identifying populations with low zinc status, although they are of limited value at the individual level. Although numerous zinc-dependent enzymes have been considered as potential biomarkers for zinc status, none have been found to be sufficiently reliable. There are preliminary reports that metallothionein monocyte mRNA concentrations may be good indicators of zinc status, but this approach has yet to be tested in field conditions *(42)*.

Conclusion

Minerals play important roles in all components of the immune system. A deficiency in an essential trace element, such as zinc, copper, or iron, or the macromineral magnesium can have severe immunomodulatory effects. Mineral deficiencies can arise through a variety of mechanisms as either primary deficiencies due to an inadequate intake or as secondary or conditioned deficiencies arising from genetic factors, interactions with other minerals, chemicals or drugs, or through stressor-induced physiological changes. Mineral deficiency-induced abnormalities in the immune system can be particularly profound when they occur during fetal and early postnatal development.

Iodine, iron, selenium, and zinc deficiency are prevalent in developing countries. Low intakes of these trace elements can markedly affect multiple components of the immune system, resulting in greater susceptibility to infectious disease. Although deficiencies in copper, magnesium, and manganese are rare, certain population groups may be susceptible to marginal deficiencies or secondary deficiencies, such as in the case of copper deficiency resulting from zinc supplementation. Marginal deficiencies can also affect an individual's overall risk for infection and contribute to chronic immune-associated disorders, such as asthma and chronic obstructive airway disease.

Given the high prevalence of mineral deficiencies in the world today, the challenge is to find effective and realistic means of reducing these deficiencies by increasing their intake though pharmaceutical supplementation and/or food fortification. This task is complex because mineral metabolism can be affected by many factors. Further research is needed to understand better the complex associations between minerals and the immune system, particularly for those groups most susceptible to immune abnormalities.

Acknowledgment

This work was supported in part by National Institutes of Health Grants AT00652; HD01743; HD26777.

References

1. Food and Nutrition Board, Institute of Medicine. (1997) *Dietary Reference Intakes for calcium, phosphorus, magnesium, vitamin D, and fluoride*. National Academy, Washington, DC.

134 Keen et al.

2. Food and Nutrition Board, Institute of Medicine. (2001) *Dietary Reference Intakes for vitamin A, vitamin K, arsenic, boron, chromium, copper, iodine, iron, manganese, molybdenum, nickel, silicon, vanadium, and zinc.* National Academy, Washington, DC.
3. World Health Organization. (1996) *Trace elements in human nutrition and health.* WHO, Geneva, p. 343.
4. Shrivastava, R., Upreti, R.K., Seth, P.K., and Chaturvedi, U.C. (2002) Effects of chromium on the immune system. *FEMS Immunol. Med. Microbiol.* **34**, 1–7.
5. Sosroseno, W. (2003) Effect of sodium fluoride on the murine splenic immune response to Porphyromonas gingivalis in vitro. *Immunopharmacol. Immunotoxicol.* **25**, 123–127.
6. Keen, C.L., Clegg, M.S., Hanna, L.A., et al. (2003) The plausibility of micronutrient deficiencies being a significant contributing factor to the occurrence of pregnancy complications. *J. Nutr.* **133**, 1597S–1605S.
7. Keen, C.L. (1996) Teratogenic effects of essential trace metals: Deficiencies and excesses, in *Toxicology of metals.* (Chang LW, Magos L, Suzuki T, eds.) CRC, New York, pp. 977–1001.
8. Danzeisen, R., Fosset, C., Chariana, Z., Page, K., David, S., and McArdle, H.J. (2002) Placental ceruloplasmin homolog is regulated by iron and copper and is implicated in iron metabolism. *Am. J. Physiol. Cell. Physiol.* **282**, C472–C478.
9. Arthur, J.R., McKenzie, R.C., and Beckett, G.J. (2003) Selenium in the immune system. *J. Nutr.* **133**, 1457S–1459S.
10. Soliman, H.M., Mercan. D., Lobo, S.S., Melot, C., and Vincent, J.L. (2003) Development of ionized hypomagnesemia is associated with higher mortality rates. *Crit. Care Med.* **31**, 1082–1087.
11. Ruz, M. and Solomons, N.W. (1990) Mineral excretion during acute, dehydrating diarrhea treated with oral rehydration therapy. *Pediatr. Res.* **27**, 170–175.
12. Walter, R.M., Uriu-Hare, J.Y., Olin, K.L., et al. (1991) Copper, zinc, manganese, and magnesium status and complications of diabetes mellitus. *Diabetes Care* **14**, 1050–1056.
13. Kupka, R. and Fawzi, W. (2002) Zinc nutrition and HIV infection. *Nutr. Rev.* **60**, 69–79.
14. Percival, S.S. (1998) Copper and immunity. *Am. J. Clin. Nutr.* **67**, 1064S–1068S.
15. Kelley, D.S., Daudu, P.A., Taylor, P.C., Mackey, B.E., and Turnlund, J.R. (1995) Effects of low-copper diets on human immune response. *Am. J. Clin. Nutr.* **62**, 412–416.
16. Prohaska, J.R. and Lukasewycz, O.A. (1989) Copper deficiency during perinatal development: effects on the immune response of mice. *J. Nutr.* **119**, 922–931.
17. Hopkins, R.G. and Failla, M.L. (1995) Chronic intake of a marginally low copper diet impairs in vitro activities of lymphocytes and neutrophils from male rats despite minimal impact on conventional indicators of copper status. *J. Nutr.* **125**, 2658–2668.
18. Hopkins, R.G. and Failla, M.L. (1999) Transcriptional regulation of interleukin-2 gene expression is impaired by copper deficiency in Jurkat human T lymphocytes. *J. Nutr.* **129**, 596–601.

19. Cerone, S.I., Sansinanea, A.S., Streitenberger, S.A., Garcia, M.C., and Auza, N.J. (1998) The effect of copper deficiency on the peripheral blood cells of cattle. *Vet. Res. Commun.* **22**, 47–57.

20. Spears, J.W. (2000) Micronutrients and immune function in cattle. *Proc. Nutr. Soc.* **59**, 587–594.

21. Nakagawa, S., Fukata, Y., Nagata, H., Miyake, M., and Hama, T. (1993) The decreased immune responses in macular mouse, a model of Menkes' kinky hair disease. *Res. Commun. Chem. Pathol. Pharmacol.* **79**, 61–73.

22. Failla, M.L., Babu, U., and Seidel, K.E. (1988) Use of immunoresponsiveness to demonstrate that the dietary requirement for copper in young rats is greater with dietary fructose than dietary starch. *J. Nutr.* **118**, 487–496.

23. Pocino, M., Baute, L., and Malave, I. (1991) Influence of the oral administration of excess copper on the immune response. *Fundam. Appl. Toxicol.* **16**, 249–256.

24. Massie, H.R., Ofosu-Appiah, W., and Aiello, V.R. (1993) Elevated serum copper is associated with reduced immune response in aging mice. *Gerontology* **39**, 136–145.

25. Weetman, A.P., McGregor, A.M., Campbell, H., Lazarus, J.H., Ibbertson, H.K., and Hall, R. (1983) Iodide enhances IgG synthesis by human peripheral blood lymphocytes in vitro. *Acta. Endocrinol. (Copenh.)* **103**, 210–215.

26. Venturi, S., Donati, F.M., Venturi, A., Venturi, M., Grossi, L., and Guidi, A. (2000) Role of iodine in evolution and carcinogenesis of thyroid, breast and stomach. *Adv. Clin. Path.* **4**, 11–17.

27. Marani, L. and Venturi, S. (1986) [Iodine and delayed immunity]. *Minerva. Med.* **77**, 805–809.

28. DeLong, G.R., Leslie, P.W., Wang, S.H., et al. (1997) Effect on infant mortality of iodination of irrigation water in a severely iodine-deficient area of China. *Lancet* **350**, 771–773.

29. Wenzel, B.E., Chow, A., Baur, R., Schleusener, H., and Wall, J.R. (1998) Natural killer cell activity in patients with Graves' disease and Hashimoto's thyroiditis. *Thyroid* **8**, 1019–1022.

30. Dai, Y.D., Rao, V.P., and Carayanniotis, G. (2002) Enhanced iodination of thyroglobulin facilitates processing and presentation of a cryptic pathogenic peptide. *J. Immunol.* **168**, 5907–5911.

31. Pedersen, I.B., Knudsen, N., Jorgensen, T., Perrild, H., Ovesen, L., and Laurberg, P. (2003) Thyroid peroxidase and thyroglobulin autoantibodies in a large survey of populations with mild and moderate iodine deficiency. *Clin. Endocrinol. (Oxf.)* **58**, 36–42.

32. Loviselli, A., Velluzzi, F., Mossa, P., et al. (2001) The Sardinian Autoimmunity Study: 3. Studies on circulating antithyroid antibodies in Sardinian schoolchildren: relationship to goiter prevalence and thyroid function. *Thyroid* **11**, 849–857.

33. Stoltzfus, R.J. Iron-deficiency anemia: reexamining the nature and magnitude of the public health problem. Summary: implications for research and programs. *J. Nutr.* **131**, 697S–700S; discussion 700S–701S.

34. Failla, M.L. (2003) Trace elements and host defense: recent advances and continuing challenges. *J. Nutr.* **133**, 1443S–1447S.
35. Gera, T. and Sachdev, H.P. (2002) Effect of iron supplementation on incidence of infectious illness in children: systematic review. *Br. Med. J.* **325**, 1142.
36. de Silva, A., Atukorala, S., Weerasinghe, I., and Ahluwalia, N. (2003) Iron supplementation improves iron status and reduces morbidity in children with or without upper respiratory tract infections: a randomized controlled study in Colombo, Sri Lanka. *Am. J. Clin. Nutr.* **77**, 234–241.
37. Nussenblatt, V. and Semba, R.D. (2002) Micronutrient malnutrition and the pathogenesis of malarial anemia. *Acta. Trop.* **82**, 321–337.
38. Afacan, Y.E., Hasan, M.S., and Omene, J.A. (2002) Iron deficiency anemia in HIV infection: immunologic and virologic response. *J. Natl. Med. Assoc.* **94**, 73–77.
39. Gordeuk, V.R., Delanghe, J.R., Langlois, M.R., and Boelaert, J.R. (2001) Iron status and the outcome of HIV infection: an overview. *J. Clin. Virol.* **20**, 111–115.
40. Totin, D., Ndugwa, C., Mmiro, F., Perry, R.T., Jackson, J.B., Semba, R.D. (2002) Iron deficiency anemia is highly prevalent among human immunodeficiency virus-infected and uninfected infants in Uganda. *J. Nutr.* **132**, 423–429.
41. Verhoef, H., West, C.E., Ndeto, P., Burema, J., Beguin, Y., Kok, F.J. (2001) Serum transferrin receptor concentration indicates increased erythropoiesis in Kenyan children with asymptomatic malaria. *Am. J. Clin. Nutr.* **74**, 767–775.
42. Hambidge M. (2003) Biomarkers of trace mineral intake and status. *J. Nutr.* **133 Suppl 3**, 948S–955S.
43. Malpuech-Brugere, C., Nowacki, W., Gueux, E., et al. (1999) Accelerated thymus involution in magnesium-deficient rats is related to enhanced apoptosis and sensitivity to oxidative stress. *Br. J. Nutr.* **81**, 405–411.
44. Ashkenazy, Y., Moshonov, S., Fischer, G., et al. (1990) Magnesium-deficient diet aggravates anaphylactic shock and promotes cardiac myolysis in guinea pigs. *Magnes. Trace Elem.* **9**, 283–288.
45. Malpuech-Brugere, C., Rock, E., Astier, C., Nowacki, W., Mazur, A., and Rayssiguier, Y. (1998) Exacerbated immune stress response during experimental magnesium deficiency results from abnormal cell calcium homeostasis. *Life Sci.* **63**, 1815–1822.
46. Malpuech-Brugere, C., Nowacki, W., Daveau, M., et al. (2000) Inflammatory response following acute magnesium deficiency in the rat. *Biochim. Biophys. Acta.* **1501**, 91–98.
47. Bussiere, F.I., Mazur, A., Fauquert, J.L., Labbe, A., Rayssiguier, Y., and Tridon, A. (2002) High magnesium concentration in vitro decreases human leukocyte activation. *Magnes. Res.* **15**, 43–48.
48. Salem, M., Kasinski, N., Munoz, R., and Chernow, B. (1995) Progressive magnesium deficiency increases mortality from endotoxin challenge: protective effects of acute magnesium replacement therapy. *Crit. Care Med.* **23**, 108–118.
49. Weglicki, W.B., Dickens, B.F., Wagner, T.L., Chmielinska, J.J., and Phillips, T.M. (1996) Immunoregulation by neuropeptides in magnesium deficiency: ex

vivo effect of enhanced substance P production on circulating T lymphocytes from magnesium-deficient mice. *Magnes. Res.* **9**, 3–11.

50. Bussiere, F.I., Gueux, E., Rock, E., et al. (2002) Increased phagocytosis and production of reactive oxygen species by neutrophils during magnesium deficiency in rats and inhibition by high magnesium concentration. *Br. J. Nutr.* **87**, 107–113.

51. Kramer, J.H., Mak, I.T., Phillips, T.M., and Weglicki, W.B. (2003) Dietary magnesium intake influences circulating pro-inflammatory neuropeptide levels and loss of myocardial tolerance to postischemic stress. *Exp. Biol. Med. (Maywood)* **228**, 665–673.

52. Petrault, I., Zimowska, W., Mathieu, J., et al. (2002) Changes in gene expression in rat thymocytes identified by cDNA array support the occurrence of oxidative stress in early magnesium deficiency. *Biochim. Biophys. Acta.* **1586**, 92–98.

53. Bussiere, F.I., Gueux, E., Rock, E., Mazur, A., and Rayssiguier, Y. (2002) Protective effect of calcium deficiency on the inflammatory response in magnesium-deficient rats. *Eur. J. Nutr.* **41**, 197–202.

54. Vormann, J., Michalski, L., and Gunther, T. (1996) Cellular and humoral immunity in rats after gestational zinc or magnesium deficiency. *J. Nutr. Biochem.* **7**, 327–332.

55. Turner, R.E., Langkamp-Henken, B., Littell, R.C., Lukowski, M.J., and Suarez, M.F. (2003) Comparing nutrient intake from food to the estimated average requirements shows middle- to upper-income pregnant women lack iron and possibly magnesium. *J. Am. Diet. Assoc.* **103**, 461–466.

56. Suitor, C.W. and Gleason, P.M. (2002) Using Dietary Reference Intake-based methods to estimate the prevalence of inadequate nutrient intake among school-aged children. *J. Am. Diet. Assoc.* **102**, 530–536.

57. Britton, J., Pavord, I., Richards, K., et al. (1994) Dietary magnesium, lung function, wheezing, and airway hyperreactivity in a random adult population sample. *Lancet* **344**, 357–362.

58. Bessmertny, O., DiGregorio, R.V., Cohen, H., et al. (2002) A randomized clinical trial of nebulized magnesium sulfate in addition to albuterol in the treatment of acute mild-to-moderate asthma exacerbations in adults. *Ann. Emerg. Med.* **39**, 585–591.

59. Porter, R.S., Nester, Braitman, L.E., Geary, U., and Dalsey, W.C. (2001) Intravenous magnesium is ineffective in adult asthma, a randomized trial. *Eur. J. Emerg. Med.* **8**, 9–15.

60. Doelman, C.J. and Bast, A. (1990) Oxygen radicals in lung pathology. *Free Radic. Biol. Med.* **9**, 381–400.

61. Keen, C.L., Ensunsa, J.L., and Clegg, M.S. (2000) Manganese metabolism in animals and humans including the toxicity of manganese. *Met. Ions. Biol. Syst.* **37**, 89–121.

62. Friedman, B.J., Freeland-Graves, J.H., Bales, C.W., et al. (1987) Manganese balance and clinical observations in young men fed a manganese-deficient diet. *J. Nutr.* **117**, 133–143.

63. Davis, C.D. and Greger, J.L. (1992) Longitudinal changes of manganese-dependent superoxide dismutase and other indexes of manganese and iron status in women. *Am. J. Clin. Nutr.* **55**, 747–752.

64. Davis, C.D., Malecki, E.A., and Greger, J.L. (1992) Interactions among dietary manganese, heme iron, and nonheme iron in women. *Am. J. Clin. Nutr.* **56**, 926–932.

65. Spillmann, C., Osorio, D., and Waugh, R. (2002) Integrin activation by divalent ions affects neutrophil homotypic adhesion. *Ann. Biomed. Eng.* **30**, 1002–1011.

66. Edwards, A.S. and Newton, A.C. (1997) Regulation of protein kinase C betaII by its C2 domain. *Biochemistry* **36**, 15615–15623.

67. Xu, X. and Hakansson, L. (2002) Degranulation of primary and secondary granules in adherent human neutrophils. *Scand. J. Immunol.* **55**, 178–188.

68. Kalb, A.J., Habash, J., Hunter, N.S., Price, H.J., Raftery, J., and Helliwell, J.R. (2000) Manganese(II) in concanavalin A and other lectin proteins. *Met. Ions. Biol. Syst.* **37**, 279–304.

69. Keen, C., Lonnerdal, B., and Hurley, L.S. (1984) Manganese, in *Biochemistry of the essential ultratrace elements.* (Frieden E, ed.) Plenum, New York, pp. 89–132.

70. Epperly, M.W., Guo, H.L., Jefferson, M., et al. (2003) Cell phenotype specific kinetics of expression of intratracheally injected manganese superoxide dismutase-plasmid/liposomes (MnSOD-PL) during lung radioprotective gene therapy. *Gene Ther.* **10**, 163–171.

71. Bertera, S., Crawford, M.L., Alexander, A.M., et al. (2003) Gene transfer of manganese superoxide dismutase extends islet graft function in a mouse model of autoimmune diabetes. *Diabetes* **52**, 387–393.

72. Zhang, Y.C., Pileggi, A., Agarwal, A., et al. (2003) Adeno-associated virus-mediated IL-10 gene therapy inhibits diabetes recurrence in syngeneic islet cell transplantation of NOD mice. *Diabetes* **52**, 708–716.

73. Srisuchart, B., Taylor, M.J., and Sharma, RP. (1987) Alteration of humoral and cellular immunity in manganese chloride-treated mice. *J. Toxicol. Environ. Health* **22**, 91–99.

74. Takagi, Y., Okada, A., Sando, K., Wasa, M., Yoshida, H., and Hirabuki, N. (2002) Evaluation of indexes of in vivo manganese status and the optimal intravenous dose for adult patients undergoing home parenteral nutrition. *Am. J. Clin. Nutr.* **75**, 112–118.

75. Kryukov, G.V. and Gladyshev, V.N. (2002) Mammalian selenoprotein gene signature: identification and functional analysis of selenoprotein genes using bioinformatics methods. *Methods Enzymol.* **347**, 84–100.

76. Lescure, A., Gautheret, D., and Krol, A. (2002) Novel selenoproteins identified from genomic sequence data. *Methods Enzymol.* **347**, 57–70.

77. Arthur, J.R. (2000) The glutathione peroxidases. *Cell. Mol. Life Sci.* **57**, 1825–1835.

78. Imai, H. and Nakagawa, Y. (2003) Biological significance of phospholipid hydroperoxide glutathione peroxidase (PHGPx, GPx4) in mammalian cells. *Free. Radical. Biol. Med.* **34**, 145–169.

79. Brigelius-Flohe, R., Banning, A., and Schnurr, K. (2003) Selenium-dependent enzymes in endothelial cell function. *Antioxidants Redox Signaling* **5**, 205–215.

80. Beck, M.A., Levander, O.A., and Handy, J. (2003) Selenium deficiency and viral infection. *J. Nutr.* **133**, 1463S–1467S.
81. Prabhu, K.S., Zamamiri-Davis, F., Stewart, J.B., Thompson, J.T., Sordillo, L.M., and Reddy, C.C. (2002) Selenium deficiency increases the expression of inducible nitric oxide synthase in RAW 264.7 macrophages: role of nuclear factor-kappa B in up-regulation. *Biochem. J.* **366**, 203–209.
82. Gartner, R., Gasnier, B.C., Dietrich, J.W., Krebs, B., Angstwurm, M.W. (2002) Selenium supplementation in patients with autoimmune thyroiditis decreases thyroid peroxidase antibodies concentrations. *J. Clin. Endocrinol. Metab.* **87**, 1687–1691.
83. Baum, M.K., Miguez-Burbano, M.J., Campa, A., and Shor-Posner, G. (2000) Selenium and interleukins in persons infected with human immunodeficiency virus type 1. *J. Infect. Dis.* **182 Suppl 1**, S69–S73.
84. Peretz, A., Neve, J., Desmedt, J., Duchateau, J., Dramaix, M., and Famaey, J.P. Lymphocyte response is enhanced by supplementation of elderly subjects with selenium-enriched yeast. *Am. J. Clin. Nutr.* **53**, 1323–1328.
85. Bonomini, M., Forster, S., De Risio, F., et al. (1995) Effects of selenium supplementation on immune parameters in chronic uraemic patients on haemodialysis. *Nephrol. Dial. Transplant.* **10**, 1654–1661.
86. Popova, N.V. (2002) Perinatal selenium exposure decreases spontaneous liver tumorogenesis in CBA mice. *Cancer. Lett.* **179**, 39–42.
87. Jackson, M.J., Broome, C.S., and McArdle, F. (2003) Marginal dietary selenium intakes in the UK: are there functional consequences? *J. Nutr.* **133**, 1557S–1559S.
88. Duffield-Lillico, A.J., Dalkin, B.L., Reid, M.E., et al. (2003) Selenium supplementation, baseline plasma selenium status and incidence of prostate cancer: an analysis of the complete treatment period of the Nutritional Prevention of Cancer Trial. *Br. J. Urol. Int.* **91**, 608–612.
89. Reid, M.E., Duffield-Lillico, A.J., Garland, L., Turnbull, B.W., Clark, L.C., and Marshall, J.R. (2002) Selenium supplementation and lung cancer incidence: an update of the nutritional prevention of cancer trial. *Cancer. Epidemiol. Biomarkers. Prev.* **11**, 1285–1291.
90. Maehira, F., Luyo, G.A., Miyagi, I., et al. (2002) Alterations of serum selenium concentrations in the acute phase of pathological conditions. *Clin. Chim. Acta.* **316**, 137–146.
91. Food and Nutrition Board, Institute of Medicine. (2000) Selenium. Dietary Reference Intakes for vitamin C, vitamin E, selenium, and carotenoids. National Academy, Washington, DC, pp. 284–324.
92. Zago, M.P. and Oteiza, P.I. (2001) The antioxidant properties of zinc: interactions with iron and antioxidants. *Free. Radic. Biol. Med.* **31**, 266–274.
93. Maret, W. (2003) Cellular zinc and redox states converge in the metallothionein/ thionein pair. *J. Nutr.* **133**, 1460S–1462S.
94. Cousins, R.J., Blanchard, R.K., Moore, J.B., et al. (2003) Regulation of zinc metabolism and genomic outcomes. *J. Nutr.* **133**, 1521S–1526S.
95. Keen, C.L. and Gershwin, M.E. (1990) Zinc deficiency and immune function. *Annu. Rev. Nutr.* **10**, 415–431.

96. Fraker, P.J., King, L.E., Laakko, T., and Vollmer, T.L. (2000) The dynamic link between the integrity of the immune system and zinc status. *J. Nutr.* **130**, 1399S–1406S.

97. Cui, L., Blanchard, R.K., and Cousins, R.J. (2003) The permissive effect of zinc deficiency on uroguanylin and inducible nitric oxide synthase gene upregulation in rat intestine induced by interleukin 1alpha is rapidly reversed by zinc repletion. *J. Nutr.* **133**, 51–56.

98. Dardenne, M. Zinc and immune function. (2002) *Eur. J. Clin. Nutr.* **56 Suppl 3**, S20–S23.

99. King, L.E., Osati-Ashtiani, F., and Fraker, P.J. (2002) Apoptosis plays a distinct role in the loss of precursor lymphocytes during zinc deficiency in mice. *J. Nutr.* **132**, 974–979.

100. Prasad, A.S. (2000) Effects of zinc deficiency on Th1 and Th2 cytokine shifts. *J. Infect. Dis.* **182 Suppl 1**, S62–S68.

101. Pinna, K., Kelley, D.S., Taylor, P.C., and King, J.C. (2002) Immune functions are maintained in healthy men with low zinc intake. *J. Nutr.* **132**, 2033–2036.

102. Ibs, K.H. and Rink, L. (2003) Zinc-altered immune function. *J. Nutr.* **133**, 1452S–1456S.

103. Osendarp, S.J., West, C.E., and Black, R.E. (2003) The need for maternal zinc supplementation in developing countries: an unresolved issue. *J. Nutr.* **133**, 817S–827S.

104. Cuevas, L.E., Almeida, L.M., Mazunder, P., et al. (2002) Effect of zinc on the tuberculin response of children exposed to adults with smear-positive tuberculosis. *Ann. Trop. Paediatr.* **22**, 313–319.

105. Shankar, A.H., Genton, B., Baisor, M., et al. (2000) The influence of zinc supplementation on morbidity due to Plasmodium falciparum: a randomized trial in preschool children in Papua New Guinea. *Am. J. Trop. Med. Hyg.* **62**, 663–669.

106. Dreyfuss, M.L. and Fawzi, W.W. (2002) Micronutrients and vertical transmission of HIV-1. *Am. J. Clin. Nutr.* **75**, 959–970.

107. Siberry, G., Ruff, A., and Black, R. (2002) Zinc and immunodeficiency virus infection. *Nutr. Res.* **22**, 527–538.

7 Dietary Fat and Immunity in Humans

Kent L. Erickson, Darshan S. Kelley, and Neil E. Hubbard

Contents

Key Points

- Results from human studies with fish and fish oils are conflicting, but generally the omega-3 fatty acids either inhibit or have no effect on immune response.
- Body fat composition can vary among subjects and is reflected by the types of fatty acids consumed.
- Moderate intakes of α-linolenic acid do not inhibit indices of immune response.
- High concentration of eicosapentaenoic acid (EPA) and docosahexaenoic acid (DHA) can inhibit neutrophil and monocyte functions that may depend on added levels of vitamin E.
- EPA and DHA may decrease proinflammatory cytokine production. Differences reported may be caused by genetic polymorphisms of the individuals. Cytokine production by lymphocytes appears to be altered more by fish oil than cytokines of macrophages.
- Supplementation with vitamin E in studies with omega-3 fatty acids alters results.
- Numerous factors may be responsible for the discrepancies in human studies including concentration and type of fat or fatty acid supplemented,

From: *Handbook of Nutrition and Immunity*
Edited by: M. E. Gershwin, P. Nestel, and C. L. Keen © Humana Press, Totowa, NJ

antioxidant status, duration of dietary manipulation, assay methods, gender, and age of subject.

Introduction

Dietary fat has diverse effects on human health based on the amounts and, more importantly, the types consumed. Dietary fat may also differentially affect certain cells, tissues, and organs depending upon their stage of development. The fatty acid composition of human tissues and organs can vary depending upon the types of fatty acids in the food consumed, and composition has been used as a biomarker for correlation with immunity and risk of disease. In addition, some dietary fatty acids can be transformed into potent biological mediators that can initiate or alter numerous processes in the body. For example, linoleic acid, a common component of some vegetable oils, can be converted by a number of different cell types into arachidonic acid, a major precursor for the potent immunomodulatory agent prostaglandin E_2 (PGE_2). Indeed, physiological levels of PGE_2 can change depending on the availability of its precursor fatty acid. Because PGE_2 has been linked to alterations in the immune system, and more recently to specific pathological processes, it is likely that dietary fat intake plays a role in human disease. This chapter focuses on recent work concerning the effects of dietary fat on the human immune system. Data from animal studies are excluded because high concentrations of single dietary fat have often been used and such diets are rarely consumed by humans. The discussion is limited to dietary omega-3 (n-3) fatty acids that are known to decrease PGE_2. Based on the studies presented herein, a case can be made for an important effect of n-3 fatty acids in the diet as a means to alter immunity.

Dietary n-3 Fatty Acids, Immune, and Inflammatory Responses

The immune system functions by an intricate network of signals that are generated intrinsically or extrinsically. Some intrinsic signals can be produced by metabolized dietary essential fatty acids. This provides a link between dietary fat intake and the alteration of immune function. This section describes the role of n-3 fatty acids in modifying human immunity. In the studies cited, individuals were usually fed experimental diets or supplements, after which several immune system parameters were evaluated typically using blood samples or skin responses. Isolated cells of the immune system were evaluated ex vivo using several different assays for function such as chemotaxis or phagocytosis.

The sources of n-3 polyunsaturated fatty acids used in human feeding trials have been flaxseed or linseed oil as sources of α-linolenic acid (ALA); fish and fish oils as sources of eicosapentaenoic acid (EPA) and docosahexaenoic acid (DHA); purified esters of EPA and DHA; or DHA triglycerides from geneti-

Table 1
Fatty Acids Used in Studies and Their Sources

Omega-3 fatty acids (n-3)
- From Fish oil
  - Eicosapentaenoic acid (EPA, 20:5n-3)
  - Docosapentaenoic acid (DHA, 22:6n-3)
- From flaxseed or linseed oil
  - α-linolenic acid (18:3n-3)

Omega-6 fatty acids (n-6)
- From vegetable oils
  - Linoleic acid (18:2n-6)
- From animal fats
  - Arachidonic acid (20:4n-6)

cally engineered algae (*see* Table 1). Only a few human studies used both flax-seed and fish oils, while several dozen studies used fish oils only.

α-Linolenic Acid

In one study, flaxseed oil was added to the diet of healthy men to increase ALA intake to 18 g/d *(1)*. Feeding the ALA diet for 8 wk significantly decreased peripheral blood mononuclear cells (PBMC) proliferation and the delayed type hypersensitivity (DTH) skin response *(1)*. The number of circulating white blood cells, granulocytes, monocytes, lymphocytes, as well as specific types were not altered with increased ALA intake. Serum concentrations of immunoglobin (Ig)G, IgA, C3 or C4, B-cell proliferation, ex vivo secretion of interleukin (IL)-2 and IL-2R also did not change. In another study, two diets based either on sunflower oil—a source of n-6 fatty acids—or flaxseed oil a source of n-3 fatty acids with 30% energy from fat, were fed to young healthy men. *(2)*. Ex vivo production of both IL-1β and tumor necrosis factor (TNF)-α was significantly reduced in the flaxseed oil group within 4 wk of feeding this diet, whereas it remained unchanged in the sunflower oil group. In a third study, a modest level of 4 g/d ALA was provided for 12 wk to healthy men *(3)*. No changes were found in neutrophil chemotaxis and superoxide production. Thus, large concentrations of ALA intake that are 10–15 times the amount normally consumed appear to inhibit both the in vivo and ex vivo indices of immune response, although lower intakes do not have the same inhibitory effects.

Fish and Fish Oil Consumption

In one study, 500 g/d of salmon containing 2.3 g EPA and 3.6 g/d DHA was fed to healthy young men *(4)*. About 25% of the energy came from fat. Feeding the salmon diet for 6 wk had no effect on a number of indices of immune response including DTH, PBMC proliferation, and the serum levels of immunoglobulins. In another study, feeding 120–188 g/d fish containing 1.23 g EPA+DHA without supplemental vitamin E to a group of elderly men and women for 24 wk significantly reduced DTH, lymphocyte proliferation, and the ex vivo production of IL-1β, IL-6, and TNF-α *(5)*. None of these parameters were inhibited in a group that received one-quarter the amount of fish. Thus, it appears that two to three servings of fish/wk should be safe even without vitamin E supplementation, but that amount may not substantially alter immune response.

A number of studies have examined the effects of fish oil supplementation on ex vivo neutrophil and monocyte chemotaxis, superoxide production, phagocytosis, lymphocyte and monocyte cytokine production, lymphocyte proliferation, and in vivo indices of immune response. The amount of fish oil supplemented ranged from 2–30 g/d containing 0.55–8.0 EPA+DHA for 4–52 wk. Many of these studies were longitudinal, in which the fish oils were added to the usual diets, but did not include parallel control groups. This study design increased not only the intake of EPA and DHA, but also total fat. Only a few studies included placebo controls and held total fat intake constant. Some studies supplemented the diet with variable amount of vitamin E, which itself affects many indices of immune response, while others did not. In most studies, fish oil supplementation inhibited or had no effect on the immune response variables measured.

Effects of EPA and DHA
Indices of Immune Status

Three studies with EPA and/or DHA have examined their effects on the number of circulating white cells *(6–8)*. One study supplemented 2.4 g EPA+DHA/d to women for 12 wk; α-tocopherol was supplemented at 6 mg/d *(6)*. The total number or the percent of circulating white blood cells remained unchanged. In another study a supplemental mixture of 3.2 g/d EPA and DHA with 200 mg/d α-tocopherol was provided to adult men and women *(7)*. No change in the numbers of circulating white blood cells was observed. In the third study, an additional 6 g/d DHA and 10 mg/d α-tocopherol were provided to healthy men *(8)*. Supplementation reduced the number of circulating white blood cells, and circulating granulocytes by 25%. In contrast to DHA, arachidonic acid caused a 25% increase in the number of circulating granulocytes. DHA supplementation did not alter serum IgG, C3, antibody titer against influenza vaccination, IL-2R, or DTH.

Table 2
EPA and DHA Alteration of Neutrophil and Monocyte Functions in Adults

Function	Amount of EPA & DHA (g/d)	Duration (wk)	Effect	Reference
Neutrophil chemotaxis	14.4	3	25–60% decrease	12*
PMN Chemotaxis	8.6	3	30–50% decrease	13*
Monocyte superoxide production	6	6	50–60% decrease	10*
PMN chemotaxis	5.4	6	70% decrease	14*
PMN chemotaxis Monocyte chemotaxis	4	8	60–70% decrease	15*
Monocyte hydrogen peroxide production	4, EPA, DHA or corn oil	7	No change	16**
PMN chemotaxis and superoxide production	2.2	12	No change	3
PMN superoxide production	2.2	4	50% decrease	9
Monocyte hydrogen peroxide production	0.6	12	No change	17

*No placebo group.
**Cells stored frozen.

Respiratory Burst, Phagocytosis, and Chemotaxis

Two studies reported about a 50% reduction in ex vivo neutrophil and monocyte superoxide production when healthy human volunteers supplemented their diet with 0.65–5.8 g/d EPA and DHA for 4–12 wk (9,10). Another study found a 64% reduction in neutrophil phagocytosis after 3.6 g/d EPA supplementation for 6 wk (11). Several studies have been published recently regarding the effects of EPA and DHA on neutrophil and monocyte chemotaxis (see Table 2). The EPA and DHA supplement in these studies ranged from 0.65 to 14.4 g/d for 3–12 wk. Neutrophil or monocyte chemotaxis was decreased in most of the studies with EPA+DHA intake of 1.3 g/d or greater. One study that reported no inhibition of chemotaxis by EPA and DHA was based on supplementation with 0.65 g/d for 12 wk (17). In contrast, neutrophil chemotaxis was inhibited after

3 wk of 8.7 g/d EPA+DHA, even after the subjects consumed extra vitamin E *(13)*. However, the amount of vitamin E intake in this study may not have been adequate to protect against the potential oxidative effects of high intakes of EPA and DHA. In the short term studies, EPA+DHA intakes below 1 g/d did not inhibit neutrophil and monocyte chemotaxis, but long-term studies are needed before firm conclusions can be made. Certainly, high concentrations of these fatty acids can inhibit neutrophil chemotaxis by 3 wk.

Inhibition of Cytokine Production by Monocytes

Numerous studies have investigated the effects of dietary EPA and DHA and ex vivo cytokine production by cells from human volunteers (*see* Table 3). The amount of EPA+DHA intake varied from 0.6 to 6.0 g/d over 4–52 wk; vitamin E supplementation ranged from 0 to 200 mg/d. Seven of these studies *(2,5,6,18–21)* reported a significant reduction in the concentration of the three proinflammatory cytokines IL-1, IL-6, or TNF-α secreted by monocytes after stimulation with lipopolysaccharide. The remaining seven studies found no reduction in monokine secretion. Four weeks was the shortest period in which EPA and DHA supplementation reduced TNF-α and IL-1 secretion. Alternatively, supplementation with about the same amount of n-3 fatty acids for 6 mo or more did not inhibit the production of those cytokines *(22)*. This was probably because the investigators did not examine cytokine secretion at any time before 6 mo; they also supplemented with 54 mg/d vitamin E. In another study, similar levels of EPA and DHA plus 200 mg/d vitamin E were given as a supplement for 12 wk; no reductions in IL-1 and TNF-α secretion were observed *(8)*. Two additional studies supplemented with DHA alone *(18,23)*. After supplementation with 700 mg/d DHA for 12 wk, no alterations in IL-1, IL-6, and TNF-α secretion were reported *(23)*. However, with 6 g/d DHA, the secretion of IL-1 and TNF-α were reduced by up to 45% *(18)*. These results suggest that high, but not low, concentrations of EPA and DHA can inhibit the secretion of select cytokines. A possible reason for the discrepancies regarding the effect of EPA and DHA on monocyte cytokine secretion may be the genetic polymorphisms of the subjects. A recent study reported that inhibition of TNF-α secretion by EPA and DHA was dependent on the polymorphism in the TNF-α gene *(21)*.

Lymphocyte and Macrophage Functions

Natural killer (NK) cell activity was examined in three studies after feeding of EPA and or DHA *(8,18,23)* or infusion with EPA-triglyceride (*see* Table 4) *(24)*. One study used 6 g/d DHA and found a significant reduction in NK cell activity after 12 wk of supplementation *(18)*. Two conflicting reports come from the same laboratory. With 3.2 g/d EPA+DHA and 200 mg/d vitamin E

Table 3
Inhibition of Monocyte Cytokine Production by EPA and DHA in Adults

Cytokine	Amount of EPA & DHA g/d	Duration (wk)	Effect	Comments	Reference
IL-1, TNF-α	6 (DHA)	13	30–45% decrease	10 mg/d vitamin E	18
IL-1, TNF-α	5.2	24	Decrease	MS patients with healthy subjects	19
IL-1, TNF-α	4.6	6	20–60% decrease	No placebo group	20
IL-1, TNF-α	3.2	12	No change	205 mg/d vitamin E	7
IL-1, TNF-α	2.7	4	70–80%	No placebo group	2
IL-1, TNF-α	2.4	12	No change	6 mg/d vitamin E	6
TNF-α	1.8	12	No change or depending on phenotype	TNF-α gene polymorphism affected response	21
IL-1, IL-6, TNF-α	1.2	24	No change	High fish and low fish diets	5
IL-1, IL-6, TNF-α	2.4	7	70–80% decrease	Cellular IL-1, not secreted IL-1 or TNF-α	6
IL, IL-1Ra, TNF-α	1.1–3.1	52	No change	5.4 IU/d vitamen E	18
TNF-α, IL-1, IL-6	0.6	12	No change	Placebo controlled	17

MS, multiple sclerosis.

supplementation for 12 wk NK cell activity was not inhibited (8). However, NK cell activity was significantly decreased with 1 g/d EPA+DHA supplementation for 12 wk, whereas 0.7 g/d DHA supplementation for the same period did not inhibit NK cell activity (23). Infusing 30 mL of EPA-triglyceride, 24 h prior to the isolation of peripheral blood mononuclear cells, reduced the NK cell activity by more than 50% (24). These studies suggest that EPA and DHA may inhibit NK cell activity. However, because of variance in experi-

Table 4
DHA and EPA Alteration of Lymphocyte Functions in Adults

Function	Amount of EPA & DHA g/d	Duration (wk)	Effect	Comments	Reference
Proliferation	7	10	80% decrease	200 mg/d vitamin E	25
Proliferation	6 (DHA)	13	No change	10 mg/d vitamin E	8
NK cell activity	6 (DHA)	13	20% decrease no change 8 wk	10 mg/d vitamin E	18
IL-2, and IFN-α secretion	5.2	24	25–30% decrease	400 mg/d vitamin E	19
IL-2 and IFN-α secretion	3.2	12	No change	205 mg/d vitamin E	7
Proliferation	3.2	12	No change	205 mg/d vitamin E	7
NK Cell activity	3.2	12	No change	205 mg/d vitamin E	7
IL-2 secretion	2.4	12	30% decrease		6
Proliferation	2.4	12	36% decrease	6 mg/d vitamin E	6
Proliferation	1.2	24	24%		5
NK cell activity	1 (DHA)	12	48% decrease	Reduction within 4 wk reversed	23
Proliferation	2.4	7	20–35% decrease wk 2 and 4	Placebo controlled	6

mental design, even with studies from the same laboratory, firm conclusions cannot be drawn.

Lymphocyte proliferation, the production of IL-2 and IFN-γ, or all were decreased in five of the nine studies in which the diets were supplemented with a mixture of EPA and DHA or DHA alone. The intake of EPA+DHA varied from 1.2 to 5.2 g/d for 6–24 wk. Two studies *(23)* that reported no alteration of lymphocyte proliferation or cytokine production used 0.7 or 6 g/d DHA supplementation for 12 wk. This indicates that the inhibition of lymphocyte proliferation and cytokine production may be caused by EPA and not DHA. The third study that reported no effect supplemented 3.2 g/d EPA+DHA for 12 wk *(8)*. The lack of inhibition observed in this study was probably as a result of the additional 200 mg/d of vitamin E. Another study showed supplementation with 200 mg/d vitamin E for 8 wk reversed the inhibition of lymphocyte proliferation caused by 15 g/d fish oil supplementation (25). The fourth study found no inhibition of lymphocyte proliferation by fish oils providing 4.6 g/d EPA+DHA for 6 wk. It is possible that more than 6 wk of fatty acid supplementation are required to inhibit lymphocyte functions, because all other studies reporting inhibition supplemented the fatty acids for 7–24 wk. The lowest concentration of EPA+DHA that was associated with inhibition of lymphocyte functions was 1.2 g/d fed for 24 wk (5); the highest concentration that did not inhibit was 3.2 g/d for 12 wk (8). The differences could be caused by the fatty acid and antioxidant composition of the basal diet, duration of feeding, the EPA to DHA ratio, or the assay methods used.

Without additional vitamin E, supplementation with 1.3–8.0 g/d EPA+DHA for 4 wk or more reduced several neutrophil functions including chemotaxis, chemiluminescence, superoxide production, and phagocytosis (9–11,12,14, 15,26). Monocyte chemotaxis and superoxide production were also decreased in two studies (10,26). However, monocyte chemotaxis and superoxide production were not reduced in one study that used a low concentration of fish oil (EPA+DHA 0.55 g/d) for 12 wk (17). In another study, supplementation with 4 g/d EPA or DHA for 7 wk did not inhibit monocyte phagocytosis (16). The effect of fish oil supplementation on the production of IL-1β and TNF-α has been examined in a number of studies. Many found a 25–75% decrease in the in vitro secretion of cytokines when 2.4 g/d or more EPA+DHA were supplemented in the diets for 4 wk or more (2,7,18,20). Thus, cytokine production by lymphocytes appears to be altered by fish oils.

Possible Reasons for Reported Differences

The many differences in both study protocols and the methods used probably contributed to the inconsistencies in results from different studies. Potentially important factors related to the study protocol include: antioxidant nutrient content of the diets; total fat and fatty acid composition; the n-6 and n-3 PUFA ratio; the amount and duration of supplementation; the amount of EPA and DHA; age, sex, and health status of the subjects; and inclusion of a control or placebo group. The methods and cells used for assessments have varied greatly and add to the variance. For example, isolated PBMC or whole blood cultured in autologous sera or fetal calf serum have been used with a wide variety of agents to stimulate the cells and to monitor their responses. Some of the assays used may have little association with human immunity. Most critical among these factors seem to be the ratio between the amounts of n-3 PUFA and vitamin E because the latter blocks the inhibition by n-3 PUFA, and the duration of supplementation.

Conclusion

Dietary fat may play an important role in modulation of the immune response in humans. Body fat composition can reflect dietary consumption, thus the potential for alteration of the immune system is great. This may be important because fatty acids may be metabolized or utilized as potent biological mediators that, in turn, can play a role in modulating the immune system. Specific fatty acids, notably those of the n-3 family, appear to selectively decrease some, but not all, lymphocyte, neutrophil, and macrophage functions. Generally, fish oils that contain n-3 fatty acids inhibit numerous responses such as proinflammatory cytokine production. The fatty acids most commonly found in fish oils—EPA and DHA—can inhibit neutrophils and monocyte function, but that may depend on the levels of supplemental vitamin E added. Even when the same lymphocyte function or cytokine profiles were assessed after dietary fat manipulation, different and sometimes divergent results have been reported by different investigators. Although a great number of animal studies have shown pronounced effects of dietary fat on immunity, these studies may not be directly comparable to human ones because high levels of a single fat source were often used; a situation quite different from human diets. Moreover, numerous factors may be responsible for the extensive differences reported in human studies, such as the amount and type of fat, fatty acid composition, antioxidant status, duration of dietary manipulation, assay methods used, and participating subjects. Nevertheless, decreasing fat consumption and an increase of n-3 fatty acids may be prudent dietary advice because no detrimental effects have been reported with respect to immunity and, in some cases, potential beneficial effects may accrue.

References

1. Kelley, D.S., Branch, L.B., Love, J.E., Taylor, P.C., Rivera, Y.M., and Iacono, J.M. (1991) Dietary alpha-linolenic acid and immunocompetence in humans. *Am. J. Clin. Nutr.* **53**, 40–46.
2. Caughey, G.E., Mantzioris, E., Gibson, R.A., Cleland, L.G., and James, M.J. (1996) The effect on human tumor necrosis factor alpha and interleukin 1 beta production of diets enriched in n-3 fatty acids from vegetable oil or fish oil. *Am. J. Clin. Nutr.* **63**, 116–122.
3. Healy, D.A., Wallace, F.A., Miles, E.A., Calder, P.C., Newsholm, P. (2000) Effect of low-to-moderate amounts of dietary fish oil on neutrophil lipid composition and function. *Lipids* **35**, 763–768.
4. Kelley, D.S., Nelson, G.J., Branch, L.B., Taylor, P.C., Rivera, Y.M., and Schmidt, PC. (1992) Salmon diet and human immune status. *Eur. J. Clin. Nutr.* **46**, 397–404.

5. Meydani, S.N., Lichtenstein, A.H., Cornwall, S., et al. (1993) Immunologic effects of national cholesterol education panel step-2 diets with and without fish-derived N-3 fatty acid enrichment. *J. Clin. Invest.* **92**, 105–113.

6. Meydani, S.N., Endres, S., Woods, M.M., et al. (1991) Oral (n-3) fatty acid supplementation suppresses cytokine production and lymphocyte proliferation: comparison between young and older women. *J. Nutr.* **121**, 547–555.

7. Yaqoob, P., Pala, H.S., Cortina-Borja, M., Newsholme, E.A., and Calder, P.C. (2000) Encapsulated fish oil enriched in alpha-tocopherol alters plasma phospholipid and mononuclear cell fatty acid compositions but not mononuclear cell functions. *Eur. J. Clin. Invest.* **30**, 260–274.

8. Kelley, D.S., Taylor, P.C., Nelson, G.J., and Mackey, B.E. (1998) Dietary docosahexaenoic acid and immunocompetence in young healthy men. *Lipids* **33**, 559–566.

9. Thompson, P.J., Misso, N.L., Passarelli, M., and Phillips, M.J. (1991) The effect of eicosapentaenoic acid consumption on human neutrophil chemiluminescence. *Lipids* **26**, 1223–1236.

10. Fisher, M., Levine, P.H., Weiner, B.H., et al. (1990) Dietary n-3 fatty acid supplementation reduces superoxide production and chemiluminescence in a monocyte-enriched preparation of leukocytes. *Am. J. Clin. Nutr.* **51**, 804–808.

11. Fisher, M., Upchurch, K.S., Levine, P.H., et al. (1986) Effects of dietary fish oil supplementation on polymorphonuclear leukocyte inflammatory potential. *Inflammation* **10**, 387–392.

12. Sperling, R.I., Benincaso, A.I., Knoell, C.T., Larkin, J.K., Austen, K.F., and Robinson, D.R. (1993) Dietary omega-3 polyunsaturated fatty acids inhibit phosphoinositide formation and chemotaxis in neutrophils. *J. Clin. Invest.* **91**, 651–660.

13. Luostarinen, R., Siegbahn, A., and Saldeen, T. (1991) Effects of dietary supplementation with vitamin E on human neutrophil chemotaxis and generation of LTB4. *Ups. J. Med. Sci.* **96**, 103–111.

14. Lee, T.H., Hoover, R.L., Williams, J.D., et al. (1985) Effect of dietary enrichment with eicosapentaenoic and docosahexaenoic acids on in vitro neutrophil and monocyte leukotriene generation and neutrophil function. *N. Engl. J. Med.* **312**, 1217–1224.

15. Payan, D.G., Wong, M.Y., Chernov-Rogan, T., et al. (1986) Alterations in human leukocyte function induced by ingestion of eicosapentaenoic acid. *J. Clin. Immunol.* **6**, 402–410.

16. Halvorsen, D.S., Hansen, J.B., Grimsgaard, S., Bonaa, K.H., Kierulf, P., and Nordoy, A. (1997) The effect of highly purified eicosapentaenoic and docosahexaenoic acids on monocyte phagocytosis in man. *Lipids* **32**, 935–942.

17. Schmidt, E.B., Varming, K., Moller, J.M., Bulow Pedersen, I., Madsen, P., Dyerberg, J. (1996) No effect of a very low dose of n-3 fatty acids on monocyte function in healthy humans. *Scand. J. Clin. Lab. Invest.* **56**, 87–92.

18. Kelley, D.S., Taylor, P.C., Nelson, G.J., et al. (1999) Docosahexaenoic acid ingestion inhibits natural killer cell activity and production of inflammatory mediators in young healthy men. *Lipids* **34**, 317–324.
19. Gallai, V., Sarchielli, P., Trequattrini, A., et al. (1995) Cytokine secretion and eicosanoid production in the peripheral blood mononuclear cells of MS patients undergoing dietary supplementation with n-3 polyunsaturated fatty acids. *J. Neuroimmunol.* **56**, 143–153.
20. Endres, S., Ghorbani, R., Kelley, V.E., et al. (1989) The effect of dietary supplementation with n-3 polyunsaturated fatty acids on the synthesis of interleukin-1 and tumor necrosis factor by mononuclear cells. *N. Engl. J. Med.* **320**, 265–271.
21. Grimble, R.F., Howell, W.M., O'Reilly, G., et al. (2002) The ability of fish oil to suppress tumor necrosis factor alpha production by peripheral blood mononuclear cells in healthy men is associated with polymorphisms in genes that influence tumor necrosis factor alpha production. *Am. J. Clin. Nutr.* **76**, 454–459.
22. Blok, W.L., Deslypere, J.P., Demacker, P.N., et al. (1997) Pro- and anti-inflammatory cytokines in healthy volunteers fed various doses of fish oil for 1 year. *Eur. J. Clin. Invest.* **27**, 1003–1008.
23. Thies, F., Nebe-von-Caron, G., Powell, J.R., Yaqoob, P., Newsholme, E.A., and Calder, P.C. (2001) Dietary supplementation with eicosapentaenoic acid, but not with other long-chain n-3 or n-6 polyunsaturated fatty acids, decreases natural killer cell activity in healthy subjects aged >55 y. *Am. J. Clin. Nutr.* **73**, 539–548.
24. Yamashita, N., Maruyama, M., Yamazaki, K., Hamazaki, T., and Yano, S. (1991) Effect of eicosapentaenoic and docosahexaenoic acid on natural killer cell activity in human peripheral blood lymphocytes. *Clin. Immunol. Immunopathol.* **59**, 335–345.
25. Kramer, T.R., Schoene, N., Douglass, L.W., et al. (1991) Increased vitamin E intake restores fish-oil-induced suppressed blastogenesis of mitogen-stimulated T lymphocytes. *Am. J. Clin. Nutr.* **54**, 896–902.
26. Schmidt, E.B., Pedersen, J.O., Varming, K., et al. (1991) n-3 fatty acids and leukocyte chemotaxis. Effects in hyperlipidemia and dose-response studies in healthy men. *Arterioscler. Thromb.* **11**, 429–435.

8 Allergies and Nutrition

CHRISTOPHER CHANG

CONTENTS

KEY POINTS

- Allergies affect more than 20% of the world's population. Food hypersensitivities affect approx 6% of children and 2–3% of adults.
- The development of allergies is the result of both genetic and environmental factors.
- The majority of adverse food reactions are not allergic in nature.
- Symptoms of food allergies include eczema, asthma, allergic rhinitis, and gastrointestinal disturbances.
- Early exposure to food allergens can lead to the development of allergies in atopic individuals.
- Crossreactivity exists within food groups, and between food allergens and environmental allergens.
- Treatment of food allergies is primarily through avoidance and awareness.
- Elimination diets are difficult to adhere to, and can have adverse effects on nutritional intake.
- Most food allergies are mediated through Type I-immunoglobulin (Ig)E-mediated hypersensitivity reactions.

From: *Handbook of Nutrition and Immunity*
Edited by: M. E. Gershwin, P. Nestel, and C. L. Keen © Humana Press, Totowa, NJ

- Food labels are frequently difficult to read or confusing, and require that the patient understand food components.
- Common foods that cause allergies include peanut, milk, eggs, fish, wheat, and soy.
- Vitamins and minerals may have antioxidant (protective) effects, but they have not been proven to be particularly useful in the treatment of asthma or allergies.
- Future developments for the treatment of food allergies include immuno-therapy, as well as genetic modification of foods to render them non-allergenic.

Introduction

Over the last 20 yr, the prevalence of allergies in most developed countries has increased and there has been a corresponding increase in the incidence of asthma. Allergies now affect 20% of the US population at some point during their lifetime. The prevalence of allergies varies greatly between countries with that in developing countries tending to be much lower than that of developed countries. For example, the prevalence in Urumqi, an underdeveloped region in China, is 2.9% whereas that in Hong Kong, where the standard of living surpasses that in many Western countries, is approx 10% (1). Whether an indi-vidual develops symptoms of allergies depends on the combined influence of a number of factors that can be genetic, environmental, infectious, physical, and/ or hormonal. The associations and interactions between these factors are not completely understood and recent information has led to the development of new theories, such as the hygiene hypothesis (2).

The state of being genetically predisposed to developing allergies is called atopy. Atopic people are prone to developing allergic symptoms when chal-lenged by a variety of external stimuli. If one parent has allergies, then the risk of an offspring having allergies is estimated to be 48%. If both parents have allergies, then the risk rises to 70%. However, data from studies of environ-mental factors and sociological patterns suggest that while the genetics of an individual are unalterable, factors early on in life may shift the balance of helper T-cell subsets to favor either a T-helper type-1 (Th1) or T-helper type-2 (Th2) response (2). A simplistic way of interpreting this is that an immune system skewed toward Th1 cell involvement is programmed to combat infections, whereas a predominantly Th2 cell-mediated immune system leads to the development of allergies and asthma.

Clinical signs of allergies usually manifest in areas of the body that are directly exposed to the environment including the skin, gastrointestinal tract, and the upper and lower respiratory tracts. External triggers for allergies can be environmental agents or food substances. In infants, the largest and initial

Table 1
Signs and Symptoms of Allergy

Head and neck
- Rhinitis
- Congestion
- Watery or itchy eyes
- Frontal headaches
- Itchy palate
- Laryngeal swelling

Chest
- Cough
- Wheezing

Gastrointestinal
- Hematemesis
- Stomach cramps (abdominal pain)
- Diarrhea
- Vomiting

Skin
- Eczema
- Urticaria
- Angioedema
- Allergic contact dermatitis
- Pruritis

Systemic
- Anaphylactic shock
- Hypotension

allergenic load is from food that will generally produce skin and gastrointestinal tract symptoms. Later on, the symptoms predominantly involve the upper and lower respiratory tract, and the eyes. Common allergy symptoms are listed in Table 1. The triggers during older childhood and adulthood are probably more often seasonal or perennial allergens that are airborne and inhaled through the nasal passages down towards the lower respiratory tract. Because of the physiological effect of allergies, allergies can also be associated with a number of comorbid conditions including asthma, sinus disease, otitis media, skin infections (secondary to eczema), anosmia, hearing loss, lack of sleep, snoring, and headache.

This chapter discusses food allergies, the treatment of food allergies, and the effect that food allergies and their treatment can have on an individual's ability to maintain a well-balanced diet. Some of the foods and food supplements that are or have been used to modify or control the development or severity of allergies or asthma are also discussed. Strategies to delay the onset of allergies are presented.

Foods That Cause Allergies
Types of Allergic Reactions

Allergic or hypersensitivity reactions are classified into four groups, Type I–IV (3). Many allergic phenomena can have components of more than one type of reaction, but common ones such as allergic rhinitis, asthma, and eczema are predominantly Type I hypersensitivity reactions that are mediated by IgE and mast cells. Other examples of Type I reactions include conjunctivitis, urticaria, angioedema, gastrointestinal anaphylactic reaction, and allergic eosinophilic gastroenteritis. A Type I hypersensitivity reaction usually occurs within minutes after exposure to stimuli, and initial allergen exposure leads to sensitization of an individual to that allergen. Sensitization occurs when allergen first presents to B-lymphocytes, leading to formation of allergen specific IgE. These IgE antibodies bind to the surface of mast cells. In subsequent exposure to the same protein, crosslinking of specific IgE on the surface of mast cells occurs and leads to the release of mast cell mediators, including histamine, into the circulation. Other molecules that are involved include vasoactive amines, lipid mediators, and cytokines. These mediators cause a number of physiologic changes, including increased membrane permeability, inflammatory cell infiltration, edema, and the disruption of mucosal surface architecture that, in turn, lead to the symptoms of an allergic reaction. A schematic of the Type I allergic reaction is shown in Fig. 1.

Type II reactions are antibody-dependent cytotoxicity reactions, in which the antibody binds to cell surface antigens leading to complement mediated lysis, phagocytosis, or killer cell activity. An example of a Type II hypersensitivity reaction to food is antibody-dependent thrombocytopenia from ingesting cow's milk. Serum-sickness-type reactions are an example of Type III immune complex-mediated hypersensitivity reactions, whereas Type IV reactions are cell-mediated hypersensitivity diseases. Type IV hypersensitivity reactions are elicited by Th1, which stimulate macrophages and other cells to produce inflammation. Type IV reactions generally take longer to manifest than Type I reactions, with an onset 2–8 h after exposure, reaching maximal effect after 24 h. Pathologic manifestations of Type IV hypersensitivity reactions include

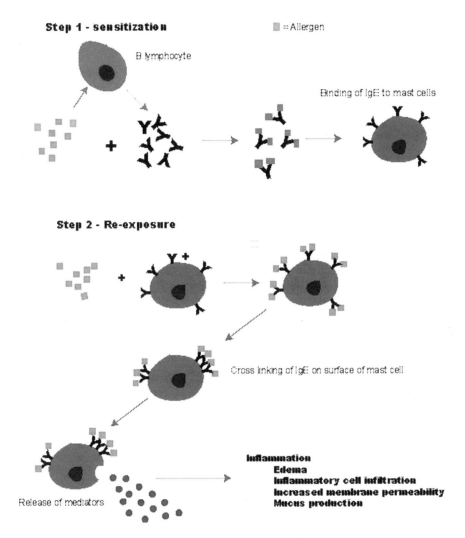

Fig. 1. Mechanism of IgE-mediated reactions.

perivascular cellular infiltration and edema. Examples of Type IV hypersensitivity reactions include allergic contact dermatitis, celiac disease, and graft rejection.

Food Allergies and Other Adverse Reactions to Foods

The prevalence of adverse food reactions and food allergies is difficult to assess owing to the frequently subjective nature of the complaints. Food intolerance was detected in 20% of 7500 households in the United Kingdom, but most were nonallergic *(4)*. In fact, many food reactions can be secondary to

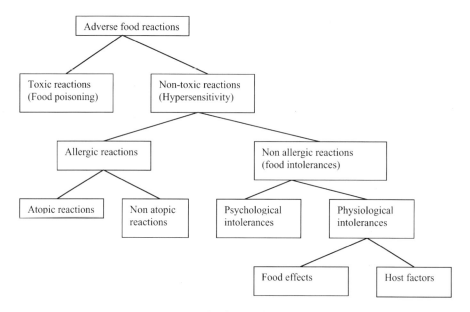

Fig. 2. Types of adverse food reactions.

chemical, pharmacological, or toxic effects, or they can be a physiological response to an otherwise normally consumed food substance (*see* Fig. 2). Some foods are not tolerated from a purely psychological standpoint, in which case they are food aversions that are not reproducible if the subject is blinded. True food allergies are estimated to affect about 6% of infants *(5)*. The characteristics of these allergies can change during a person's lifetime, and by adulthood only 1–2% of people have food allergies *(4)*.

Food allergies are either IgE-mediated (atopic) or non-IgE-mediated (nonatopic). IgE-mediated ones are responsible for a variety of different symptoms that generally appear soon after eating the food. Skin reactions can be urticarial or a nonspecific maculopapular rash. Eczema is another dermatologic manifestation of food allergy, especially in young infants. Pruritis (itching) usually accompanies any rashes related to food allergy. In the oral allergy syndrome (described later), the rash can be more consistent with an allergic contact dermatitis. Gastrointestinal symptoms include vomiting and diarrhea, with accompanying abdominal pain and nausea. Food allergies can also result in the typical upper and lower allergy constellation of symptoms including asthma symptoms such as cough, dyspnea, or wheezing. Nasal pruritis, congestion, sneezing, rhinorrhea, and ocular symptoms can also result from food allergy. The most extreme result of a food allergy is anaphylaxis that sometimes ends in death.

Non-IgE-mediated food allergies include celiac disease, food-induced enterocolitis syndrome, food-induced pulmonary hemosiderosis (Heiner's syndrome), dermatitis herpetiformis, and cow's milk-induced intestinal blood loss. Celiac disease involves a T-cell dependent inflammatory response that leads to villous atrophy and an inflammatory cell infiltrate. Food triggers in celiac disease include gliadin, an alcohol-soluble portion of gluten that is found in grains such as oat, rye, barley, and wheat.

Nonallergic food hypersensitivities and adverse food effects account for most food intolerances. These reactions can be owing to a pharmacological effect of a food component or a failure to digest food substances, such as lactose in milk intolerance. Adverse food reactions can also be a result of food poisoning, in which case the cause may be a bacterial endotoxin. A more complete list of non-IgE-mediated food hypersensitivities and nonallergic food reactions is shown in Table 2.

Whether a food reaction is allergic or not is sometimes impossible to discern based on clinical presentation. For example, intolerance to cow's milk may be caused by a number of etiologies including IgE-mediated allergies, non-IgE-mediated allergy, or lactose intolerance. In a patient with a food hypersensitivity presenting with gastrointestinal symptoms, (e.g., vomiting, nausea, diarrhea, or abdominal pain), the likelihood of the hypersensitivity being IgE mediated is only about 5%. The percentage is probably higher for food hypersensitivity patients presenting with skin symptoms or asthma.

Food Allergens

Almost any food substance can cause allergies, but 90% are caused by eight foods (*see* Table 3). Geographical variation exists, depending on what people are exposed to. For example, Asians tend to have a higher incidence of allergy to rice. Most food allergens are proteins or glycoproteins, and many foods contain multiple proteins that can cause allergies. The allergens can be classified into major and minor allergens. A protein that causes allergies in 50% or more of allergic patients is a major allergen. A list of common food allergens is shown in Table 4.

Common Foods That Cause Allergies

Cow's Milk

The two main groups of cow's milk proteins that cause allergenic sensitization are the casein and whey proteins. Caseins comprise the largest group of proteins. Cow's milk allergy is very common in young infants, but a large percentage outgrow their allergy by early childhood. Because cow's milk is a common ingredient in many other foods, care must be taken to read labels

Table 2
Examples of Non-IgE-Mediated Adverse Food Reactions

Non-IgE mediated food allergies
- Allergic eosinophilic gastroenteritis
- Enterocolitis syndrome
- Food-induced enterocolitis syndrome
- Food-induced eosinophilic proctocolitis
- Food protein-induced enteropathy
- Celiac disease
- Allergic eosinophilic gastroenteritis
- Food-induced pulmonary hemosiderosis
- Dermatitis herpetiformis

Non-allergic food intolerances
- Enzyme deficiency
  - Milk intolerance—disaccharide deficiency
  - Pancreatic insufficiency
  - Phenylketonuria
  - Alcohol—aldehyde dehydrogenase
  - Galactosemia—galactose-1-phosphate uridyl transferase
- Food poisonings
  - Bacterial endotoxins
  - Parasitic infestations
- Pharmacologic effect of food component
  - Tyramine in cheese
  - Caffeine in coffee
  - Capsaicin in peppers
  - Alcohol
  - Histamine release triggered by certain foods, for example, wine, cheese
- Host dependent factors
  - Food aversions—psychologic
  - Anorexia nervosa
  - Bulemia

carefully. Terms that are used to describe the components of cow's milk on food labels include casein, whey, dairy, or simply the symbol "D." Significant crossreactivity to goat's milk also exists, meaning a person allergic to cow's milk is usually also allergic to goat's milk.

Table 3
Common Foods that Cause Allergies

The eight major groups of common food allergies and % allergic individuals affected
- Egg   73%
- Fish   55%
- Milk   50%
- Peanut   49%
- Soy   28%
- Wheat   22%
- Tree nuts
- Crustacea (shellfish)

Other foods/food groups that can cause allergies
- Rice
- Fruits
  - Rosaceae fruits
  - Kiwi
  - Mango
  - Banana
  - Apple
- Spices
- Food additives
  - Coloring
  - Artificial flavoring
  - Sulfites
  - Preservatives
  - Fillers
  - Contaminants
- Vegetables
  - Celery

Egg

Egg allergy is the most common allergy in food allergic individuals (73%) *(6)*. The allergenic proteins are listed in Table 4. Egg yolk is generally not as allergenic as egg white. There is strong crossreactivity between chicken egg and duck egg. Although there is homology between egg allergens and chicken allergens, clinical crossreactivity does not appear to occur.

Table 4
Common Food Allergens[a]

Group 1	Group 2	Group 3	Group 4	Group 5
Milk, yogurt and cheese	Meat, poultry, fish, dry beans, egg, nut	Vegetable	Fruits	Bread, cereal, rice, pasta
Milk	*Egg*	*Mustard*	*Kiwi*	*Rice*
Casein α$_s$ β, κ, and γ (Bos d 8)	Ovalbumin (Gal d 1)	Sin a 1	Act c 1 (Actinidin)	α-amylase trypsin inhibitor
Whey:	Ovomucoid (Gal d 2)	Bra j 1	TLP	
α-lactalbumin,	Ovotransferrin (Gal d 3)			Ric c 1
β-lactoglobulin (Bos d 4)	Lysozyme (Gal d 4)			Ric c 3
β-lactoglobulin (Bos d 5)	α-livetin			
Immunoglobulins (Bos d 7)	Antigen 22			
Bovine serum albumin				
Other smaller peptide fractions				
	Peanut	*Potato*	*Pear*	*Wheat*
	Ara h 1	Sol t 1	Pyr c 1	α-amylase inhibitor
	Ara h 2		Pyr c 4	
	Ara h 3			
	Ara h 5			

162

Soybean	Celery	Apple	Barley
Gly m 1	Api g 1	Mal d 1	Hor v 1
Trypsin inhibitor	Api g 4		
Brazil nut	Carrot	Cherry	Buckwheat
Ber m 1	Dau c 1	Pru a 1	Fag e 1
	Pru a 2		
Fish			
Gad c 1 (Allergen M)			
Sal s 1 (Salmon)			
Shrimp			
Pen a 1			
Antigen 1			
Antigen 2			
Met e 1			
Chicken			
α-livetin			

[a]Allergens are named according to the first three letters of the genus of their origin, followed by a space and the first letter (in lower case) of the species of origin, then a space, and then a number (in Arabic format) representing the order of discovery of that allergen for that genus and species.

163

Peanut

Until recently, it was generally thought that peanut allergy was one of the few food allergies that persists throughout life. However, a recent study showed that over 20% of peanut allergic patients lose their allergy after several years *(7)*. Peanut allergies can be very severe, and symptoms include angioedema and urticaria, difficult swallowing, severe itching, hoarseness, and anaphylaxis. Several peanut proteins have been characterized *(see* Table 4). Peanut oil is not a significant hazard to peanut allergic patients, although contamination with peanut protein is possible. Thresholds for subjective reactions to peanut range from 100 µg to 1 g of protein *(8)*, whereas those for objective symptoms range from 10 to 30 mg. Peanut allergies are increasing in the Western world, nearly doubling in prevalence from 0.5% in 1989 to 1% in 2002, which has been attributed to the increase in the number of health-conscious people shifting to a vegetarian diet and increasing their consumption of peanuts *(9)*.

Wheat

Allergy to grains is quite common and wheat is the most common allergen in this food group. The major allergenic component of wheat appears to be a 14-kDa α-amylase inhibitor. This protein may be responsible for the development of an occupational asthma disease called Baker's asthma. There is known homology and crossreactivity between wheat α-amylase inhibitor and a 14-kDa glycoprotein component of rice. In addition, there is extensive crossreactivity among wheat, barley, and rye.

Fish

Individuals with fish allergy are usually allergic to multiple species of fish. The most common allergen is Gad c 1, which was first isolated from codfish. Fish allergen appears to be susceptible to different methods of processing: some individuals allergic to cooked fish are able to tolerate canned fish of the same species. Some people are allergic only to one species of fish and, for these individuals, the current recommendations for avoidance does not require that all varieties of fish be completely eliminated from the diet.

Soy

Soy is a common food alternative for infants and children with cow's milk allergy. However, soy allergy is also quite common; more than 15 protein components of the bean are allergenic. Three major allergenic proteins associated with atopic dermatitis have been characterized: Gly m Bd 60K, a component of a storage protein; Gly mBd 30K, an oil-body associated protein with homology to the major dust mite allergenic determinant Der p 1; and Gly m Bd 28K, a vicilin-like glycoprotein. Two other low-molecular weight soybean hull allergens, Gly m1 and Gly m 2, have been associated with asthma outbreaks.

Other

Other commonly seen food allergies relate to fruits, vegetables, shrimp and other crustaceans, and food additives. The major allergenic determinants for lobster, shrimp, mollusks, oysters, crab, abalone, and squid have been identified and characterized (10). The characteristics and patterns of crossreactivity of some major food allergens are shown in Table 5. The allergenic proteins can be structural proteins, storage proteins, transfer proteins, or enzymes. Exposure to large amounts of a specific food type, such as rice in Asian countries, leads to increased sensitization rates. There is a great deal of homology across species, and patients who have been previously exposed to pollen allergens that carry similar structure to certain foods may then become allergic to these foods.

Crossreactivity of Food and Environmental Allergies

Crossreactivity within classes of foods is quite common. For example, crossreactivity between cow's and goat's milk is more than 50%. Homology between proteins occurring in nature causes patients to show crossreactivity between various food and pollen allergens. For example, individuals allergic to birch may also be allergic to raw potatoes, carrots, apples, hazelnuts, kiwi, or celery. Those allergic to ragweed pollen may also exhibit signs of allergy to melons and bananas. These patterns of crossreactivity have given rise to several syndromes, including the oral allergy syndrome, the latex fruit syndrome, and the tree nut syndrome.

The Oral Allergy Syndrome

The oral allergy syndrome is a contact allergy involving the lips, tongue, palate, and structures of the mouth, throat, and perioral area that leads to pruritis, rash, and angioedema. It is more common in individuals with pollen allergies, specifically against birch or ragweed, in which the primary sensitizer is probably the pollen. In the oral allergy syndrome, individuals who are allergic to birch react to Roasaceae fruits (peach, apple, almond, plum, apricot, pear, and strawberry) as well as potatoes, carrots, hazelnuts, celery, and kiwifruit, whereas those with ragweed allergy react to melons, including watermelon, cantaloupe, and honeydew. Mugwort allergic patients can react to celery.

Table 5
Classification and Characteristics of Proteins That Cause Food Allergies

Protein	Name derivation	Source	Classification	Size (kd)	Homology/cross reactivity	Comments
Act c 1	Actinidin	Kiwi	Thiol-protease	30	Birch, latex, avocado, banana	Glycoprotein
Api g 1	Apium graveolens	Celery		16.2	Mugwort	Also sensitization by birch
Api g 4	Apium graveolens		Profilin	14.3		
Ara h 1	Arachis hypogaea	Peanut		63.5	Tree nuts, legumes	
Ara h 2	Arachis hypogaea	Peanut		17	Tree nuts, legumes	
Ara h 3	Arachis hypogaea	Peanut		14.3	Hazelnut, other legumes	IgE epitopes same as soybean
Ber e 1	Bertholletia excelsa	Brazil nut	Seed storage protein			Methionine rich 2S albumin
Bra j 1	Brassica juncea	Mustard	2S albumin	16	Sin a 1	
Cha f 1	Charybdis feriatus	Crab	Tropomyosin	34	Met e 1	
Cor a 9	Croylus avellana	Hazelnut	11S globulin storage protein	40	Ara h 3	
Cra g 1.03	Crassostrea gigas	Oyster	Tropomyosin	59	Shellfish	
Dau c 1	Daucas carota	Carrot		18	Birch, celery	
Fag e 1	Fagopyrum esculentum	Buckwheat	Globulin protein	24	Rice	
G2 glycinin	Glycine max	Soybean	Storage protein	22		
Gad c 1	Gadus callarias	Codfish	Muscular parvalbumin	12.3	Other fish	Heat and digestion resistant
Gal d 1	Gallus domesticus	Egg	Ovomucoid	28	Duck eggs	
Gal d 2	Gallus domesticus	Egg	Ovalbumin	45	Duck eggs	
Gal d 3	Gallus domesticus	Egg	Ovotransferrin	77.7	Duck eggs	
Gal d 4	Gallus domesticus	Egg	Lysozyme	14.3	Duck eggs	
Gly m 1	Glycine max	Soybean	Trypsin inhibitor	30		
Hal m 1	Halliotis midae	Abalone	Tropomyosin	49	Crustaceae	

Allergen	Species	Common name	Protein	MW	Cross-reactivity	Comments
Hom a 1	Homarus americanus	Lobster	Tropomyosin	34	Shrimp	
Hor v 1	Hordeum vulgare	Barley	α-amylase inhibitor	14.5		Methionine rich 2S albumin
Jug r 1	Juglans regia	Walnut	Seed storage protein		Ber e 1	
Mal d 1	Malus domestica	Apple		17.7	Bet v 1 (birch)	
Met e 1	Metapenaeus ensis	Shrimp	Tropomyosin	34	Other shellfish, dust mite	Major heat labile shrimp allergen
Pan s 1	Panulirus stimpsoni	Lobster	Tropomyosin	34	Shrimp, other shellfish	cDNA cloned
Pen a 1	Penaeus aztecus	Shrimp	Tropomyosin	36	Dust mites	cDNA cloned
Pru a 1	Prunus avium 1	Cherry	Lipid transfer protein	18	Birch	
Pru a 2	Prunus avium 2	Cherry	Lipid transfer protein	23		
Pyr c 1	Pyrus communis	Pear			Bet v 1, Mal d 1	
Pyr c 4	Pyrus communis	Pear	Profilin		Pru a 4, Bet v 2, Api g 4	Profilin is pan-allergen in many fruits
Ric c 1	Ricinus communis	Castor bean	2S albumin			Albumin storage protein
Ric c 3	Ricinus communis	Castor bean	2S albumin			Albumin storage protein
Sal s 1	Salmo salar	Salmon	Parvalbumin			
Sin a 1	Sinapis alba	Mustard	Seed storage protein	14	Bra j 1	2S albumin, resistant to trypsin digestion
Sol t 1	Solanum tuberosum	Potato	Soybean trypsin inhibitor, storage protein	43	Latex	Also called patatin, cross reacts with latex Hev b 7
TLP	Thaumatin-like protein	Kiwi		24		Concavalin A-binding, antifungal effects
Tod p 1	Todarodes pacificus	Squid	Tropomyosin	38	Other shellfish, dust mite	
Trypsin inhibitor		Maize	Trypsin inhibitor	9	Peach, grass, wheat, barley, rice	
α-amylase inhibitor		Wheat	α-amylase inhibitor	15		Role in Baker's asthma disease?

The Latex Fruit Syndrome

Cross-sensitization between fruits and latex fruits has been clearly demonstrated and include papaya, avocado, banana, chestnut, passion fruit, fig, melon, mango, kiwi, pineapple, peach, and tomato. The crossreacting protein responsible has been proposed to be chitinase 1, which has been identified as being a "pan-allergen" for the above fruits.

The Tree Nut Syndrome

Patients allergic to peanuts may exhibit crossreactivity to other legumes or tree nuts. In this condition, peanuts may contain the sensitizing allergen. Peanut allergic subjects can be allergic to hazelnut, brazilnut, or both. Other nuts demonstrating crossreactivity include cashews and walnuts.

The Effects of Food Preparation on Allergenicity

Most foods allergens tend to be fairly stable during food preparation and processing. Some are resistant to heat, while others are denatured in cooking. For example, both heat-stable and heat-labile allergenic proteins are found in shrimp. To be allergenic, foods must also be able to survive the digestive process and cross the intestinal mucosa in an immunologically intact form. The absorption of foods can be affected by other components "consumed" at the same time, for example, ethanol, cigarette smoking, and antacids. Ethanol can increase gastric permeability to sucrose, whereas cigarette smoking has the opposite effect *(11)*. Exercise causes body temperature to increase, which increases sensitization to an ingested antigen in some people. Other cofactors that may regulate or affect the severity of symptoms of a food allergy include resistance to digestive enzymes, differential expression of allergens during pregnancy, and food preparation and processing.

The Diagnosis and Treatment of Food Allergies
Diagnosis of Food Allergies
History and Physical

Taking a good history is always the first step toward diagnosing a food allergy. Like all medical histories, the physician needs to know the who, when, how, where, and what of the clinical reaction to a food. "Who" refers to the characteristics of the patient, including their family history of allergy. "When" refers to the time between eating the food and the onset of the reaction as well as the number of recurrences that have occurred. "What" refers to the amount of food consumed, as well as other foods consumed along with the suspected agent. "How" refers to how the patient manifests symptoms of the food intolerance, and may help to distinguish whether or not the reaction is a true allergy

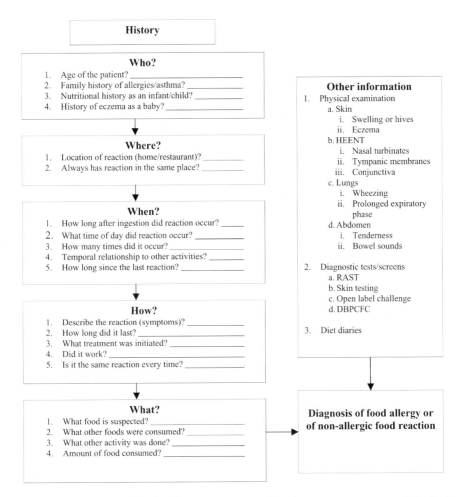

Fig. 3. Diagnosing food allergies. HEENT, head, eyes, ears, nose, blind placebo controlled food challenge.

or a different type of adverse food reaction. "Where" helps to identify concurrent exposures that may be confusing the picture. Once obtained, this information can be assimilated to help with a diagnosis. Figure 3 shows some of the specific questions to be asked in taking a food allergy history. Other information to be collected includes accompanying events or activities, such as exercise-induced food anaphylaxis. The degree of severity of the reaction will help direct the type of treatment to use. Patients may find it difficult to identify an offending food from a diverse diet, and factors that affect sensitization can frequently cause confusion. A patient's medical history is dependent on their memory, which may not be accurate when trying to isolate a specific food.

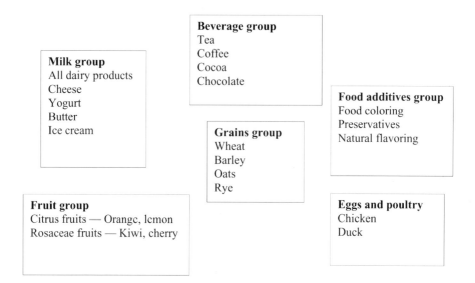

Fig. 4. An example of the food groups to avoid in an elimination diet. This is an example of the food groups that can be used to construct an elimination diet. Patients must remember to strictly adhere to the diet and it will be necessary for them to understand how to read labels, as many of the constituents of foods may not be obvious at first.

Food Diaries

The limitations of memory recall can be overcome by using a food diary, which has the advantage of being proactive. The information recorded needs to be as detailed as possible, and include when and how much food was eaten, how it was prepared, as well as other events occurring around the time of eating and the onset of the reaction.

Elimination Diets

Elimination diets can be used to diagnose allergies, and their use depends on the type or number of foods suspected. They tend to take a long time to complete and are notoriously difficult to adhere to. A common method of instituting an elimination diet is to divide foods into food groups (e.g., as in Fig. 4). All the foods in one group are eliminated for 6 d and on the seventh day one food is reintroduced. If the individual is asymptomatic during the initial 6 d, and symptoms reappear on the seventh day after reintroduction of the food, the likelihood that the patient is allergic to that specific food is high. Because only one food group can be studied at a time, the whole process can take a long time to complete.

The Double-Blind Placebo-Controlled Food Challenge (DBPCFC)

The double-blind placebo-controlled food challenge is the gold standard for testing for food allergies. However, there are limitations to using the DBPCFC. First, performing a DBPCFC requires that the endpoint occurs immediately (within a few minutes) after ingestion. Second, the endpoint must be measured objectively and accurately. To perform a DBPCFC, some knowledge of what to test for must exist. Identifying the foods to be tested can be based on history, diet diaries, radioallergosorbent testing (RAST), or skin testing. Because of the preparation needed, DBPCFC are not always feasible for detecting food allergies in most outpatient settings. To do a DBPCFC properly, the subject must have avoided exposure to the food under investigation for at least 2 wk, been off antihistamines for at least a few days, and fasted prior to the challenge. The test must be conducted as scientifically as possible, with food and placebo doses being administered in equal amounts in an equal number of doses. The test and placebo foods must taste, look, and smell the same and also have the same texture. Foods must be as pure as possible, without contaminants or confounding foods that may cause symptoms themselves. The total dose administered should be 10 g over 1 h. Starting doses can be variable, but a safe DBPCFC is conducted using the minimal threshold dose for anaphylactic reactions previously recorded *(12)*. Scoring of symptoms must be standardized. At the end of the test all subjects undergo open challenge under observation, meaning the patient ingests a full serving of the food in question under close observation by medical staff.

Immunoassays and Radioallergosorbent Testing (RAST)

Serum immunoassays for specific IgE exist *(12)*. Moreover, improved automation and the development of a high-capacity ImmunoCAP has allowed for the standardization of RAST testing for allergen specific IgE. The current "UniCAP" system by Pharmacia can detect allergen specific IgE with a sensitivity and specificity of 89 and 91%, respectively, compared with clinical diagnosis or DBPCFC *(6)*. RAST testing results can be reported in several ways, including units/mL, percentage of a control value, or by class ranges (generally zero to six) with six representing the higher amounts of allergen specific IgE detected.

Skin Testing

Skin-prick testing, in which a small amount of allergen is epicutaneously applied to the skin and the patient is observed for development of a wheal and flare reaction, is used for food allergy testing. Both in vivo and in vitro food testing have good positive and negative predictive values *(14)*. Skin testing in particular has been shown to diminish the need for DBPCFC *(15)*. The advantages of skin-prick testing are that results can be obtained immediately, and a wheal and flare reaction gives more information about the patient's in vivo response to allergen. The disadvantages of skin-prick testing, compared to RAST, are that more pricks are done and the procedure is potentially more traumatic-especially for children. Skin testing is contraindicated in a number of conditions, including the use of β-blockers, skin conditions such as eczema or hives, a history of anaphylaxis, and the use of antihistamines (that can invalidate the results of the skin testing). Intradermal testing is not generally used in testing for food allergies because of the high frequency of false positives and lack of specificity.

Open-Label Challenge

An open label challenge is carried out in a clinic setting where there is emergency equipment available for potential systemic side effects. In this case, both the patient and the physician are aware of the food substance being tested. Although not as objective as the DBPCFC, an open-label challenge can provide valuable information under specific circumstances. The allergy signs and symptoms must be visible and be as objective as possible, such as hives, angioedema, or asthma symptoms. The time between administration of the food and onset of symptoms must be short and the test must be reproducible. Open-label testing will not work for vague symptoms, and testing foods containing complex ingredients confuses the picture further.

Other Assays

Several other assays are also available, but these are not routinely used in diagnosing food allergies. Basophil histamine release assay uses whole blood to determine the histamine response to antigen challenge. Results are comparable to RAST. The intestinal mast cell histamine release assay is an in vitro test that measures the response to food antigens using biopsy specimens.

Treatment of Food Allergies

Prevention of Allergies

As mentioned earlier, the onset and severity of allergies depends both on genetic and environmental factors. Because the genetic factors that predispose an individual to allergies cannot be altered, prevention must be done at the environmental level. Identifying infants who may be at high risk for allergies is important, because this helps to determine how much intervention is needed in early infancy. The risk factors for the development of allergies are shown in Table 6. The extent to which the onset of allergies can be delayed or the sever-

Table 6
Possible Risk Factors for Atopy in Children and Factors
That Counteract Increased Risk of Developing Food Allergies

Risk factors
- Family history
- Elevated cord blood IgE
- Elevated serum IgE in early childhood
- Early exposure to foods
- Concurrent exposure to environmental allergies
- Exposure to cigarette smoke
- Blood or nasal eosinophilia
- Decreased cord blood platelets
- Decreased CD8 T-cells
- The lambdaMS.51 marker on chromosome 11q
- Increased monocyte phosphodiesterase activity
- Increased arachidonia acid pathway metabolites

Factors to counteract increased risk of developing food allergies
- Delayed introduction of solid foods
  - Eggs
  - Fish
  - Nuts
  - Soybean
- Avoidance of inhalant allergens
  - Dust mite
  - Cat
  - Dog
  - Cockroach
- Maternal avoidance during lactation
  - Milk
  - Peanut
  - Egg
  - Fish
- Prolonged exclusive breast feeding
- Use of hydrolyzed milk formula

ity of asthma, eczema, and allergic rhinitis can be decreased remains controversial. For those at-risk of atopic diseases, avoidance of highly allergic foods by both the mother and young infant can help to delay the onset of allergic diseases (*see* Table 6) *(16)*. Avoidance of foods by pregnant mothers is generally not recommended except for peanuts.

Breast Milk and Milk Formula

Prolonged breastfeeding is recommended for infants at risk of allergies because breast milk contains protective antibodies. Soy-based milk formulas contain several allergenic proteins. Hypoallergenic formulas are now available, in which the cow's milk protein components have been hydrolyzed to produce smaller peptide units. The tertiary structure is thus changed so that these peptide units are, theoretically, no longer allergenic, leading to less exposure to allergenic determinants. Casein hydrolysates contain peptide fragments that are less than 1.5 kDa and have low immunogenicity. Whey hydrolysates contain peptides that are larger, and potentially retain their immunogenicity. Both casein and whey hydrolysates have been effective in preventing eczema, but not allergic rhinitis or asthma symptoms *(17)*. Amino acid-based formulas are also available. They have been shown to be nutritionally adequate and to decrease allergic reactions in 31 allergic infants, including 14 with allergic eosinophilic gastroenteritis *(18)*. Studies that compared the effect of using of soy milk vs cow's milk-based formula to decrease symptoms of asthma or eczema found the outcomes to be similar *(19)*.

Breast milk contains high concentrations of nucleotides that may play a role in immunization-induced antibody production, although whether or not the nucleotide content of breast milk and formulas has any role in the development of atopy is not known. New and better infant formulas are constantly being developed to mimic breast milk, and newer molecular biology and cloning techniques are being used to create formula that will be truly nonallergenic while maintaining good nutrition content.

Avoidance

The cornerstone of treatment of food allergies involves eliminating the offending allergen. However, foods are complex mixtures of numerous components and people with multiple food allergies often have a difficult time managing their diet in the face of multiple food allergies. In the case of a single offending food, elimination of that food from the diet should not lead to any nutritional deficiency. In addition, some foods are easier to avoid than others. Peanut allergic patients can usually avoid peanuts with some degree of confidence, but it is more difficult to avoid foods such as milk, wheat, or corn because they are ingredients in many processed foods. Sometimes it is necessary to eliminate an entire food group at a time. Alternative foods that can be used to replace the nutrients found in common foods allergens are shown in Table 7. Occasionally, a vitamin or mineral supplement may be advised. It is possible to become overzealous in the management of a food allergy. Fear of developing an asthma attack or making a child's eczema worse can lead some

Table 7
Alternative Foods Sources of Nutrients for People With Food Allergies

Nutrient	Usual source	Alternative sources
Calcium	Milk	Cheese, yogurt, soy or rice beverage, infant formula
Iron	Meat	Bread, legume, fruit, vegetables
Protein	Meat	Tofu, beans
Selenium	Cereal products	Meat, seafood
Thiamine	Nuts, seeds	Meats
Vitamin A	Plant carotenoids	Liver, fish, potato
Vitamin B_{12}	Milk and eggs	Fish and seafood, meats
Vitamin B_6	Eggs	Meat and cereals
Vitamin C	Fruit and fruit juices	Vegetables, peppers
Vitamin D	Milk	Milk substitute products, egg yolk, fish oil
Vitamin E	Seeds, whole grain products	Vegetable oils, leafy green vegetables
Zinc	Nuts, legumes	Whole grain products, meats, fish, shellfish

people to take avoidance to an unreasonable extreme. A common sense approach to diet is of utmost importance in managing food allergies.

Elimination Diets for the Treatment of Allergies

Elimination diets are a structured way of practicing avoidance. Their use in the treatment of allergies is fairly simple if there are only a few foods or a single food that must be eliminated from the diet. In this case, the risk of compromising nutritional status is low, and alternative sources of nutrients can be used. If the offending allergen has not been clearly defined, or if RAST or skin testing yields a high number of positive sensitivities, then using an elimination diet becomes more complicated and, indeed, more controversial. The ultimate elimination diet is an elemental diet, but the more drastic the diet the greater the likelihood of compromising nutritional status. Elemental formulas such as "Nutramigen" or "Pregestamil" are available for infants. Elemental diets are also available for children and adolescents, and can be effective in treating eosinophilic eosophagitis.

Current Labeling Laws

Many countries do not have food labeling laws or guidelines. Good avoidance measures involve careful reading of labels. Labeling laws have evolved in the United States under the direction of the Food and Drug Administration, while the Food Standards Agency handles labeling guidelines in the United Kingdom. Food labels are not always easy to read, nor are they always accurate or complete. Even with labeling guidelines, labels can be confusing and the food content is sometimes disguised by the use of ambiguous terminology or chemical terms that the general public does not understand. In a study conducted in the United States, the correct identification of food ingredients and components from food labels by parents of children on a restrictive diet was poor. Most of the problems were associated with foods containing milk, soy, and peanut; recognition of the components of egg and wheat was fairly good *(20)*. Clearly labeling practices have to be revised to facilitate easy, quick, and accurate identification of all potential offending allergens by the public at large.

Pharmacologic

ANTIHISTAMINES

Antihistamines block the H_1-histamine receptors, thus preventing the physiological effects of histamine. Antihistamines have been used since the 1950s and, until about 20 yr ago, all of them were sedating. Since then, the nonsedating second generation histamines have been developed. Antihistamines are useful in the treatment of allergen-induced urticaria, asthma, allergic rhinitis, and conjunctivitis. Antihistamines can also help decrease the pruritis associated with atopic dermatitis.

LEUKOTRIENE ANTAGONISTS

Leukotrienes are powerful mediators of inflammation. Pharmacologic agents that counteract these effects are either leukotriene receptor antagonists or inhibitors of the leukotriene synthesis. Currently, the leukotriene receptor antagonists are more widely used. Leukotriene antagonists are very safe, and can be taken once or twice daily. They are used in the treatment of allergic rhinitis, asthma, urticaria, and atopic dermatitis.

STEROID CREAMS AND INHALED STEROIDS

The profound antiinflammatory effects of corticosteroids have led to the development of topical preparations that do not carry the serious side effects of long-term systemic corticosteroid use. Topical steroid creams and ointments are the mainstay for treating atopic dermatitis. Side effects include thinning of the skin and, where overused, absorption of corticosteroids into the systemic circulation. Inhaled steroids are the first-line treatment for asthma, and nasal steroids are the most effective method for treating allergic rhinitis. Although the issue is still controversial, inhaled steroids have not been generally found to cause permanent growth retardation or suppression of hypothalamic–pituitary axis in children *(21)*.

TOPICAL IMMUNOMODULATORY AGENTS

The newer topical immunomodulatory agents include tacrolimus and pimecrolimus. These agents inhibit the upregulation of cytokine production following T-cell activation and decreased Fc epsilon RI expression on dendritic antigen-presenting cells in skin. Other effects of tacrolimus include inhibition of cytokines that participate in the early immune response and the pathogenesis of atopic dermatitis, including interleukins (IL)-2 IL-3, IL-4, IL-5, interferon (IFN)-γ, tumor necrosis factor (TNF)-α, and granulocyte-macrophage colony-stimulating factor. A double-blind vehicle controlled study in 351 children (age 2–15 years) with severe atopic dermatitis, affecting a mean of 47.7% body surface area, found that significantly more patients in the tacrolimus treated group had a 90% improvement (itching, body surface area involvement, appearance) after 12 wk compared with the placebo group *(22)*. In addition, adverse effects were no greater in the tacrolimus-treated group. This class of immunomodulatory agents has been found to be safe and efficacious in the treatment of atopic dermatitis.

ORAL CORTICOSTEROIDS

Oral corticosteroids have been important medication for treating asthma exacerbation, and are also sometimes used in the treatment of hives, eczema, and angioedema secondary to food allergies. Oral corticosteroids are usually prescribed for short-term treatment of these conditions, because long-term use of corticosteroid have potentially severe side effects including osteonecrosis of the hip, osteoporosis, hypertension, diabetes, hirsutism, growth retardation in children, and suppression of the hypothalamic–pituitary axis. Fortunately, with the recent advances in the treatment of asthma and atopic dermatitis, the use of oral steroids on a chronic basis has been much curtailed.

ANTI-IgE

The anti-IgE drug TNX-901 has been studied in peanut allergy and found to increase the threshold for developing an allergic reaction from an average of 0.5 peanuts to 6 peanuts. A concomitant decrease in total IgE levels was also observed. Anti-IgE is administered monthly by injection. It is not considered a curative measure, but it will protect against the accidental exposure of one or two peanuts worth of peanut allergen. An anti-IgE antibody has been found to inhibit both the early and late phase reactions to allergic stimuli *(23)*. It decreases asthma exacerbation rates and severity, and also nasal and ocular symptom scores, and reduces the need for antihistamines in patients with seasonal allergic rhinitis.

In patients who have anaphylaxis to foods, epinephrine, administered subcutaneously can be a life-saving measure. These patients are instructed to carry their epinephrine with them at all times, and this is usually in the form of an Epi-pen or Epi-pen Jr. autoinjector device. Schoolchildren may need to obtain written permission from their parents or physicians to carry their epinephrine on their person. School policies vary, but a recent survey conducted by the US Food Allergy and Anaphylaxis Network revealed that 9 out of 10 schools permit their school nurse to administer epinephrine, and about 50% allow students to carry their Epi-pen with them. Other school personnel are allowed to administer Epi-pen in 80% of schools, provided they have been properly trained by the school nurse. Patients with a history of anaphylaxis should also be allowed to carry their Epi-pen on board a commercial airliner, with a permission slip from their physician.

The Effects of Foods on Allergies and Asthma
Minerals, Vitamins, and Antioxidants

An association between minerals or vitamins intake and the development of atopy is not known to exist. However, the association between the development of allergies and asthma, and the presence of oxygen free radicals, is a topic of discussion. It is postulated that an allergic response to antigen challenge, including inflammatory cell infiltration, results in the generation and release of reactive oxygen species. These species (superoxide and hydrogen peroxide) are further metabolized to hypochlorous acid and the hydroxyl radical by neutrophil myeloperoxidase and ferrous ion reduction, respectively. These oxygen free radicals lead to bronchoconstriction, increased mucus secretion, and microvascular leakage *(24)*.

Minerals and trace elements are components of naturally occurring compounds superoxide dismutase (zinc and copper or manganese) and glutathione peroxidase (selenium). Other naturally occurring compounds are catalase, β-carotene, coenzyme Q10. These substances protect the airway against oxygen free-radical-mediated airway hyperresponsiveness. In asthmatic airways, the activity levels of these enzymes is decreased, and treatment with inhaled corticosteroids appears to reverse this and, thus, treat the inflammation *(25)*. Much research has been conducted on the effects of minerals and vitamins on the allergic response. Zinc is a component of many creams and ointments used to treat irritating rashes and eczema. Because low levels of serum zinc levels have been detected in children with eczema *(26)*, treating these children with oral zinc supplementation has not proffered any benefit *(27)*. Magnesium picolinate has been studied in the treatment of allergic rhinitis and, in a small cohort of 38 patients, was beneficial in diminishing symptoms of rhinorrhea, watery eyes, number of Kleenex used, and number of sneezes *(28)*. One week of magnesium supplementation led to an improvement in asthma symptom scores in 17 asthmatic patients subjected to low dietary magnesium for two 3-wk periods *(29)*. A larger study of 2633 patients in the United Kingdom found that magnesium supplements increased forced expiratory volume (FEV)$_1$ by an average of 27.7 L/min *(30)*. Selenium, a component of glutathione peroxidase, and copper have also been studied. Selenium-rich yeast supplements in 60 subjects had no significant clinical effect on atopic dermatitis *(31)*. Manganese is thought to play a role in IL-5 regulated eosinophilic recruitment, but clinical studies of the effects of manganese on allergic rhinitis are lacking. Low dietary intake of manganese has been associated with higher increased risk of bronchial hyperreactivity *(32)*.

Vitamins C and E are antioxidants that may play a role in preventing or protecting against asthma or allergic inflammation. Vitamin C supplementation in 12 patients with exercise-induced asthma, improved forced vital capacity (FVC) and FEV$_1$ compared with placebo *(33)*. However, the study population was too small to draw any definite conclusions regarding the role of vitamin C in asthma. In a large retrospective study on 77,866 women aged 34–68 yr, vitamin E had a protective effect on the development of asthma (relative risk 0.53) *(34)*. Vitamin C has not been shown to have any inhibitory effect on skin or nasal hypersensitivity to histamine or allergen challenge *(35)*.

Fish Oil

The role of the arachidonic acid pathway intermediates in asthma and atopic dermatitis is a subject of particular interest. Arachidonic acid is metabolized to a class of compounds known as leukotrienes by the enzymatic action of 5-lipoxygenase. Leukotrienes are mediators of inflammation that lead to increased vascular permeability, neutrophil chemotaxis, and activation of inflammatory cells. Physiologic consequences of these histocellular events include bronchial constriction, edema, and mucus plugging. Arachadonic acid is also metabolized by cyclooxygenase to produce prostaglandins PGD_2, PGE_2, PGI_2, PGF_{2a} and thromboxane A_2. These compounds also have inflammatory effects, as illustrated in Table 8.

With increasing awareness about the adverse health effects of consuming large amounts of saturated fats, diets in developed countries has shifted toward foods high in vegetable oils. Linoleic acid is a component of these vegetable

Table 8
Antiinflammatory Effects of Lipid Mediators

Lipid mediator or metabolite	Pathway	Inflammatory effects
Leukotriene B4	Lipooxygenase	Neutrophil chemotaxis
Leukotriene C4	Lipooxygenase	Bronchoconstriction, increased airway secretions, microvascular leakage, bronchial hyperresponsiveness
PGD_2	Cyclooxygenase	Bronchoconstriction, increased airway secretions, vasodilation, bronchial hyperresponsiveness
PGE_2	Cyclooxygenase	Increased airway secretions, chemotaxis, vasodilation, increased vascular permeability
PGF_{2a}	Cyclooxygenase	Bronchoconstriction, vascular constriction
PGI_2	Cyclooxygenase	Vasodilation, increased vascular permeability
Platelet activating factor	Acyl-CoA acyltransferase pathway	Bronchoconstriction, increased airway secretions, microvascular leakage, eosinophil chemotaxis, bronchial hyperresponsiveness, vascular smooth muscle relaxation, inflammatory leukocyte activation, endothelial retraction
Thromboxane A2	Cyclooxygenase	Bronchoconstriction, increased airway hyperresponsiveness, vasoconstriction, platelet aggregation
Eicosapentaenoic acid	Substrate competitor of arachidonic acid	Decreases active cystinyl-leukotriene products of lipooxygenase pathway

Source: Adapted from ref. 45.

oils, and increased ingestion of this precursor of arachidonic acid synthesis may lead to a higher production of leukotrienes, theoretically increasing the severity of asthma and allergies. A treatment for both allergies and asthma is the use of leukotriene pathway inhibitors, as described earlier. Fish oil contains a competitor of arachidonic acid in the form of eicosapentanoic acid. Eicosapentanoic acid is metabolized by the catalytic action of 5-lipoxygenase to a number of inactive or partially active metabolites that do not possess the same inflammatory activity as the leukotrienes. Multiple studies have been conducted to see if the theoretical benefit of fish oil consumption translates to a clinical improvement of asthma. One epidemiological study on 574 children, which was based on the responses to food diaries and symptom questionnaires, demonstrated that fish oil consumption led to a significantly decreased risk of asthma symptoms *(36)*. This was supported by a study in 2526 adults that showed a positive effect of dietary fish intake on FEV_1 *(37)*. In addition, a fish oil lipid extract inhibited an allergen-induced late phase asthmatic response in 12 of the 17 subjects, although other parameters of allergic inflammation such as total serum IgE and airway conductance were unchanged *(38)*. Because significant effects of fish oil on nasal symptomatology have not been observed, a diet that included a daily intake of eicosapentanoic acid of 3.5 g/d for 8 wk led to a decrease in the number of eosinophils in nasal secretions and a reduction in nasal blood flow as measured by laser Doppler probe technique *(39)*. In contrast, in a study of 145 patients with moderate to severe atopic dermatitis, a diet rich in n-3 unsaturated fatty acids showed no clinical benefits over a corn oil diet for the treatment of atopic dermatitis *(40)*.

Onion

Whereas allergy to onion exists, onions also possess antiasthmatic activity. Onions contain alk(en)ylsulfinothioic acid alk(en)yl-esters, which inhibit histamine release from polymorphonuclear leukocytes, 5-lipooxygenase of porcine leukocytes, leukotriene B4 and C4 synthesis by human neutrophils, and thromboxane-B2 biosynthesis by human platelets in vitro. Onion esters also counteract platelet activity factor and allergen-induced bronchial obstruction in guinea pigs in vivo *(41)*.

The Hygiene Hypothesis As It Relates to Food Allergy

The hygiene hypothesis states that exposure to infections and microbial agents early in life can protect against the development of allergic diseases or asthma. As society advances, the benefits of "clean" or "sterile" habitats become more apparent, with an accompanying reduction in exposure to viral and bacterial agents or products. The hygiene hypothesis has conventionally been discussed in terms of viral agents or bacterial endotoxins being protective against the development of hay fever symptoms and atopic asthma. However, exposure to gastrointestinal pathogens such as Toxoplasma, Helicobacter, and Shistosoma may protect against the development of food sensitivies; thus leading to a decrease in the incidence of atopic dermatitis in the young child. Indeed, the type and distribution of bacteria present in the gastrointestinal tract may effect the development of atopy. In one study, infants with atopic dermatitis and allergen sensitization by 2 yr of age were found to have more clostridia species and Staphylococcus species in their stool and less enterococci and bifidobacteria *(42)*. The association between overall hygiene, food intake, bacterial colonization of the gastrointestinal tract, exposure to environmental allergens, and the balance between Th1 and Th2 subsets is still not completely clear.

Conclusions

Allergies affect a large portion of the population in developed countries. Food allergies are common in children and are a cause of atopic dermatitis and asthma. Many food intolerances are not allergic in nature, and can be because of a variety of other mechanisms. A mainstay of treatment of food allergies, and also food intolerances, is avoidance or elimination of the offending food. However, if the food to be eliminated is one containing crucial nutrients, or if there are multiple food allergies, then the treatment of food allergies can compromise good nutritional intake and status. Patients need to understand what and how to avoid the allergen. Avoidance requires being able to read food labels. However, food label guidelines do not necessarily ensure that labels are easily understandable, and food allergy patients have to understand the constituents of common foods and alternate names that are frequently used to describe food constituents.

Establishing the diagnosis of food allergies by skin prick, RAST testing, or DBPCFC is important, so that patients do not avoid a food type unnecessarily. Once an elimination diet is put into play, great care must be taken to ensure that nutrient requirements are met. Alternative sources for nutrients must be recognized, and sometimes vitamin and mineral supplements can be beneficial. With the widespread dissemination of information made possible by the internet, patients and their caregivers have a tremendous amount of resources at their disposal.

Other methods for treating food allergies include delaying the onset of symptoms by restricting exposure of high-risk foods to high-risk infants. The natural history of food allergies is such that, except for peanut and some tree nut allergy, most food allergies are not persistent throughout life *(43)*. For example, a milk allergy can cause of severe eczema in a child, but as the child grows older he or she may find that tolerance improves. Immunotherapy for the treatment of food allergies is not currently widely used, but recent studies suggest a role for immunotherapy in the treatment of peanut allergy *(44)*. Other treatment methodologies under investigation include immunization with DNA or with immunostimulatory sequences. In addition, the genetic modification of foods to render food protein components nonallergenic may provide a solution to maintaining good nutrition in the face of food allergens.

References

1. Zhao, T., Wang, A., Chen, Y., et al. (2000) Prevalence of childhood asthma, allergic rhinitis and eczema in Urumqi and Beijing. *J. Paediatr. Child Health* **36**, 128–133.
2. Lui, A. and Murphy, J. (2003) Hygiene hypothesis: fact or fiction? *J. Allergy Clin. Immunol.* **111**, 471–478.

3. Gell, P. and Coombs, R. (1975) Classification of allergic reactions responsible for hypersensitivity and disease, in *Clinical Aspects of Immunology.* (Gell, P., Coombs, R., Lachmann, P., eds.) Blackwell, Oxford.
4. Young, E., Stoneham, M., Petruckevitch, A., et al. (1994) A population study of food intolerance. *Lancet* **343**, 1127–1130.
5. Bock, S. (1987) Prospective appraisal of complaints of adverse reactions to foods in children during the first 3 years of life. *J. Pediatr.* **79**, 683–688.
6. Sampson, H. and Ho, D. (1997) Relationship between food-specific IgE concentrations and the risk of positive food challenges in children and adolescents. *J. Allergy Clin. Immunol.* **100**, 444–451.
7. Hourihane, J. (2002) Recent advances in peanut allergy. *Curr. Opin. Allergy Clin. Immunol.* **2**, 227–231.
8. Wensing, M., Penninks, A., Hefle, S., Koppelman, S., Bruijnzeel-Koomen, C., and Knulst, A. (2002) The distribution of individual threshold doses eliciting allergic reactions in a population with peanut allergy. *J. Allergy Clin. Immunol.* **110**, 915–920.
9. Grundy, J., Matthews, S., Bateman, B., Dean, T., and Arshad, S. (2002) Rising prevalence of allergy to peanut in children: Data from 2 sequential cohorts. *J. Allergy Clin. Immunol.* **110**, 784–789.
10. Leung, P., Chen, Y., and Chu, K. (1999) Seafood Allergy: tropomyosins and beyond. *J. Microbiol. Immunol. Infect.* **32**, 143–154.
11. Gotteland, M., Cruchet, S., Frau, V., et al. (2002) Effect of acute cigarette smoking, alone or with alcohol, on gastric barrier function in healthy volunteers. *Dig. Liver Dis.* **34**, 702–706.
12. Taylor, S., Hefle, S., Bindslev-Jensen, C., et al. (2002) Factors affecting the determination of threshold doses for allergenic foods: how much is too much? *J. Allergy Clin. Immunol.* **109**, 24–30.
13. Wide, L., Bennich, H., and Johansson, S. (1967) Diagnosis of allergy by an in vitro test for allergen antibodies. *Lancet* **2**, 1105–1107.
14. Williams, L. (2001) Skin testing and food challenges for the evaluation of food allergy. *Curr. Allergy Rep.* **1**, 61–66.
15. Hill, D., Hosking, C., and Reyes-Benito, L. (2001) Reducing the need for food allergen challenges in young children: a comparison of in vitro with in vivo tests. *Clin. Exp. Allergy* **31**, 1031–1035.
16. Chandra, R. (2000) Food allergy and nutrition in early life: implications for later health. *Proc. Nutr. Soc.* **59**, 273–277.
17. Mallet, E. and Henocq, A. (1992) Long term prevention of allergic disease by using protein hydrolysate formula in at-risk infants. *J. Pediatr.* **121**, S95–S100.
18. Sicherer, S., Noone, S., Barnes Koerner, C., Christie, L., Burks, A., and Sampson, H. (2001) Hypoallergenicity and efficacy of an amino acid-based formula in children with cow's milk and multiple food hypersensitivities. *J. Pediatr.* **138**, 688–693.
19. Kjellman, N. and Johansson, S. (1979) Soy versus cow's milk in infants with a biparental history of atopic disease: development of atopoic disease and immunoglobulins from birth to 4 years of age. *Clin. Allergy* **9**, 347–358.

20. Joshi, P., Mofidi, S., and Sicherer, S. (2002) Interpretation of commercial food ingredient labels by parents of food-allergic children. *J. Allergy Clin. Immunol.* **109**, 1019–1021.
21. Turktas, I., Ozkaya, O., Bostanci, I., Bidcci, A., and Cinaz, P. (2001) Safety of inhaled corticosteroid therapy in young children with asthma. *Ann. Allergy Asthma Immunol.* **86**, 649–654.
22. Paller, A., Eichenfield, L., Leung, D., Stewart, D., and Appell, M. (2001) A 12-week study of tacrolimus ointment for the treatment of atopic dermatitis in pediatric patients. *J. Am. Acad. Dermatol.* **44**, S47–S57.
23. Fahy, J., Fleming, H., Wong, H., et al. (1997) The effect of an anti-IgE monoclonal antibody on the early- and late-phase responses to allergen inhalation in asthmatic subjects. *Am. J. Respir. Crit. Care Med.* **155**, 1828–1834.
24. Doleman, C. and Bast, A. (1990) Oxygen radical in lung pathology. *Free Radical Biol. Med.* **9**, 381–400.
25. De Raeve, H., Thunnissen, F., Kaneko, F., et al. (1997) Decreased Cu,Zn-SOD activity in asthmatic airway epithelium: correction by inhaled corticosteroid in vivo. *Am. J. Physiol.* **272**, L148–L154.
26. David, T., Gibbs, A., Sharpe, T., and Wells, F. (1984) Low serum zinc in children with atopic eczema. *Br. J. Dermatol.* **111**, 597–601.
27. Ewing, C., David, T., Ashcroft, C., and Gibbs, A. (1991) Failure of oral zinc supplementation in atopic eczema. *Eur. J. Clin. Nutr.* **45**, 507–510.
28. Cipolla, C., D'Antuono, G., Lugo, G., Orciara, P., and Occhionero, T. (1990) Magnesium picolate in the treatment of seasonal allergic rhinitis. Preliminary data. *Magnesium Res.* **3**, 109–112.
29. Hill, J., Britton, J., Lewis, S., and Mickelwright, A. (1997) Investigation of the effect of short term change in dietary magnesium intake in asthma. *Eur. Respir. J.* **10**, 2225–2229.
30. Britton, J., Weiss, S., Tattersfield, A., et al. (1994) Dietary magnesium, lung function, wheezing, and airway hyperreactivity in a random adult population sample. *Lancet* **344**, 357–362.
31. Fairris, G., Perkins, P., Lloyd, B., Hinks, L., and Clayton, B. (1989) The effect on atopic dermatitis of supplementation with selenium and vitamin E. *Acta. Derm. Venereol.* **69**, 359–362.
32. Soutar, A., Seaton, A., and Brown, K. (1997) Bronchial reactivity and dietary antioxidants. *Thorax* **52**, 166–170.
33. Schachter, E. and Schlesinger, A. (1982) The attenuation of exercise-induced bronchospasm by ascorbic acid. *Ann. Allergy* **49**, 146–151.
34. Troisi, R., Willett, W., Weiss, S., Trichopoulos, D., Rosner, B., and Speizer, F. (1995) A prospective study of diet and adult-onset asthma. *Am. J. Respir. Crit. Care Med.* **151**, 1401–1408.
35. Fortner, B.J., Danziger, R., Rabinowitz, P., and Nelson, H. (1982) The effect of ascorbic acid on cutaneous and nasal response to histamine and allergen. *J. Allergy Clin. Immunol.* **69**, 484–488.

36. Hodge, L., Salome, C., Peat, J., Haby, M., Xuan, W., and Woolcock, A. (1996) Consumption of oily fish and childhood asthma risk. *Med. J. Aust.* **164**, 137–140.
37. Schwartz, J. and Weiss, S. (1994) The relationship of dietary fish intake to level of pulmonary function in the first National Health and Nutrition Survey (NHANES 1). *Eur. Respir. J.* **7**, 1821–1824.
38. Arm, J., Horton, C., Spur, B., Mencia-Huerta, J., and Lee, T. (1989) The effects of dietary supplementation with fish oil lipids on the airway response to inhaled allergen in bronchial asthma. *Am. Rev. Respir. Dis.* **139**, 1395–1400.
39. Rangi, S., Servonska, M., Lenathan, G., et al. (1990) Suppression by ingested eicosapentaenoic acid of the increases in nasal mucosal blood flow and eosinophilia of ryegrass-allergic reactions. *J. Allergy Clin. Immunol.* **85**, 484–489.
40. Soyland, E., Funk, J., Rajka, G., et al. (1994) Dietary supplementation with very long-chain n-3 fatty acids in patients with atopic dermatitis. A double-blind, multicentre study. *Br. J. Dermatol.* **130**, 757–764.
41. Dorsch, W., Wagner, H., Bayer, T., et al. (1988) Anti-asthmatic effects of onions. Alk(en)ylsulfinothioic acid alk(en)yl-esters inhibit histamine release, leukotriene and thromboxane biosynthesis in vitro and counteract PAF and allergen-induced bronchial obstruction in vivo. *Biochem. Pharmacol.* **37**, 4479–4486.
42. Bjorksten, B., Sepp, E., Julge, K., Voor, T., and Mikelsaar, M. (2001) Allergy development and the intestinal microflora during the first year of life. *J. Allergy Clin. Immunol.* **108**, 516–520.
43. Bock, S. (1982) The natural history of food sensitivity. J Allergy Clin Immunol **69**, 113–117.
44. Wild, L. and Lehrer, S. (2001) Immunotherapy for food allergies. *Curr. Allergy Rep.* **1**, 48–53.
45. Chang, C. and Gershwin, M. (2000) Nutrition and allergy, in *Nutrition and immunology.* (Gershwin, M., German, J., Keen, C., eds.) Humana, Totowa, NJ, pp. 221–232.

9 Antioxidant Nutrition and Immunity

Laurence S. Harbige and M. Eric Gershwin

Contents

Key Points

- Nutritional antioxidants have enhancing nonspecific effects on both innate and adaptive immune responses, and appear to be essential for immune functions.
- Nutritional antioxidants have effects on the immune system, that appear independent of their classical antioxidant functions.
- There are synergistic effects of dietary antioxidants on immune function.
- Simply measuring plasma antioxidant status may not parallel or be sufficient to predict immunological changes.
- Low antioxidant status is linked to infection, certain cancers, and atherosclerosis.

From: *Handbook of Nutrition and Immunity*
Edited by: M. E. Gershwin, P. Nestel, and C. L. Keen © Humana Press, Totowa, NJ

- Supplementation can increase resistance to certain viral, bacterial and parasitic infections (animal studies), cancers, and free radical-mediated pathologies.
- Controlled trials are required to test whether the observed protective effects of nutritional antioxidant supplementation on infection in animals also apply to humans.
- Outcome measures of a supplementation program may be influenced by the initial antioxidant status of a population, which could affect interstudy comparisons.
- Under certain circumstances, nutritional antioxidants may be useful as less toxic alternatives to other nutrients/therapies for their immunopotentiating capacity.
- Interactions with other nutrients such as polyunsaturated fats and selenium are important when studying antioxidants, immune functions, and disease.

Introduction

Many fundamental principles in nutritional immunology have emerged over the years and provide the basis for analysis of antioxidant nutrition and immunity. These include the following:

1. Nutrition can affect innate immunity such as barriers to infection, mucosal surfaces, complement, natural killer (NK), and polymorphonuclear cell functions.
2. Nutrients can also effect a decrease or increase and therefore imbalance in the ratio of T- to B-cells, their subsets, e.g., CD4+ to CD8+ ratio, lymphoproliferation, cytokine balance, and antibody production and function.
3. Lymphoid tissues and cells are particularly vulnerable to environmental (e.g., nutritional) insult during fetal and neonatal growth and differentiation (vulnerable period), which can have short- as well as longterm consequences.
4. Pathological nutritional deficits can impact the immune response in both developed and developing countries. For example, infection can induce similar immunological changes to that observed under different nutritional states, and can induce metabolic effects on nutritional status, e.g., the effect of measles on vitamin A, Epstein-Barr virus infection (and HIV) on essential fatty acid status *(1–3)*.
5. The nutrition-immunity-infection model has been classically considered a more-or-less "one way" model, but there is also evidence for reverse flow, that is, nutrients can affect genotype and virulence *(4,5)* and possibly vertical transmission of pathogens *(6)*. The nutrition-immunity-infection model is, therefore, more complex than originally thought *(see* Fig 1).

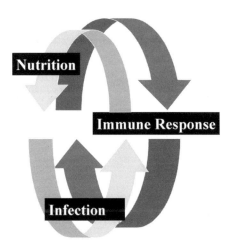

Fig 1. Bi-cyclic models of nutrition, infection, and immunity interactions.

Nutritional Biochemistry and Physiology of Dietary Antioxidants

Free radicals are chemical species that contain one or more unpaired electrons, making them reactive. They are produced constantly in vivo under physiological conditions and can be further enhanced under pathological conditions. Free radicals can attack DNA (which has a repair system for such oxidative damage), proteins (which are degraded once damaged), and lipids (which results in lipid peroxidation products). Antioxidant defenses have, therefore, evolved to protect organisms against the damaging effects of free radicals. These defenses include endogenous gene-regulated antioxidant enzymes such as superoxide dismutase (SOD) enzymes that remove superoxide radicals $O_2{}^{\bullet-}$, converting it to hydrogen peroxide (H_2O_2), which is mostly removed by other endogenous antioxidant enzymes, e.g., catalase and glutathione peroxidase (GSH). Glutathione is a tripeptide of γ-glutamyl-cysteinyl-glycine present in all cells at millimolar concentrations, it exists in the thiol-reduced form (GSH) and disulphide oxidized form (GSSG).

There are also molecules that remove free radicals by reacting directly with them in a noncatalytic way such as α-tocopherol (vitamin E), β-carotene, ascorbate, and reduced glutathione (GSH). The diet being a major source of many of these "free radical scavengers." The trace metals, manganese, copper, and zinc, are important components of SOD as is selenium for GSH. Thus, it is not unexpected that these associated nutrients are also linked in some of their biological effects to the nutritional antioxidants. Indeed, some authors characterize them as nutritional antioxidants.

There is also a demonstrable critical interaction between polyunsaturated fatty acids and antioxidants, e.g., vitamin E, particularly in relation to omega-

3 polyunsaturated fatty acids, where vitamin E often reverses their immunologic effects *(7)*; and selenium and vitamin E, which may spare one another's
effects *(4,8)*. The latter differences in "sparing" probably reflects the action of
vitamin E in lipid membranes of the cell, which is inaccessible to the selenium
containing cytoplasmic glutathione and visa versa. It is important to be mind-
ful of these additional interacting nutritional factors when investigating
antioxidants, immune functions, and infection whether in the field or the laboratory. In recent years measurements of total antioxidant status have become
popular e.g., total radical-trapping antioxidant parameter (TRAP) or oxygen-
radical absorbing capacity (ORAC). This approach could be applicable to the
field situation as an initial screen to assess the "general antioxidant status" of
populations and individuals using small volumes of body fluids, e.g., microli-
ter amounts of plasma or saliva. The methods of analysis are relatively simple,
sensitive, and reliable, e.g., chemiluminescent assays, and can also be automated. This initial screen could then, if necessary or possible, be followed by
more refined biochemical investigations to identify any individual antioxidant
problem.

Fruits and vegetables are the major dietary sources of the antioxidants ascorbate, tocopherols (saturated side chains), tocotrienols (unsaturated side chains),
and carotenoids, e.g., lycopene, lutein, cryptoxanthin, and canthaxanthin (*see*
Fig. 2) and other important antioxidant compounds such as polyphenolic antioxidants, e.g., flavonoids (more than 4000 have been identified in plants). The
full biological significance of most of these compounds is, at present, poorly
understood or unknown. Moreover, in relation to the previously mentioned
measurement of total antioxidant status, flavonoids may mask the effects of
the classical antioxidants and some appear to have opposing functions, e.g.,
quercetin has antiproliferative effects; thus, despite being antioxidants, they
may have different effects on immune functions. Not unexpectedly, there are
large differences between and within populations in blood levels of these
dietary antioxidants. Doyle et al. *(9)* reported that school children in East London had a high percentage of marginal to deficient blood levels of vitamin E
and β-carotene. Furthermore, seasonal (e.g., rainy vs dry), changes in dietary
antioxidants have been observed in the Gambia and Cuba *(10,11)*. These findings demonstrate that populations can vary in their antioxidant nutrient status
that may influence the clinical, immunological, and biochemical outcome measures of a nutritional intervention program.

Antioxidants and Immune Functions

Experimental studies have demonstrated that high vitamin E intakes (10–50
times the normal intake) in laboratory rodents enhance antibody responses (particularly, immunoglobins [Ig]G_2), NK cell activity, B- and T-cell mitogenic

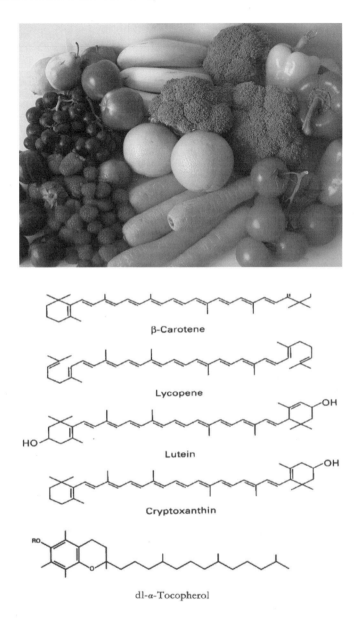

Fig 2. Some commonly occurring dietary antioxidants and their food sources.

responses, T-helper (Th) activity, and phagocytic functions *(12,13)*. However, very high intakes of vitamin E have been reported to suppress some of these functions and to be toxic *(12)*. Increased activation of macrophages induced by vitamin E feeding is a result of the production of macrophage activating factor

(MAF) *(13)*; the principle MAF produced by T-helper cells (Th1 cells) is interferon (IFN)-γ. Consistent with the above studies, aged mice (aging is associated with a decrease in immune functions) show enhanced T- and B-cell mitogenic responses, interleukin (IL)-2 production, and improved delayed-type hypersensitivity (DTH) response with increased vitamin E intake (20 times the normal intake) *(14)*. Human studies are also consistent with the foregoing experimental animal findings. Consumption of a carotenoid-rich diet in man (40 mg lycopene/d, 1.5 mg β-carotene/d) resulted in increased secretion of IL-2 (Th1-like) and IL-4 (Th2-like) by Con A stimulated peripheral blood mononuclear cells (PBMCs) compared with a low carotenoid diet *(15)*. Furthermore, the low carotenoid diet had lower T-cell proliferative responses *(15)*. Importantly, the plasma carotenoid concentrations were not correlated with the above changes in T-cell functions *(15)* and indicate that simply measuring plasma antioxidant status cannot be used as a proxy for prediction of certain immune function changes. Some of these immunological effects of nutritional antioxidants may be linked to increased peripheral blood CD4[+] T cells, to be described later in this chapter.

Increasing the intake of β-carotene has been reported by Watson et al. *(16)* to be associated with an increase in lymphocyte surface receptor expression IL-2R and CD71 (transferrin receptor). Furthermore, supplementing the diet of healthy volunteers with a dietary achievable level of β-carotene demonstrated significant increases in the percentage of monocytes expressing HLA-DR (MHC class II molecule), and adhesion molecules ICAM-1 and LFA-3 *(17)*. In both animal and human studies, vitamin E deficiency is associated with impaired NK cell activity, and oral administration of tocopherol increases the activity of NK cells as measured in tumorolytic assays; this has also been replicated in vitro *(18)*. Interestingly, tocotrienol increases NK cell activity, but at much lower doses than tocopherol *(18)*.

Healthy adult volunteers supplemented with vitamin C (1 g/d) and E (400 mg/d) for 28 d had synergistic effects, increasing the in vitro PBMC production of IL-1β and TNF-α *(19)* compared with vitamin E or vitamins C alone. Synergistic effects have also been reported with vitamin C (400 mg/d) and vitamin E (100 mg/d) on IgG and complement C3 levels in healthy elderly women *(20)*. Utilizing a high dose of vitamin E, Meydani et al. *(21)* observed increased plasma vitamin E levels, mitogenic responses (Con A), IL-2 production, and DTH in healthy elderly men and women supplemented with 800 mg dL-α-tocopherol for 30 d.

One explanation for some of the above immune-enhancing effects of antioxidants is that neutrophils and macrophages inhibit lymphocyte functions through production of reactive oxygen intermediates, prostaglandin E_2, and nitric oxide production *(7)*, but this inhibitory effect is lost when antioxidant levels are increased. There are, however, other possibilities including a specific effect on lymphopoiesis. Studies with vitamin E and β-carotene, as well as antioxidant mixtures in humans, have shown increases in the CD4$^+$ T-cell count (22–24). Consistent with this observation intracellular glutathione, another antioxidant, correlates with both CD4$^+$ and CD8$^+$ T-cell numbers and oral ingestion of cysteine (as N-acetyl-cysteine), a substrate for glutathione biosynthesis, can increase the CD4$^+$ T-cell number in humans (25). There is a high rate of renewal of CD4$^+$ T-cells (about 5% of the CD4$^+$ cell population per day). Thus, there are several possibilities for the specific effect of these antioxidants on CD4$^+$ T-cells. For example, there may be stimulation of the production of CD4$^+$ T-cells from primary lymphoid sites, e.g., thymus, a delay in the rate at which aged CD4$^+$ T-cells are cleared and/or a high level of sensitivity of CD4$^+$ T-cells to apoptotic activity induced by oxidative stress. In relation to the previously mentioned association of glutathione with CD4$^+$ T-cells, lymphocyte GSH and GSSG levels are important for immune cell function and a moderate depletion of GSH has important consequences particularly for lymphocyte function (26). For example, the proliferative response of lymphocytes and the induction of several immune responses appear to be dependent on a relatively high intracellular GSH level (27). The concentration of GSH and ascorbic acid in lymphocytes of healthy adults are correlated ($r = 0.62, p < 0.001; n = 240$) suggesting a reciprocal sparing effect of these two antioxidants (28). Furthermore, ascorbic acid supplementation (500 mg/d) of healthy individuals with low plasma ascorbate status significantly increases lymphocyte GSH (29).

Taken together, the above findings demonstrate that nutritional antioxidants, particularly when consumed in combination, as would be the case in the natural food chain where a range of antioxidants would be found, enhance both adaptive and innate immunity. They can increase the CD4$^+$ T-cell count, enhance lymphoproliferative, Th1 and Th2 cytokine and antibody responses, NK cell, and phagocytic functions. It could be argued, therefore, that dietary antioxidants are an essential requirement for the normal functioning of the immune system. Figure 3 illustrates schematically the potential effects of nutritional antioxidants on immune functions.

Antioxidants and Infection

Robert Tengerdy, Rollin Heinzerling, Cheryl Nockels, and their co-workers, were the first to show protective effects of vitamin E against infection. They found that Vitamin E protected chicks against experimental Escherichia coli (E. coli) infection using three and six times the normal dietary intake. Futuremore, these observations were associated with increased antibody titer to E. coli antigen (30,31). Increased resistance to infection by supplemental

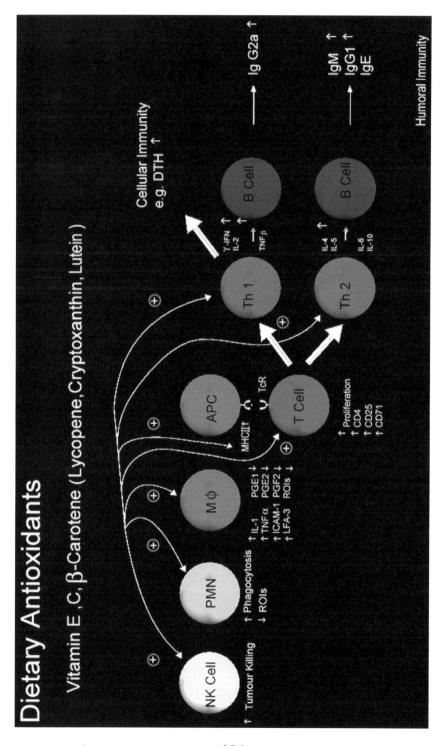

Fig. 3. The effects of nutritional antioxidants on immune functions.

vitamin E was later found experimentally for *Eimeria tenella* and *Histamonas meleacridis* in chicks and turkeys, *Chlamydia* in sheep and lambs, *E. coli* and *Treponema hyodysenteriae* in pigs, and *Diplococcus pneumoniae* and *Mycoplasma pulmonis* in rodents *(32,33)*. Many of these studies showed that increased vitamin E intake enhanced the antibody response (IgG and IgA) and the phagocytic function of polymorphonuclear cells *(33)*. Vitamin E has also been shown to markedly enhance antigen-specific antibody responses in field trials with *Brucella ovis* and *Clostridium perfringens* vaccines in sheep *(33)*. Protection of livestock against certain infections, for example, RNA viruses, is not only important for the supply of dietary protein, but also because livestock are a reservoir of potential infection for man (zoonosis) and the emergence of new viral strains (subtypes) that can have important consequences for human populations. The latter can be a serious global problem, as seen with the recent severe acute respiratory syndrome (SARS) virus. However, the factors that influence the emergence of these new viral subtypes are not well understood. Antioxidant status is thought to be one important factor in this phenomenon.

Beck et al. *(4)* have shown that selenium-deficient mice inoculated with avirulent Coxsackievirus B3 develop myocardial lesions *(4)*. Moreover, Coxsackievirus B3 recovered from the hearts of selenium-deficient mice when transferred to adequately fed mice causes significant heart pathology owing to virus nucleotide changes and, therefore, mutation to a virulent strain *(4)*. Selenium acts as an antioxidant and deficiency produces a prooxidant state in the host, and it is by this means that the nutritionally induced genetic changes are thought to occur *(5)*. These findings may be important in relation to a cardiomyopathy in humans known as Keshan disease, which is associated with selenium deficiency and Coxsackievirus infection. Similar findings have also been reported for an enterovirus-like virus in humans *(5)*.

There can be increased pathological damage during infection with concomitant vitamin E deficiency. Mice fed a vitamin E-deficient diet develop myocarditis when infected with the normally avirulent Coxsackievirus B3 strain, which is consistent with the previously described findings for selenium deficiency *(5)*. In contrast, vitamin E is known to reduce the protective effects of fish oil in malaria although the mechanisms are not well understood *(7)*. Oral treatment with *N*-acetyl-cysteine (NAC), a substrate for glutathione biosynthesis, improved histopathological lesions in a murine model of Leishmaniasis *(34)*. This protective effect of NAC in Leishmaniasis was associated with an increased frequency of TNF-α- and IFN-γ-producing cells (Th1-like response), which are factors known to be important in the resistance to the parasite. The authors concluded that NAC can induce changes in the cytokine microenvironment that can allow for a more efficient control of parasite replication at the site of infection. In murine AIDS, vitamin E has been shown to restore IL-2 and IFN-γ production, lymphoproliferation, and NK cell activity, which is normally suppressed by the retrovirus infection *(35)*.

Many human studies have reported the effects of infections such as malaria and influenza virus on plasma antioxidant status, e.g., vitamins E and C demonstrating a reduction *(36)*. This effect appears indirect and linked to changes in lipoproteins and the acute phase response *(36)*. There are few reports on the effects of supplemental antioxidants such as vitamin E and β-carotene on infection in humans. Nevertheless, these studies do indicate that beneficial effects are likely. Clausen *(37)* demonstrated that children given β-carotene-rich foods had increased resistance to bacterial infections; although the author concluded that the effect was caused by vitamin A rather than the provitamin β-carotene. In a large trial conducted in Nepal, maternal deaths resulting from infection were found to be fewer with β-carotene supplementation compared with vitamin A or placebo treatment *(38)*. Futhermore, in a retrospective study in an elderly population, Chavance et al. *(39)* found that vitamin E was negatively associated to the number of infections. However, it could be argued that the infections may have influenced the vitamin E status rather than the other way around. A better understanding of antioxidants in relation to immunity and infection has come from the increased research impetus brought about by the global HIV/AIDS problem.

Antioxidants and HIV Infection

Epidemiological research on the association between dietary nutrient intake and the progression of HIV to AIDS suggests that increased levels of intake (both from food and supplements) of riboflain (B_2), thiamin (B_1), iron, and vitamins C and E are associated with a significantly decreased progression rate to AIDS *(40,41)*. In addition, studies by Tang et al. *(42)* have shown that the serum levels of vitamin E may be associated with a slower HIV disease progression. These findings may well indicate that some nutrients decrease progression of HIV disease and others enhance it but, conversely, disease progression may influence the nutrient status. Decreased plasma levels of vitamins C and B_{12}, carotenes, pyridoxine, copper, and selenium occur in early and early asymptomatic HIV^+ patients *(43–45)*. Futhermore, despite higher intake of pyridoxine, vitamins B_{12}, A, and E, and zinc in early HIV^+ compared with HIV^- homosexual men, the former had similar if not lower plasma levels of these nutrients *(46)*. HIV^+ individuals who had had opportunistic infections, neoplasms, chronic diarrhea, and wasting syndrome also had decreased blood nutrient levels, particularly vitamins A, pyridoxine, C, D, carotene, and glutathione *(47,48)*. Both in early HIV-infection and in patients without diarrhea, the low serum carotene levels may therefore indicate fat malabsorption *(49)*.

Many of the latter studies indicate that early on in HIV-infection disturbance of nutrient status exists, but whether this predates HIV-infection and/or can adversely affect disease course is not clear. There was a weak correlation between percentage CD4$^+$ cells, CD4$^+$ count, and CD4$^+$/CD8$^+$ ratio with serum carotene concentration in a clinically heterogenous group of HIV$^+$ subjects *(49)*. Trials to test the efficacy of β-carotene to increase CD4$^+$ counts and other leukocyte markers in HIV$^+$ subjects have been undertaken *(50,51)*. In the first trial, no changes in total lymphocyte count or in the proportion of cells expressing CD11$^+$, CD8$^+$, or CD4$^+$ markers were recorded *(50)*. However, in the second trial treatment with β-carotene resulted in significant increases in total white blood cell counts, the CD4$^+$/CD8$^+$ ratio, and increased percentage CD4$^+$ cells, B cells (although not significant), and CD4$^+$ count *(51)*. Important differences in the dosage (60 mg/d vs 180 mg/d) and scheduling (4 mo vs 4 wk) of treatment are apparent between the two trials, and the magnitude of change in serum β-carotene was lower in asymptomatic HIV$^+$ patients *(51)* compared with healthy subjects with the same dose and timing of treatment *(22)*, which suggests a higher (>180 mg/d) β-carotene dosage maybe required in HIV. More recent studies by Silverman et al. *(52)* and Nimmagadda et al. *(53)*, using 60–120 mg/d of β-carotene and 180 mg/d of β-carotene, respectively, in HIV infected individuals have reported no benefit on CD4$^+$, CD8$^+$, plasma HIV RNA titers, and chronic candidiasis. Total antioxidant capacity is reduced in HIV infection *(54)* and a positive correlation between CD4$^+$ T-cell counts and the SOD activities of plasma and mononuclear cells have been recorded *(45)*. Furthermore, a reduced viral load and oxidative stress has been reported in a study where HIV-infected subjects were supplemented with vitamins E and C *(55)*. There are a number of oxidative stress and disease situations that are associated with reduced levels of total GSH+GSSG, or GSH, or a decreased ratio of GSH:GSSG. HIV infection, in particular, is associated with reduced blood GSH, including reduced concentrations in peripheral blood mononuclear cells; T-, B-, and NK-cells; and monocytes, the reduction increasing with severity of the disease *(26,27,56,57)*. Furthermore, the extent of reduction is predictive of survival *(58–61)*. Consistent with the latter, Aukrust et al. *(62)* found a marked and specific increase in oxidized glutathione and decreased ratio of reduced to total glutathione in the CD4$^+$CD45RA$^+$ and CD8$^+$CD45RA$^+$ subsets in patients with HIV infection. Furthermore, it was the CD4$^+$CD45RA$^+$ subset that was preferentially depleted. CD4$^+$ T-cells, which play such a central and critical role in immunoregulation, have a high proportion of membrane arachidonic acid *(7)*. In contrast, HIV-patient CD4$^+$ T-cells have depleted membrane arachidonic acid levels *(63)*, which may be linked to low antioxidant status and loss of immunoregulation.

HIV infection is associated with catabolism of cysteine to sulphate and the high ratio of loss of sulphur to nitrogen in the urine indicates a loss of cysteine from GSH (mainly from muscle cells) rather than from muscle protein *(64)*. In addition to loss of cysteine and GSH in HIV⁺ individuals, there is also a decrease in synthesis of GSH *(65)*. Dietary supply of cystine, methionine, or *N*-acetyl-cysteine (NAC) can restore cellular GSH concentrations and increase synthesis *(65)*. Dietary NAC increased blood GSH in HIV-positive subjects and prolonged survival during the period of supplementation *(59)*. In two other trials, supplementation with NAC reversed the impairment of immune functions caused by HIV infection, significantly improving T-cell response and NK cell activity *(66)*. De Rosa et al. *(67)* reported, in an 8-wk double-blind study, that NAC increased blood and CD4⁺ and CD8⁺ T-cell GSH of HIV⁺ subjects. However, no effect was found on CD4⁺ T-cell count or viral load. In an open extension of the latter trial to 24 wk, NAC increased survival. Muller et al. *(68)* examined a very high dose of NAC over 6 d (3 d continuous intravenous infusion at 300 mg/kg W/24 h followed by 5 g perorally every 6 h) in conjunction with a high dose of vitamin C in eight HIV⁺ subjects and found an increased CD4⁺ T-cell count and reduced viral load in the five patients with the most advanced disease (CD4 counts less than 200×10^6/L). However, NAC may have dose-limiting toxic profiles, significant side effects, and only short-term effects in raising GSH levels, thus any approach that can increase cystine supply might be useful. One particularly good source of cysteine and methionine, i.e., 2.7 g/100 g protein and 2.5 g/100 g protein, respectively (the total sulphur amino acids being 5.2% of protein), is whey protein isolate. Whey protein is also an excellent source of all essential amino acids. A daily supply of 45 g could meet all the essential amino acid requirements of the adult with smaller amounts meeting the requirements of infants and children, which in relation to HIV infection in women, infants, and during pregnancy and poor nutrition in many African countries is important. Supplementing the diet of normal healthy adults with 20 g/d of whey protein isolate for 3 mo resulted in a 35% increase in lymphocyte GSH and giving whey protein isolate to HIV⁺ patients has been shown to increase GSH levels *(69–71)*. Furthermore, Bounos et al. *(69)*, also reported improved body weight in some of the study HIV⁺ subjects, but Micke et al. *(71)* reported no change in body weight or T-cell count.

Despite the present lack of controlled human studies on nutritional antioxidants in relation to infection, except for HIV infection, the evidence for a beneficial effect on infection in experimental animals and the enhancing effects on immune functions in humans suggests strongly that there is a potentially beneficial impact of antioxidant supplementation on reducing infection in man. Well controlled studies using different dietary antioxidant regimes and cock-

Table 1
Range of Infectious Organisms in Animals Where Antioxidants are Beneficial

Bacterial	Viral	Parasitic
Escherichia coli	Influenza	*Eimeria tenella*
Clostridium perfringens	Rhinotracheitis virus	*Leishmania* sp
Streptococci sp	Coxsackievirus	*Histamonas meleacridis*
Staphylococci sp	Retrovirus	
Treponema hyodysenteriae		
Pseudomonas aeruginosa .		
Diplococcus pneumoniae		
Chlamydia sp		
Mycoplasma pulmonis		

Sources: Bendich 1990 *(32)*, Han and Meydani 1999 *(106)*.

tails are needed to test the effects of nutritional antioxidants on infection in humans. The range of different infectious organisms known to be affected by dietary antioxidants is summarized in Table 1.

Antioxidant Nutrition and Developmental Immunology

Lymphoid organs and tissues have a relatively fast and high degree of growth, expansion, and both pre- and postnatal development *(72)*, which in man continues until around 10 yr of age (*see* Fig. 4). In gestation, lactation, and infancy, various cell types proliferate and differentiate during the formation of lymphoid tissues. In this period, lymphoid tissues and cells are vulnerable to nutritional effects (perhaps analogous to nutritional effects on brain development, for which there is a good deal of evidence), which appear to have longer lasting consequences. Recent studies in mice have shown that the anti-oxidants β-carotene and lycopene can affect the development of the immune system during these "critical developmental periods" *(73)*. Garcia et al. *(73)* found that dietary β-carotene and lycopene increased the T- and B-cell numbers and that β-carotene had a specific enhancing effect on serum IgG level in neonate mice *(73)*. These findings are important because they demonstrate an effect of antioxidant nutrition on early immune development (boosting or accelerating lymphocyte numbers and immunoglobulin levels), which has wider implications to human immune system development. There is also evidence that breastfeeding, compared with feeding cow's or formula milk, increases the absorption and bioavailability of antioxidants such as vitamin E *(74)*. Detailed studies in low-birth-weight (LBW), and premature babies have shown multiple micronutrient deficiencies, particularly vitamins A and E and copper *(74)*. In a large randomized trial designed to examine the effects of

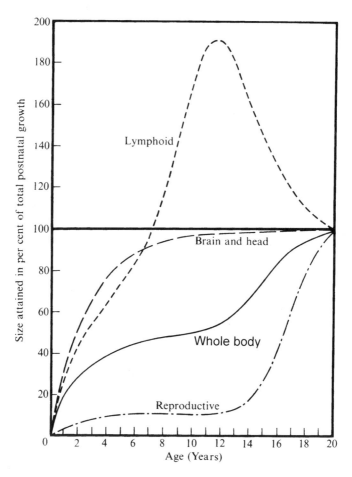

Fig 4. Growth curves for human lymphoid tissue, reproductive, brain, and whole body shown as a percentage of total gain from birth to 20 yr. Note the growth of lymphoid tissue up until 10 yr.

vitamin supplementation on pregnancy outcomes and T-cell counts in HIV-infected women in Tanzania, multivitamin supplementation (vitamins E and C, B_1, B_2, B_6, niacin, B_{12}, and folic acid) decreased the risk of LBW and premature birth and increased the $CD4^+$, $CD8^+$, and $CD3^+$ counts, whereas vitamin A alone had no effect (75). These Tanzania findings are, or are likely to be, linked to LBW, prematurity, and intrauterine growth retardation and the causally associated effects of maternal nutrient deficits and infection. Infants born small are known to exhibit thymus atrophy and functional defects in innate and adaptive cellular and humoral immunity (76–80). Thus, they are born with a very limited structural and functional, i.e., immature, immune system. Improving both the immune system and the response through maternal nutritional interventions (including lactation), which might also result in longer gestation times, would ensure the integrity of the neonate immune system at birth and early postnatally. This may be the causal pathway in the recently reported beneficial clinical outcomes reported by Fawzi et al. *(81)*. Clearly, nutrients other than antioxidants are critical in this interaction and must also be taken into account.

Accumulated pre- and postnatal nutrient deficits may have longer term consequences on the immune system and immunity. For example, there is evidence from the Gambia to suggest that poor nutrition during fetal development can permanently affect the immune system causing a higher mortality rate from infectious disease in later life *(82)*. Similar observations in relation to immune function and zinc have also been found in experimental animals by Beach, Gershwin, and Hurley *(83)*. From an immunological and nutritional perspective the pre- and postnatal period is uniquely vulnerable and complicated by the interplay of several factors. Transfer of nutrients and immunity from the mother is taking place, and the demand for nutrients is high owing to rapid growth and development of fetal tissues, including those of the immune system. Thus, the maternal nutritional state and the ability to transfer immunity are critical. Even without the burden of nutritional and immunological deficits transferred from the mother (or further deficits following birth), the newborn is immunologically susceptible because there is a decline in maternal antibodies, which is not fully compensated for by the infant antibodies for about 3–6 mo. The effect of maternal nutrition and nutrition intervention on the duration of this hypogammaglobulinaemia and the transfer of maternal regulatory and effector cells in infants is not known and requires investigation. It is probable that, like the central nervous system, there is a window of opportunity where nutritional intervention is effective in reversing immune system deficits, but once passed the damage is irreversible leading to adverse long-term consequences. Research is needed to identify precisely the vulnerable period and the window of opportunity.

Antioxidants and Autoimmune Disease

Autoimmunity and autoimmune disease are closely connected with infectious disease as it is thought that the immune system recognizes self-determinants through "molecular mimicry" with microbial antigens *(84)*. The resultant immune-effector systems deployed during infection is counterproductive in autoimmune disease. However, this is only one of several mechanisms put forward to account for autoimmune disease. There are limited data on the effects of nutritional antioxidants in experimental autoimmune disease. However, vitamin E plus fish oil has been found to have a synergistic effect in delaying the onset of disease in MRL/lpr mice *(85)*. Plasma levels of vitamin E have been reported to be low in some but not all patients with rheumatoid arthritis (RA) *(86)* and multiple sclerosis (MS) *(87)*. A decreased glutathione peroxidase (GSH-Px) activity has been documented by Jensen et al. *(88)* and Shukla et al. *(89)* in the erythrocytes and leucocytes of Danish MS patients. Interestingly, Jensen and Clausen *(90)* were able to correct these GSH-Px abnormalities with antioxidant treatment in the form of supplemental vitamins E, C, and sodium selenite. However, other investigators have not found such changes in GSH-Px in different MS populations *(91,92)*. The plasma concentration of selenium in RA has been observed to be low in a number of studies *(93)*, and epidemiological studies appear to support this finding *(94)*, although the full significance of these observations are unclear.

Dietary Antioxidants, Cancer, and Atherosclerosis

Many epidemiological studies have noted a strong and consistent link between lower risk of cancer (particularly gastrointestinal cancers) in people whose diets include a relatively large amount of vegetables and fruits *(95)*. Among the many compounds in fruit and vegetables that might possess anticarcinogenic properties, the carotenoids, a group of highly pigmented, fat-soluble antioxidants (*see* Fig. 2), have received much interest. β-carotene, in particular, received attention since Peto et al. *(96)* highlighted the possibility that it might be a potent anticancer agent. β-carotene was shown to be particularly effective in preventing experimentally induced cancer in animals; this may be linked, at least in part, to β-carotene's effect on enhancing immune cell activity. The Carotene and Retinol Efficacy Trial (CARET), however, found that a combination of β-carotene and vitamin A had no benefit and may, in fact, have had an adverse effect on the incidence of lung cancer and death *(97)*, indicating that the single-nutrient approach to antioxidant nutrition (rather than food) must be approached far more cautiously for cancer. Low plasma antioxidant concentrations are associated with cardiovascular disease and a wealth of evidence exists to show that oxidative modification of apo-lipoprotein B100 plays a key role in the recognition of low-density lipoprotein (LDL) and that oxidized LDL uptake by scavenger receptors (CD36) on macrophages leads to foam-cell formation and atherosclerotic plaques *(98–100)*. In addition, there is an early immunologic (possibly autoimmune) involvement in atherosclerosis and an association with infection *(99–102)*, both of which can be influenced by antioxidant nutrition as outlined in this overview. Research linking the above immunologic and infection factors in atherosclerosis with antioxidants is clearly warranted.

Sources of Dietary Antioxidants

How to provide nutritional antioxidants both in developing and developed countries is clearly an important issue. This can involve advice to eat more fruit and vegetables, fortification of staple foods and milk formula, genetically engineered foods (e.g., staple cereals or grains, pharamaceutical), supplementation, or introduction of new foods. In developing countries, important and practical sources of specific and mixed antioxidants such as carotenes and tocopherols include indigenous fruits and vegetables, tomato paste, dried tomato constitute, palm oil, spirulina and carotino oil, whereas whey and soya proteins can provide nutritional precursors for GSH. Vitamin A, but not β-carotene, is toxic at pharmacologically high doses (150,000–300,000 IU) *(103)*, and toxicity can be avoided through low intakes of β-carotene. By including the provitamin β-carotene within a nutritional antioxidant supplement (to avoid vitamin A insufficiency), we would suggest consideration be given to the use of such regimes in developing countries (given that the appropriate research be undertaken) and that under certain circumstances, it be used as an alternative to the WHO/UNICEF *(104)* recommendation to use vitamin A (100,000–200,000 IU) alone as an adjunct therapy for measles, vaccination, and thus avoid any potential toxicity and possible lack of seroconversion *(105)*. Furthermore, as with vitamin A, nutritional antioxidant intervention could lead to a reduction in the number of vaccine failures that occur in developing countries. Research is clearly needed to establish the efficacy of using antioxidant supplements as adjunct therapy in relation to the common child morbidities.

Conclusions and Perspectives

Nutritional antioxidants generally stimulate innate and adaptive immunity. Studies in humans and other animals have shown that dietary antioxidants can increase the CD4+ T-cell count, MHC class II and adhesion molecule expression, enhance lympho-proliferative, Th1 and Th2 cytokine and antibody responses, NK cell, and phagocytic functions, and appear to be an essential requirement for the normal functioning of the immune system. Antioxidants synergistically effect immune functions, but data are limited at present and increased research in this area is clearly warranted. Moreover, the synergistic effects of nutritional antioxidants demonstrate the importance of interactions and interdependence among nutrients during digestion, absorption, and metabolism and, therefore, caution must be exercised when adopting the single nutrient approach. There are demonstrable interactions between vitamin E and selenium, as well as polyunsaturated fatty acids and vitamin E in relation to immunity and infection. In addition to the classical view that antioxidant mechanisms underlie the effects of dietary antioxidants on the immune system, some nutritional antioxidants appear to have an important role in lymphopoie-

204   Harbige and Gershwin

sis. Many of the observations made on the effects of nutritional antioxidants on immune functions in health are relevant to the effects of these antioxidant nutrients on infection. Much evidence exists demonstrating protective effects against a range of viral, bacterial, and parasitic infections in experimental animals, which is consistent with the general immunopotentiating effects of nutritional antioxidants. However, human studies on the effects of nutritional antioxidants on infection are lacking and further work is clearly needed in this area before recommendations can be made.

Poor antioxidant status can also lead to the emergence of new virulent viral subtypes, but the importance in human viral infections such as influenza and HIV is unclear. In relation to HIV infection, a good deal of evidence exists for reduced antioxidant capacity within the immune system that impacts on immune functions. Trials of antioxidant supplementation to correct these deficits in HIV infection have been generally disappointing. However, these studies have been limited in their approach and further studies are needed using higher dosages and different antioxidant cocktails. Studies on whey protein isolate, presumably acting by providing the necessary precursors for GSH synthesis, appear promising and more nutritional and immunological research is required in this area. Dietary antioxidants in relation to developmental immunology appear to be important and may have important implications for low birth weight and prematurity and immune development. Nutritional antioxidant effects on immune functions in relation to the pathogenesis of cancer and atherosclerosis deserves increased research effort, given their effect on mortality and morbidity. Clearly both developed and developing countries will benefit from increased research in the field of antioxidant nutrition and immunology.

Acknowledgment

The authors wish to thank Dr. Eric L. Miller, Nutrition Laboratory, University of Cambridge, U.K., for bringing to their attention the importance of whey protein isolate.

References

1. Frieden, T.R., Sowell, A.L., Henning, K.J., Huff, D.L., and Gunn, R.A. (1992) Vitamin A levels and severity of measles. New York City. *Am. J. Dis. Child.* **146**, 182–186.
2. Williams, L.L., Doody, D.M., and Horrocks, L.A. Serum fatty acid proportions are altered during the year following acute Epstein-Barr virus infection. *Lipids* **23**, 981–988.
3. Agostoni, C., Riva, E., Esposito, S., Ferraris, G., Principi, N., and Zuccotti, G.V.

(2000) Fatty acid composition of plasma lipids in HIV-infected children. Comparison with seroreverters. *Acta Paediatr.* **89**, 172–176.

4. Beck, M.A. (1999) Selenium and host defence towards viruses. *Proc. Nutr. Soc.* **58**, 707–711.

5. Beck, M.A., Shi, Q., Morris, V.C., and Levander, O.A. (1995) Rapid genomic evolution of a non-virulent coxsackievirus B3 in selenium-deficient mice results in selection of identical virulent isolates. *Nat. Med.* **1**, 433–436.

6. Semba, R.D., Miotti, P.G., Chiphangwi, J.D., et al. (1994) Maternal vitamin A deficiency and mother-to-child transmission of HIV-1. *Lancet* **343**, 1593–1597.

7. Harbige, L.S. (2003) Fatty acids, the immune response, and autoimmunity: a question of n-6 essentiality and the balance between n-6 and n-3. *Lipids* **38**, 323–341.

8. Levander, O.A., Ager, A.L., Jr., and Beck, M.A. (1995) Vitamin E and selenium: contrasting and interacting nutritional determinants of host resistance to parasitic and viral infections. *Proc. Nutr. Soc.* **54**, 475–487.

9. Doyle, W., Jenkins, S., Crawford, M.A., and Puvandendran, K. (1994) Nutritional status of schoolchildren in an inner city area. *Arch. Dis. Child.* **70**, 376–381.

10. Bates, C.J., Prentice, A.M., and Paul, A.A. (1994) Seasonal variations in vitamins A, C, riboflavin and folate intakes and status of pregnant and lactating women in a rural Gambian community: some possible implications. *Eur. J. Clin. Nutr.* **48**, 660–668.

11. Arnaud, J., Fleites, P., Chassagne, M., et al. (2001) Seasonal variations of antioxidant imbalance in Cuban healthy men. *Eur. J. Clin. Nutr.* **55**, 29–38.

12. Yasunaga, T., Kato, H., Ohgaki, K., Inamoto, T., and Hikasa, Y. (1982) Effect of vitamin E as an immunopotentiation agent for mice at optimal dosage and its toxicity at high dosage. *J. Nutr.* **112**, 1075–1084.

13. Moriguchi, S., Kobayashi, N., and Kishino, Y. (1990) High dietary intakes of vitamin E and cellular immune functions in rats. *J. Nutr.* **120**, 1096–1102.

14. Meydani, S.N., Meydani, M., Verdon, C.P., Shapiro, A.A., Blumberg, J.B., and Hayes, K.C. (1986) Vitamin E supplementation suppresses prostaglandin E synthesis and enhances the immune response of aged mice. *Mech. Ageing Dev.* **34**, 191–201.

15. Watzl, B., Bub, A., Brandstetter, B.R., and Rechkemmer, G. (1999) Modulation of human T-lymphocyte functions by the consumption of carotenoid-rich vegetables. *Brit. J. Nutr.* **82**, 383–389.

16. Watson, R.R., Prabhala, R.H., Plezia, P.M., and Alberts, D.S. (1991) Effect of beta-carotene on lymphocyte subpopulations in elderly humans: evidence for a dose-response relationship. *Am. J. Clin. Nutr.* **53**, 90–94.

17. Hughes, D.A. (1999) Effects of carotenoids on human immune function. *Proc. Nutr. Soc.* **58**, 713–718.

18. Ashfaq, M.K., Zuberi, H.S., and Anwar Waqar, M. (2000) Vitamin E and beta-carotene affect natural killer cell function. *Int. J. Food Sci. Nutr.* **51 Suppl**, S13–S20.

19. Jeng, K.C., Yang, C.S., Siu, W.Y., Tsai, Y.S., Liao, W.J., and Kuo, J.S. (1996)

Supplementation with vitamins C and E enhances cytokine production by peripheral blood mononuclear cells in healthy adults. *Am. J. Clin. Nutr.* **64**, 960–965.

20. Ziemianski, S., Wartanowicz, M., Klos, A., Raczka, A., and Klos, M. (1986) The effect of ascorbic acid and alpha-tocopherol supplementation on serum proteins and immunoglobulin concentration in the elderly. *Nutr. Int.* **2**, 1–5.

21. Meydani, S.N., Barklund, M.P., Liu, S., et al. (1990) Vitamin E supplementation enhances cell-mediated immunity in healthy elderly subjects. *Am. J. Clin. Nutr.* **52**, 557–563.

22. Alexander, M., Newmark, H., and Miller, R.G. (1985) Oral beta-carotene can increase the number of OKT4+ cells in human blood. *Immunol. Lett.* **9**, 221–224.

23. Purkins, L., Penn, N.D., Kelleher, J., and Heatley, R.V. (1990) Vitamin E alters T cell subsets in elderly patients. *Proc. Nutr. Soc.* **49**, 29A.

24. Kelleher, J. (1991) Vitamin E and the immune response. *Proc. Nutr. Soc.* **50**, 245–249.

25. Kinscherf, R., Fischbach, T., Mihm, S., et al. (1994) Effect of glutathione depletion and oral N-acetyl-cysteine treatment on CD4+ and CD8+ cells. *Faseb. J.* **8**, 448–451.

26. Droge, W. and Breitkreutz, R. (2000) Glutathione and immune function. *Proc. Nutr. Soc.* **59**, 595–600.

27. Droge, W. (2002) Free radicals in the physiological control of cell function. *Physiol. Rev.* **82**, 47–95.

28. Lenton, K.J., Therriault, H., Cantin, A.M., Fulop, T., Payette, H., and Wagner, J.R. (2000) Direct correlation of glutathione and ascorbate and their dependence on age and season in human lymphocytes. *Am. J. Clin. Nutr.* **71**, 1194–1200.

29. Lenton, K.J., Sane, A.T., Therriault, H., Cantin, A.M., Payette, H., and Wagner, J.R. (2003) Vitamin C augments lymphocyte glutathione in subjects with ascorbate deficiency. *Am. J. Clin. Nutr.* **77**, 189–195.

30. Heinzerling, R.H., Nockels, C.F., Quarles, C.L., and Tengerdy, R.P. (1974) Protection of chicks against E. coli infection by dietary supplementation with vitamin E. *Proc. Soc. Exp. Biol. Med.* **146**, 279–283.

31. Tengerdy, R.P. and Brown, J.C. (1977) Effect of vitamin E and A on humoral immunity and phagocytosis in E. coli infected chicken. *Poult. Sci.* **56**, 957–963.

32. Bendich, A. (1990) Antioxidant vitamins and their functions in immune responses. *Adv. Exp. Med. Biol.* **262**, 35–55.

33. Tengerdy, R.P. Immunity and disease resistance in farm animals fed vitamin E supplement. *Adv. Exp. Med. Biol.* **262**, 103–110.

34. Rocha-Vieira, E., Ferreira, E., Vianna, P., et al. (2003) Histopathological outcome of Leishmania major-infected BALB/c mice is improved by oral treatment with N-acetyl-l-cysteine. *Immunology* **108**, 401–408.

35. Wang, J.Y., Liang, B., and Watson, R.R. (1995) Vitamin E supplementation with interferon-gamma administration retards immune dysfunction during murine retrovirus infection. *J. Leukoc. Biol.* **58**, 698–703.

36. Thurnham, D.I. (1997) Impact of disease on markers of micronutrient status.

Proc. Nutr. Soc. **56**, 421–431.

37. Clausen, S. (1931) Carotenemia and resistance to infection. *Trans. Am. Ped. Soc.* **43**, 27–30.

38. Villar, J., Merialdi, M., Gulmerzoglu, A.M., et al. (2003) Nutritional interventions during pregnancy for the prevention or treatment of maternal morbidity and preterm delivery: an overviw of randomized controlled trials. *J. Nutr.* **133**, 1606S–1625S.

39. Chavance, M., Herbeth, B., Fournier, C., Janot, C., and Vernhes, G. (1989) Vitamin status, immunity and infections in an elderly population. *Eur. J. Clin. Nutr.* **43**, 827–835.

40. Abrams, B., Duncan, D., and Hertz-Picciotto, I. (1993) A prospective study of dietary intake and acquired immune deficiency syndrome in HIV-seropositive homosexual men. *J. Acquir. Immune Defic. Syndr.* **6**, 949–958.

41. Tang, A.M., Graham, N.M., Kirby, A.J., McCall, L.D., Willett, W.C., and Saah, A.J. (1993) Dietary micronutrient intake and risk of progression to acquired immunodeficiency syndrome (AIDS) in human immunodeficiency virus type 1 (HIV-1)-infected homosexual men. *Am. J. Epidemiol.* **138**, 937–951.

42. Tang, A.M., Graham, N.M., Semba, R.D., and Saah, A.J. (1997) Association between serum vitamin A and E levels and HIV-1 disease progression. *AIDS* **11**, 613–620.

43. Beach, R.S., Mantero-Atienza, E., Shor-Posner, G., et al. (1992) Specific nutrient abnormalities in asymptomatic HIV-1 infection. *AIDS* **6**, 701–708.

44. Lacey, C.J., Murphy, M.E., Sanderson, M.J., Monteiro, E.F., Vail, A., and Schorah, C.J. (1996) Antioxidant-micronutrients and HIV infection. *Int. J. Std AIDS* **7**, 485–489.

45. Treitinger, A., Spada, C., Verdi, J.C., et al. (2000) Decreased antioxidant defence in individuals infected by the human immunodeficiency virus. *Eur. J. Clin. Invest.* **30**, 454–459.

46. Baum, M., Cassetti, L., Bonvehi, P., Shor-Posner, G., Lu, Y., and Sauberlich, H. (1994) Inadequate dietary intake and altered nutrition status in early HIV-1 infection. *Nutrition* **10**, 16–20.

47. Coodley, G.O., Coodley, M.K., Nelson, H.D., and Loveless, M.O. (1993) Micronutrient concentrations in the HIV wasting syndrome. *AIDS* **7**, 1595–1600.

48. Ward, B.J., Humphrey, J.H., and Clement, L. (1993) Vitamin A status in HIV infection. *Nutr. Res.* **13**, 157–166.

49. Ullrich, R., Schneider, T., Heise, W., et al. (1994) Serum carotene deficiency in HIV-infected patients. Berlin Diarrhoea/Wasting Syndrome Study Group. *AIDS* **8**, 661–665.

50. Garewal, H.S., Ampel, N.M., Watson, R.R., Prabhala, R.H., and Dols, C.L. (1992) A preliminary trial of beta-carotene in subjects infected with the human immunodeficiency virus. *J. Nutr.* **122**, 728–732.

51. Coodley, G.O., Nelson, H.D., Loveless, M.O., and Folk, C. (1993) beta-Carotene in HIV infection. *J. Acquir. Immune Defic.* **6**, 277–276.

52. Silverman, S., Jr., Kaugars, G.E., Gallo, J., et al. (1994) Clinical and lympho-

cyte responses to beta-carotene supplementation in 11 HIV-positive patients with chronic oral candidiasis. *Oral. Surg. Oral. Med. Oral. Pathol.* **78**, 442–447.

53. Nimmagadda, A.P., Burri, B.J., Neidlinger, T., O'Brien, W.A., and Goetz, M.B. (1998) Effect of oral beta-carotene supplementation on plasma human immunodeficiency virus (HIV) RNA levels and CD4+ cell counts in HIV-infected patients. *Clin. Infect. Dis.* **27**, 1311–1313.

54. McLemore, J.L., Beeley, P., Thorton, K., Morrisroe, K., Blackwell, W., and Dasgupta, A. (1998) Rapid automated determination of lipid hydroperoxide concentrations and total antioxidant status of serum samples from patients infected with HIV: elevated lipid hydroperoxide concentrations and depleted total antioxidant capacity of serum samples. *Am. J. Clin. Pathol.* **109**, 268–273.

55. Allard, J.P., Aghdassi, E., Chau, J., et al. (1998) Effects of vitamin E and C supplementation on oxidative stress and viral load in HIV-infected subjects. *AIDS* **12**, 1653–1659.

56. Roederer, M., Staal, F.J., Osada, H., and Herzenberg, L.A. (1991) CD4 and CD8 T cells with high intracellular glutathione levels are selectively lost as the HIV infection progresses. *Int. Immunol.* **3**, 933–937.

57. Droge, W. and Holm, E. (1997) Role of cysteine and glutathione in HIV infection and other diseases associated with muscle wasting and immunological dysfunction. *Faseb. J.* **11**, 1077–1089.

58. Buhl, R., Jaffe, H.A., Holroyd, K.J., et al. (1989) Systemic glutathione deficiency in symptom-free HIV-seropositive individuals. *Lancet* **2**, 1294–1298.

59. Staal, F.J., Ela, S.W., Roederer, M., Anderson, M.T., and Herzenberg, L.A. (1992) Glutathione deficiency and human immunodeficiency virus infection. *Lancet* **339**, 909–912.

60. Herzenberg, L.A., De Rosa, S.C., Dubs, J.G., et al. (1997) Glutathione deficiency is associated with impaired survival in HIV disease. *Proc. Natl. Acad. Sci. USA* **94**, 1967–1972.

61. Marmor, M., Alcabes, P., Titus, S., et al. (1997) Low serum thiol levels predict shorter times-to-death among HIV-infected injecting drug users. *AIDS* **11**, 1389–1393.

62. Aukrust, P., Svardal, A.M., Muller, F., Lunden, B., Nordoy, I., and Froland, S.S. (1996) Markedly disturbed glutathione redox status in CD45RA+CD4+ lymphocytes in human immunodeficiency virus type 1 infection is associated with selective depletion of this lymphocyte subset. *Blood* **88**, 2626–2633.

63. Klein, A., Bruser, B., Bast, M., and Rachlis, A. Progress of HIV infection and changes in the lipid membrane structure of CD4+ cells. *AIDS* **6**, 332–333.

64. Breitkreutz, R., Holm, S., Pittack, N., et al. (2000) Massive loss of sulfur in HIV infection. *AIDS Res. Hum. Retroviruses* **16**, 203–209.

65. Jahoor, F., Jackson, A., Gazzard, B., et al. (1999) Erythrocyte glutathione deficiency in symptom-free HIV infection is associated with decreased synthesis rate. *Am. J. Physiol.* **276**, E205–E211.

66. Breitkreutz, R., Pittack, N., Nebe, C.T., et al. (2000) Improvement of immune

functions in HIV infection by sulfur supplementation: two randomized trials. *J. Mol. Med.* **78**, 55–62.

67. De Rosa, S.C., Zaretsky, M.D., Dubs, J.G., et al. (2000) N-acetylcysteine replenishes glutathione in HIV infection. *Eur. J. Clin. Invest.* **30**, 841–842.

68. Muller, F., Svardal, A.M., Nordoy, I., Berge, R.K., Aukrust, P., and Froland, S.S. (2000) Virological and immunological effects of antioxidant treatment in patients with HIV infection. *Eur. J. Clin. Invest.* **30**, 905–914.

69. Bounous, G., Baruchel, S., Falutz, J., and Gold, P. (1993) Whey proteins as a food supplement in HIV-seropositive individuals. *Clin. Invest. Med.* **16**, 204–209.

70. Micke, P., Beeh, K.M., Schlaak, J.F., and Buhl, R. (2001) Oral supplementation with whey proteins increases plasma glutathione levels of HIV-infected patients. *Eur. J. Clin. Invest.* **31**, 171–178.

71. Micke, P., Beeh, K.M., and Buhl, R. (2002) Effects of long-term supplementation with whey proteins on plasma glutathione levels of HIV-infected patients. *Eur. J. Nutr.* **41**, 12–18.

72. Young, J.Z. (1971) *An introduction to the study of man.* Oxford, Oxford University Press, 1971; pp. 219–225.

73. Garcia, A.L., Ruhl, R., Herz, U., Koebnick, C., Schweigert, F.J., and Worm, M. (2003) Retinoid and carotenoid enriched diets influence the ontogenesis of the immune system in mice. *Immunology* **110**, 180–187.

74. Ghebremeskel, K., Burns, L., Costeloe, K., et al. (1999) Plasma vitamin A and E in preterm babies fed on breast milk or formula milk with or without long-chain polyunsaturated fatty acids. *Int. J. Vitam. Nutr. Res.* **69**, 83–91.

75. Fawzi, W.W., Msamanga, G.I., Spiegelman, D., et al. (1998) Randomised trial of effects of vitamin supplements on pregnancy outcomes and T cell counts in HIV-1-infected women in Tanzania. *Lancet* **351**, 1477–1482.

76. Watts, T. (1969) Thymus weights in malnourished children. *J. Trop. Pediatr.* **15**, 155–158.

77. Naeye, R.L., Diener, M.M., Harcke, H.T., and Blanc, W.A. (1971) Relation of poverty and race to birth weight and organ and cell structure in the newborn. *Pediat. Res.* **5**, 17–22.

78. Chandra, R.K. (1976) Nutrition as a critical determinant in susceptibility to infection. *World Rev. Nutr. Diet* **25**, 166–188.

79. Moscatelli, P., Bricarelli, F.D., Piccinini, A., Tomatis, C., and Dufour, M.A. (1976) Defective immunocompetence in foetal undernutrition. *Helv. Paediatr. Acta 31*, 241–247.

82. Payne, N.R., Frestedt, J., Hunkeler, N., and Gehrz, R. (1993) Cell-surface expression of immunoglobulin G receptors on the polymorphonuclear leukocytes and monocytes of extremely premature infants. *Pediatr. Res.* **33**, 452–457.

81. Fawzi, W.W., Msamanga, G.I., Wei, R., et al. (2003) Effect of providing vitamin supplements to human immunodeficiency virus-infected, lactating mothers on the child's morbidity and CD4+ cell counts. *Clin. Infect. Dis.* **36**, 1053–1062.

82. Moore, S.E., Cole, T.J., Poskitt, E.M., et al. (1997) Season of birth predicts mortality in rural Gambia. *Nature* **388**, 434.

83. Beach, R.S., Gershwin, M.E., and Hurley, L.S. (1982) Gestational zinc depriva-

tion in mice: persistence of immunodeficiency for three generations. *Science* **218**, 469–471.

84. Baum, H., Davies, H., and Peakman, M. (1996) Molecular mimicry in the MHC: hidden clues to autoimmunity? *Immunol. Today* **17**, 64–70.

85. Venkatraman, J.T. and Chu, W.C. (1999) Effects of dietary omega-3 and omega-6 lipids and vitamin E on serum cytokines, lipid mediators and anti-DNA antibodies in a mouse model for rheumatoid arthritis. *J. Am. Coll. Nutr.* **18**, 602–613.

86. Honkanen, V., Konttinen, Y.T., and Mussalo-Rauhamaa, H. (1989) Vitamins A and E, retinol binding protein and zinc in rheumatoid arthritis. *Clin. Exp. Rheumatol.* **7**, 465–469.

87. Ghebremeskel, K., Williams, G., Harbige, L.S., and Forti, A.D. (1986) Plasma retinol and alpha-tocopherol concentrations in supplemented and unsupplemented multiple sclerosis. *Clin. Biochem. Nutr.* **5**, 81–85.

88. Jensen, G.E., Gissel-Nielsen, G., and Clausen, J. (1980) Leucocyte glutathione peroxidase activity and selenium level in multiple sclerosis. *J. Neurol. Sci.* **48**, 61–67.

89. Shukla, V.K., Jensen, G.E., and Clausen, J. (1997) Erythrocyte glutathione perioxidase deficiency in multiple sclerosis. *Acta Neurol. Scand.* **56**, 542–550.

90. Jensen, G.E. and Clausen, J. (1986) Glutathione peroxidase activity, associated enzymes and substrates in blood cells from patients with multiple sclerosis—effects of antioxidant supplementation. *Acta Pharmacol. Toxicol. (Copenh.)* **59 (Suppl 7)**, 450–453.

91. Zachara, B., Gromadzinska, J., Czernicki, J., Maciejek, Z., and Chmielewski, H. (1984) Red blood cell glutathione peroxidase activity in multiple sclerosis. *Klin. Wochenschr.* **62**, 179–182.

92. Simonarson, B., Eiriksdottir, G., Benedikz, J.E., Gudmundsson, G., and Thorsteinsson, T. (1987) Glutathione peroxidase and selenium in multiple sclerosis, in (Rice-Evans C, ed.) *Free Radicals, Oxidant Stress and Drug Action.* Richelieu, London, pp. 399–418.

93. Adam, O. (1995) Anti-inflammatory diet in rheumatic diseases. *Eur. J. Clin. Nutr.* **49**, 703–17.

94. Heliovaara, M., Knekt, P., Aho, K., Aaran, R.K., Alfthan, G., and Aromaa, A. (1994) Serum antioxidants and risk of rheumatoid arthritis. *Ann. Rheum. Dis.* **53**, 51–53.

95. Block, G., Patterson, B., and Subar, A. (1992) Fruit, vegetables, and cancer prevention: a review of the epidemiological evidence. *Nutr. Cancer* **18**, 1–29.

96. Peto, R., Doll, R., Buckley, J.D., and Sporn, M.B. (1981) Can dietary beta-carotene materially reduce human cancer rates? *Nature* **290**, 201–208.

97. Omenn, G.S., Goodman, G.E., Thornquist, M.D., et al. (1996) Effects of a combination of beta carotene and vitamin A on lung cancer and cardiovascular disease. *N. Engl. J. Med.* **334**, 1150–1155.

98. Gey, K.F. (1995) Ten year retrospective on the antioxidant hypothesis of arteriosclerosis: threshold plasma levels of antioxidant micronutrients related to minimum cardiovascular risk. *J. Nutr. Biochem.* **6**, 206–236.

99. Ross, R. (1993) The pathogenesis of atherosclerosis: a perspective for the 1990s. *Nature* **362**, 801–809.
100. Ames, B.N., Shigenaga, M.K., and Hagen, T.M. (1993) Oxidants, antioxidants, and the degenerative diseases of aging. *Proc. Natl. Acad. Sci. USA* **90**, 7915–7922.
101. Ross, R. Atherosclerosis—an inflammatory disease. *N. Engl. J. Med.* **340**, 115–126.
102. Greaves, D.R. and Channon, K.M. (2002) Inflammation and immune reponses in atherosclerosis. *Trends Immunol.* **23**, 535–541.
103. Stephensen, C.B., Franchi, L.M., Hernandez, H., Campos, M., Gilman, R.H., and Alvarez, J.O. (1998) Adverse effects of high-dose vitamin A supplements in children hospitalized with pneumonia. *Pediatrics* **101**, E3.
104. WHO/UNICEF. (1987) Statement on vitamin A for measles. *Weekly Epidm. Rec.* **62**, 133–134.
105. Semba, R.D., Munasir, Z., Beeler, J., et al. (1995) Reduced seroconversion to measles in infants given vitamin A with measles vaccination. *Lancet* **345**, 1330–1332.
106. Han, S.N. and Meydani, S.N. (1999) Vitamin E and infectious diseases in the aged. *Proc. Nutri. Soc.* **58**, 697–705.

10 Probiotics and Prebiotics

ANDREA T. BORCHERS, CARL L. KEEN, AND M. ERIC GERSHWIN

CONTENTS

KEY POINTS

- Probiotics can be defined as live microorganisms which, when administered in adequate amounts, confer a health benefit on the host. Numerous other definitions have been proposed.
- Prebiotics are defined as nondigestible food ingredients that improve host health by selectively stimulating the growth and/or activity of one or a limited number of bacteria in the colon.
- The most commonly used probiotic bacterial strains are lactobacilli and bifidobacteria; representatives of both genera are part of the indigenous intestinal microflora.

From: *Handbook of Nutrition and Immunity*
Edited by: M. E. Gershwin, P. Nestel, and C. L. Keen © Humana Press, Totowa, NJ

- The functions of exogenous bacterial supplements are thought to resemble those of commensal bacteria, which play a pivotal role not only in enhancing the barrier function of the intestinal mucosa but also in the development and maintenance of a fully functional and balanced immune system, including tolerance towards food antigens and intestinal microbes.
- Several probiotics have been used successfully in the prevention and treatment of various forms of diarrhea; treatment is most effective when started early during rehydration therapy.
- The antidiarrheal effects of many probiotics appear to be at least partly mediated by enhancement of cellular and nonspecific immune responses.
- Probiotics have also been shown to be very effective in modulating the immune response of neonates and infants, thereby preventing food allergies and atopic disease in a large proportion of high-risk populations
- The minimal effective dose appears to be 10^9 colony-forming units for most probiotics, but the existing data on dose response are extremely limited.
- Some probiotics applied intravaginally or orally can maintain and/or restore a normal lactobacillus-dominated vaginal microflora.
- A normal vaginal microflora may provide some protection against HIV-1 infection.
- Available probiotics are generally considered safe, but close observation is recommended in the case of immunocompromised patients supplemented with probiotics.
- The need to refrigerate most probiotic preparations and their short shelf lives may limit their use in developing countries.
- Nonviable bacteria exert the same anti-diarrheal, but not the same immunomodulating, effects as viable bacteria and may offer a more stable alternative in some situations.
- Another approach to probiotic supplementation in developing countries may be their incorporation into the starter cultures of traditional lactic acid-fermented foods in current use in many African, South American, and Asian countries.

Definitions
Probiotics

Cultured dairy products, along with other lactic acid-fermented foods, have been part of the human diet for thousands of years and are still considered therapeutic food during sickness in many cultures. The Nobel laureate and director of the Pasteur Institute in Paris, Elie Metchnikoff, is generally credited with having formulated a hypothesis explaining the health benefits of yogurt bacteria in the early part of the 20th century. Studies with yogurt starter culture and other lactic acid bacteria were conducted throughout the last century. It has only been in recent decades, however, that reproducible data began to accumulate indicating that some microbial preparations can beneficially affect human health.

The term "probiotic" was originally used by Lilley and Stillwell in 1965 as an antonym to "antibiotics." Its redefinition by Fuller *(1)* as "live microbial feed supplement which beneficially affects the host animal by improving its intestinal microbial balance" has become widely established. The definition has been broadened since then to include human use for organs and tissues other than the gastrointestinal (GI) tract and to encompass effects not directly mediated by the microflora (*see* Table 1). In view of evidence that nonviable microbes can exert health benefits, several recent definitions no longer require that microbes have to be alive in order to qualify as probiotics. Table 2 lists desirable properties generally thought to be relevant for any potential probiotic microorganism, although an individual bacterial strain does not necessarily have to fulfill all of these requirements.

Prebiotics

The concept of "prebiotics" was proposed by Gibson and Roberfroid *(2)*, who defined a prebiotic as "a nondigestible food ingredient that beneficially affects the host by selectively stimulating the growth and/or activity of one or a limited number of bacteria in the colon, and thus improves host health." Any food constituent that reaches the colon undigested has the potential to be a prebiotic. To date, however, beneficial effects arising from colonic bacterial fermentation of nondigestible lipids as well as peptides and proteins have not been established. Resistant starch and nonstarch polysaccharides (plant cell wall polysaccharides, hemicellulose, pectins, gums) stimulate bacterial growth and metabolism nonspecifically, i.e., of both potentially harmful and beneficial species. Hence, they do not meet the requirement of metabolic selectivity for one or a limited number of beneficial bacteria. Thus, ultimately, only nondigestible oligosacharides (NDO), in particular fructooligosaccharides (FOS), fulfill the criteria of prebiotics. Depending on the degree of polymerization (DP), FOS are referred to as either oligofructose (DP < 9) or as inulin (DP $\geq$ 9 and < 60) *(2)*. Additional candidates are lactulose and oligosaccharides containing galactose, xylose, and mannose.

The bacterial species most likely to benefit from prebiotics are bifidobacteria and lactobacilli, but most research efforts have focused on their bifidogenic effect. In vitro and animal studies have demonstrated that endogenous bifidobacteria can inhibit the growth of potentially pathogenic microbes, partly by producing acetate and lactate and, hence, lowering the pH of the colon and partly by producing growth-inhibitory substances *(2)*. They were also reported

Table 1
Definitions of Probiotics

Definition	Source
A live microbial feed supplement that beneficially affects the host animal by improving is intestinal microbial balance	Fuller 1989 (1)
Mono- or mixed-culture of live microorganisms which, applied to animal or man, beneficially affects the host by improving the properties of the indigenous microflora	Huis in't Veld and Havenaar 1992 (38)
Living microorganisms, which upon ingestion in certain numbers, exert health benefits beyond inherent basic nutrition	LABIP workshop (39)
Live microorganisms that when administered in adequate amounts confer a health benefit on the host	FAO/WHO expert consultation (40)
Microbial cell preparations or components of microbial cells that have a beneficial effect on the health and well-being of the host	Salminen et al. (41)
Microbial feed supplements that, when ingested, have a positive effect on the prevention or treatment of a specific pathological condition	Saavedra (42)

Table 2
Criteria of Probiotics for Human Use *(1,4,88)*

Human origin
Identity at the genus and species level
   Identity needs to be established by DNA–DNA hybridization and rRNA
      sequence determination
   Strain needs to be deposited in international culture collection
Safe for food and clinical use
   Nonpathogenic
   Not degrading the intestinal mucosa
   Not carrying transferable antibiotic resistance genes
   Not conjugating bile acids
Able to survive intestinal transit
   Acid and bile tolerant*
Able to adhere to mucosal surfaces
Able to colonize the human intestine or vagina (at least temporarily)
Producing antimicrobial substances
Able to antagonize pathogenic bacteria
Resistant to spermicides (for those probiotics destined for vaginal use)
Possessing clinically documentd and validated health effects
   At least one phase 2 study, preferably independent confirmation of results
   by another center
Stable during processing and storage

*In the case of a vaginal probiotic, this characteristic is important only if the preparation is to be taken orally.

to be able to counteract the disturbances of the intestinal flora produced by antibiotic therapy. In addition, they produce certain B vitamins.

Synbiotics

Synbiotics are defined as a mixture of probiotics and prebiotics that beneficially affect the host by improving the survival and implantation of live microbial dietary supplements in the gastrointestinal tract, selectively stimulating the growth, and/or activating the metabolism of one or a limited number of health-promoting bacteria, and thus improving host welfare *(2)*.

The Human Intestinal Microflora, the Mucosa, and the Gut-Associated Lymphoid Tissue (GALT)

Most human mucosal surfaces—GI, urogenital tract, and upper respiratory tracts—are colonized by bacteria that form a symbiotic interaction with the host. To date, pro- and prebiotic research has focused mostly on the modulation of the composition and function of the microflora associated with the GI tract with the aim of improving the intestinal microbial balance. Few attempts, however, have been made to define what constitutes a balanced, normal micro-flora. One of the few existing definitions, a microbiota in which the so-called beneficial strains predominate over the potentially harmful species (2), reveals the underlying assumption that the types and proportions of microbial species of the intestinal microflora are not only known, but also characterized. Even though the human microflora represents one of the most intensively studied microbial ecosystems, knowledge of its composition is still extremely limited.

Composition of the Human Intestinal Microflora

The adult human intestinal microflora is estimated to comprise approx 10^{14} microbes representing 300–500 cultivable species from numerous genera of mostly anaerobic bacteria along with smaller numbers of aerobic bacteria. The density of colonization increases from the stomach to the distal colon, the latter containing $10^{10}–10^{12}$ CFU/g. Classical culture methods indentified *Bacteroides*, *Eubacterium*, *Bifidobacterium*, *Clostridium*, *Fusobacterium*, *Ruminococcus*, *Peptococcus*, and *Peptostreptococcus* as the predominant genera. Some of these findings have recently been confirmed with molecular methods, but the contribution of bifidobacteria appears to have been signifi-cantly overestimated using classic culture enumeration methods and current estimates are that bifidobacteria represent at most 3–4% of total bacteria. The genus *Lactobacillus* accounts for an even smaller portion (<1%) and is gener-ally detectable in ≤ 80% of subjects. Molecular methods and microscopic counts further indicate that a vast majority of intestinal microorganisms cannot be cultured in vitro.

Development of the Microflora After Birth

At birth, the gut is sterile, but it is rapidly colonized by bacteria from the mother's birth canal and the environment. In caesarian births, environmental microorganisms from equipment, air, and other infants that are transferred by nurses constitute the major early colonizers. Although not an entirely consis-tent finding, a majority of studies indicate that the microflora of breastfed in-fants differs from that of formula-fed infants, the major difference being a higher number of bifidobacteria, lower *Bacteroides* count, and almost com-plete absence of clostridia in breastfed infants. Overall, the microflora of breastfed infants appears to be somewhat less complex than that of formula-fed infants. A recent study that used a molecular method essentially confirmed these findings, although the proportion of bacteroides and bifidobacteria in breastfed infants differed less dramatically than had been reported in studies using culture-based method. It has repeatedly been claimed that the differences in intestinal microflora between breastfed and formula-fed infants account for the lower incidence of infections in breastfed compared with formula-fed infants. However, breast milk is known to contain a variety of factors, most importantly antibodies, that provide protection from various infections.

With the introduction of solid foods, the microflora of infants becomes more complex and resembles that of adults by the second year of life. Subsequently, the species composition of the intestinal microflora generally appears to be quite stable within a given individual in the absence of factors that disturb this balance. One of the most important factors influencing the stability of the intestinal microflora is the intake of antimicrobial agents, but changes in dietary habits, stress, age, and particularly infections and diseases can all affect the absolute and relative numbers of microorganisms in the GI tract. Ingestion of certain pro- and prebiotics has also been shown to alter the numbers and/or proportions of certain groups of intestinal and vaginal bacteria. These changes are almost invariably transient, persisting only for days or weeks after supplementation ends. However, intestinal colonization is commonly assessed from the fecal recovery of bacteria, but colonic biopsies have demonstrated the persistence of supplemented bacteria at times when they could no longer be recovered from the feces of the same subject.

Probiotic Genera and Strains

The two most commonly used probiotic genera are bifidobacteria and lactobacilli, but other lactic acid bacteria and even yeast strains also qualify (*see* Table 3). It has only been after the development of molecular biology methods that many of the individual bacterial strains were identified unambiguously. The taxonomic changes that have resulted from the introduction of such methods are illustrated by two examples of frequently studied bacteria. *Lactobacillus acidophilus* (*L. acidophilus*) was divided into six species: *L. acidophilus*, *L. amylovorus*, *L. crispatus*, *L. gallinarum*, *L. gasseri*, *L. johnsonii*; and what is commonly referred to as *Lactobacillus* GG (LGG, ATCC 53103) was originally identified as *L. acidophilus* and later named *L. casei* GG, but was recently identified as *L. rhamnosus* GG.

Lactobacilli are gram-positive, non-spore-forming, microaerophilic rods that produce abundant lactate as an end product and can be H_2O_2-producing or not. Several recent studies using molecular biology techniques on fecal samples indicate that the intestinal lactobacillus population of each individual is unique, with *L. plantarum*, *L. rhamnosus*, and *L. paracasei* ssp. *paracasei* representing the most frequently detected taxa. In some subjects, the lactobacillus population is quite simple with one or two strains predominating over several months. In others, it is markedly more complex, consisting of up to 11 different strains of which none is truly dominant. Considerable fluctuation in the strain composition and size of the lactobacillus population have been observed in some individuals. Interestingly, exogenously supplied lactobacillus may become

Table 3
Species Used as Probiotics *(88,90)*

Genus	Species	Strain
Lactobacillus	*lactis*	
	*plantarum**	
	*rhamnosus**	GG, HN110
	johnsonii	LJ-1 (LA-1), NCFB 1748
	*reuteri**	ATCC 55730
	*casei**	Shirota
	*gasseri**	
Bidifobacterium	*bifidum**	Bb-12
	longum	
	breve	
	infantis	
	*lactis**	HN019
	adolescentis	
Streptococcus	*thermophilus*	
Enterococcus	*faecalis*	
	faecium	
Escherischia	*coli*	
Bacillus	*cereus*	
Saccharomyces	*boulardii*	

*With evidence from clinical trials.

transiently established as the predominant lactobacillus species but only in subjects with fluctuations in their endogenous lactobacillus population. Among the latter, a 6-mo supplementation period resulted in permanent changes in the lactobacillus strain composition during the posttest period, i.e., at a time when the supplemented lactobacillus could no longer be detected in the feces.

Bifidobacteria are strictly anaerobic gram-positive rods, often shaped in the "Y" or bifid form. They possess a special metabolic pathway that allows them to produce acetic as well as lactic acid. Both classical culture method and recent molecular biology studies have shown that the pattern of bifidobacteria is unique for each human host. Data are somewhat conflicting on the stability of the total numbers and numbers of different strains of bifidobacteria present in individual subjects. Both parameters seem to fluctuate in some humans, but not in others; whereas only one or two species of bifidobacteria are detected in some individuals, others harbor up to seven different strains.

In a recent study of fecal samples from 48 healthy Japanese adults, *B. catenulatum* represented the most common taxon (92% of samples) followed by *B. longum* (65%) and *B. adolescentis* (60%). Similar findings were reported from a small group of British volunteers, except that *B. angulatum* was the most frequently detected species. Fecal samples of 22–46-d-old breast fed infants contained up to seven different species, with *B. breve* (70%), *B. infantis* (41%), and *B. longum* (37%) constituting the dominant species.

Commensal Bacteria and the Immune System (3)

The GI tract constitutes the interface between the environment and the host, and as such has the important dual role of excluding potential pathogens while facilitating the passage of nutrients. Intestinal epithelial cells, which are joined by tight junctions that prevent passage between cells, and the mucus they produce form a physical barrier against pathogens. Increasing evidence from studies with gnotobiotic animals suggest that initial colonization with commensal bacteria constitutes a vital stimulus for the synthesis of substances that fortify the mucosal barrier and decreases intestinal permeability. In addition, commensal bacteria play a vital role in colonization resistance. This term was originally introduced only in reference to the ability of the indigenous microflora to inhibit colonization by exogenous potentially pathogenic microorganisms. It has since been broadened to include the prevention of overgrowth of indigenous microorganisms that have the potential to become pathogenic. Anatomical and physiological factors such as an intact mucosa, salivation, swallowing, normal gastrointestinal motility, production of gastric acids, and secretion of IgA contribute to colonization resistance, but are ineffective in the absence of a normal undisturbed flora. Mechanisms of colonization resistance include production of antimicrobial substances and toxic metabolic end products, competition for nutrients required for growth of pathogens, competitive inhibition of adhesion of pathogens, modification of toxins or toxin receptors, and stimulation of the immune system.

In addition to the nonimmunological barrier of the intestinal mucosa, the GALT plays a vital role in immune exclusion. GALT is the largest lymphoid tissue of the human body and its hallmark is the production of secretory IgA which, in contrast to serum IgA, is dimeric or polymeric and resistant to proteolysis in the intestinal lumen and does not activate inflammatory responses. Colonization with commensal bacteria is essential for the development of a fully functional and balanced immune system, including not only the development and maturation of IgA plasmocytes and IgA production, but also the development of tolerance towards food antigens and intestinal microbes. Interactions between the intestinal microflora and GALT are also thought to be vital for maintaining the intestinal immune system in a state of permanent low-level activation, or physiological inflammation, that is considered to be important in host defense against pathogens. It appears to be generally assumed that supplementation with exogenous bacteria will exert similar effects, and by similar mechanisms, as those observed during initial colonization. This is supported to some extent by observations in experimental animals, and human data are beginning to accumulate.

Probiotics in Diarrhea Treatment and Prevention

Diarrheal diseases still constitute a major cause of morbidity and mortality in infants and young children in developing and developed countries causing millions of deaths each year *(4)*. Rotavirus is the predominant causative agent of severe dehydrating diarrhea in children up to age 2 worldwide. In addition, acute diarrhea is often caused by bacteria, such as enterotoxigenic *E. coli*, *Shigella*, *Salmonella*, cytotoxigenic *Clostridium difficile*, and *Campylobacter* species.

In recent years, several groups of investigators have demonstrated that supplementation with some bacterial strains can shorten the duration of acute diarrhea in infants and children (*see* Table 4). A number of well designed randomized controlled trials have established the efficacy of particularly LGG (ATCC 53103) to control rotavirus-induced diarrhea, whereas an effect of this strain on diarrhea of bacterial etiology has only rarely been documented. Several studies have also demonstrated a beneficial effect of *Saccharomyces boulardii* administration on acute and chronic diarrhea both in pediatric patients and in adult HIV patients *(5)*. Evidence for a role of other strains or combination of strains in shortening acute diarrhea is more limited, and much of it is awaiting independent confirmation. In earlier trials, probiotic supplementation was started after the completion of oral rehydration, but recent studies indicate that earlier administration of probiotics via incorporation into the rehydration solution may be even more effective. Throughout the world, but particularly in developing countries, children with diarrhea are frequently and inappropriately treated with antibiotics. The WHO has warned that antibiotic resistance has become a major public health problem worldwide and has urged that the use of probiotics instead of antimicrobial agents be considered.

The ability of a variety of microbial preparations to prevent diarrhea, including nosocomial and antibiotic-induced diarrhea, has also been documented in a number of RCTs *(6,7)*. *Saccharomyces boulardii* has been shown to reduce the recurrence of *Clostridium difficile* disease, and the frequency of recurrence was inversely correlated with the stool concentration of *S. boulardii (8)*.

Gastrointestinal infections can cause disturbances of the intestinal microflora and increase intestinal permeability, thereby weakening the barrier effect that is provided by the mucosa in association with its flora. Balancing the microflora in order to reestablish mucosal integrity has been one of the prime objectives of bacterial therapy in acute diarrhea. Exogenous bacteria can, at least temporarily, colonize the intestine even during acute diarrhea *(9,10)*, although *C. difficile* patients supplemented with *S. boulardii* were found to exhibit lower counts of this probiotic during periods of acute diarrhea *(8)*. The rapidity with which probiotic supplementation becomes effective in acute diarrhea suggests they exert a pharmacological rather than, or in addition to, a biological effect. This is also supported by the finding that both nonviable and viable bacteria can shorten diarrhea to a comparable extent *(11)*.

Although both live and heat-inactivated LGG were clinically effective, only ingestion of viable LGG was associated with a significantly enhanced nonspecific and specific humoral immune response compared with the placebo group in children with rotavirus-induced diarrhea *(11)*. Thus, rotavirus-specific IgA-secreting cells were detected at convalescence in 10 of the 12 infants treated with live LGG, but only 2 of the 13 infants treated with inactivated LGG. The same group had previously reported that 90% of children treated with LGG during acute rotavirus-induced diarrhea, but only 46% of the placebo-treated children, had IgA antibody-secreting cells (ASC) specific for rotavirus 3 wk after recovery, although the number of IgA sASC during the acute phase had been similar. This effect appears to be somewhat specific to LGG since higher numbers of specific IgA ASC were detected in children with rotavirus-induced diarrhea treated with LGG than in those receiving either *L. casei* subsp. *rhamnosus* or a combination of *S. thermophilus* and *L. delbrueckii* subsp. *Bulgaricus (12)*. Serum rotavirus IgA antibody levels were also higher in the LGG group compared with the other groups. A higher rate of rotavirus IgA seroconversion was also observed in infants given an oral rotavirus vaccine together with *L. casei* GG than in those receiving the vaccine plus placebo *(13)*. However, that a clear role for IgA in the recovery from rotavirus infection and/or protection from future recurrence has not been established.

In contrast, 30 volunteers who consumed either 4×10^{10} CFU *LGG* (ATCC 53103), 3.4×10^{10} CFU *Lactococcus lactis*, or placebo for 7 d starting on the day of the first dose of an attenuated *S. typhi* Ty21a vaccine, showed only a trend toward a greater increase in specific IgA in the LGG group, and the numbers of IgA-, IgG-, and IgM-secreting cells did not differ significantly among the three groups *(14)*. Meanwhile, volunteers who consumed fermented milk containing *L. acidophilus* La1 (now: *L. johnsonii* La1) and bifidobacteria (3.75×10^9 to 3.75×10^{10} CFU/d) before, during, and after the administration of an

Table 4

Probiotics in the Treatment of Acute Diarrhea in Infants and Children (Ref. 6 and Other Studies)

| Bacteria | Etiology | | | Locations | Outcome |
	HRV	Bacterial	Undetermined		
LGG	82		18	Finland	Significant shortening of the duration of diarrhea
	35	24	100 40	Finland Poland, Egypt, Croatia, Italy, Slovenia, Holland, Greece, Israel, UK, Portugal	
	28 100	21	51	Russia Finland	Significant shortening of diarrhea duration
			100	Finland	Shortened duration of diarrhea compared with *L. casei* subsp. *rhamnosus* or a combination of *S. thermo philus* and *L. delbrueckii* subsp. *bulgaricus*
	92			Finland	One early dose of LGG given together with hypotonic ORS significantly shortened the duration of diarrhea compared with placebo and to a greater extent than LGG administered during later phases
	61			Italy	Significant shortening of the

224

Organism				Country	Result
	ND			Pakistan	duration of mild diarrhea in both rotavirus-positive and -negative children
					In children with nonbloody diarrhea, a significantly smaller percentage had watery diarrhea at 48 h; no difference in those with bloody diarrhea
L. reuteri	75			Finland	Significant shortening of diarrhea duration
L. acidophilus LB	100 ND			Finland France	Significant shortening of diarrhea duration
Heat-killed L. acidophilus LB	48	ND		Thailand	Significant shortening of diarrhea duration
L. rhammosus + L. reuteri	66 58 % HRV only*	10 6% bacterial only*	29	Denmark	Shortening of diarrhea duration, difference to placebo significant only in those with diarrhea of <60 h duration at initiation of therapy

HRV = human rotavirus
ORS = oral rehydration solution
*8.7% were coinfected with HRV and a bacterial pathogen

225

attenuated *S. typhi* Ty21a vaccine exhibited enhanced responses in specific serum IgA compared with the group that did not consume fermented milk products *(15)*.

Some of the discrepancies in the results of these studies may be owing to different levels of crossreactivity between antibodies to probiotic bacteria and pathogens. Humoral immune responses to commensal bacteria have been described repeatedly, including a genus rather than species-specific response to both lactobacilli and bifidobacteria *(16)*. Some of the antibodies against commensal and/or probiotic strains exhibit crossreactivity with enteropathogens. Based on these findings, it has been suggested that some of the increased IgA responses reported after supplementation with various lactobacilli may at least partially reflect such cross-reactivity. Conversely, the absence of cross-reactivity may account for the failure of some probiotic strains to induce enhanced humoral responses to certain antigens. In addition, the type of delivery vehicle (fermented milk product versus capsules containing freeze-dried bacteria), dose schedule, and duration of probiotic intake may have contributed to the observed differences.

Probiotics and Nonspecific Immune Responses

It has variously been suggested that modulation of nonspecific immunity may also play a role in the beneficial effect of various probiotics on diarrheal disease. This issue has not been assessed directly; there are, however, studies demonstrating the ability of various probiotics to enhance nonspecific immune functions. The design of most of these studies is to administer a milk product to subjects for a 2–3-wk adaptation period, then provide milk containing the test probiotic to all of the subjects, and finally switch back to unsupplemented milk for a follow-up period. The immune functions are measured at the end of each period and the group mean responses are compared. As summarized in Table 5, all studies using this design and one double-blind placebo controlled trial showed enhanced phagocytosis and increased natural killer (NK) activity after supplementation with a variety of probiotic strains. Generally, these activities started to decline soon after the end of probiotic supplementation, but frequently remained elevated compared with baseline for up to 4 wk.

The results of the trial investigating the effects of *L. casei* on a variety of immune parameters differ markedly from those reported from other similar investigations *(17)*. This randomized placebo-controlled trial was unique in that the subjects were kept on a controlled diet before, during, and after administration of a commercially available lactic acid-fermented product. It also assessed a much wider range of immune functions than any of the other studies, including lymphocyte subsets, NK activity, phagocyte function, delayed type hypersensitivity responses, cytokine production by LPS- and Con A-stimulated peripheral blood mononuclear cells, and immunoglobulin levels. Supplementation with 3×10^{11} CFU of *L. casei* strain Shirota in three daily doses for 4 wk did not significantly affect any of the immune parameters measured, even though fecal *L. casei* strain Shirota, total lactobacillus, and bifidobacterium counts significantly increased.

The well-designed and carefully controlled nature of this trial lends additional weight to the finding that *L. casei* Shirota does not exert any immunomodulatory effects in healthy adults and makes it likely that the disparity in the results between this and other studies is attributable to an inherent difference between *L. casei* Shirota and other lactobacilli. However, immunomodulating effects of probiotic ingestion may not be easily detectable in healthy subjects whose immune system is functioning at or near optimal levels. This is supported to some extent by the finding in a group of elderly (>60 yr old) volunteers that *B. lactis* HN019 supplementation induced significantly greater enhancement of polymorphonuclear leukocyte (PMN) and mononuclear cell phagocytosis in subjects who exhibited poor preintervention immunity than in those with adequate immunity at baseline, while the difference in NK activity improvement did not reach statistical significance *(18)*.

A study involving both healthy and milk-hypersensitive subjects suggests that probiotics may have differential immunomodulatory effects depending on the activation state of the immune cells under investigation *(19)*. Compared with consumption of milk only, ingestion of milk containing 2.6×10^8 CFU LGG for 1 wk resulted in a significant upregulation of phagocytosis receptor (CR1, CR3, FcγPI, and FcαR) expression on neutrophils in healthy subjects. Only statistically nonsignificant increases of these receptors were detected on monocytes. In contrast, in milk-hypersensitive subjects, there was considerably higher expression of all of these receptors on monocytes and neutrophils during milk consumption. Addition of LGG to the milk, however, counteracted this increase and receptor expression did not differ significantly from that seen before milk challenge.

Probiotics in Allergy and Atopic Disease

Some of the most convincing evidence for an immunomodulatory effect of probiotic ingestion comes from studies in infants with food allergies and atopic eczema. Allergic diseases are characterized by a polarization of the immune response towards a helper-T-cell (Th)2-type response. During pregnancy, the maternal-fetal interface is markedly skewed towards a Th2-type pattern to avoid rejection of the fetus. This pattern is maintained in the neonate, as evidenced by the polarization towards a Th2-type cytokine profile of the immune responses of virtually all neonates, whether they subsequently become atopic or not.

Table 5

Effects of Probiotics on Nonspecific Immunity in Healthy Human Volunteers

Probiotic	Study Design	Dose (CFU/d)	n	Age range	Outcomes
B. lactis HN019	Randomized, double-blind, placebo-controlled; also comparison of pre- and postintervention values	3×10^{11}	25	60–83	Enhanced mitogen-stimulated IFN-α production by PBMC and increased PMN phagocytosis compared to placebo and to own pre-intervention values Increase in bactericidal activity in both B. lactis and control groups
B. lactis HN019	Comparison of pre- and postintervention;	5×10^{9} or 5×10^{10}	30	63–84	Increase in proportion of CD3$^+$, CD4$^+$, CD56$^+$ cells Increase in PMN and mononuclear cell phagocytosis Increase in NK activity (measured as above)
B. lactis HN019	Comparison of pre- and postintervention B. lactis either in low-fat milk (LFM) or in lactose hydrolyzed low-fat milk	5×10^{10}	50	41–81	Increased PMN phagocytosis Increased NK activity Increases greater in group receiving B. lactis in lactose-hydrolyzed milk (significant difference in NK activity)
B. lactis HN019 or L. rhamnosus HN001	Comparison of pre- and postintervention	5×10^{9}	27	60–84	Small, but significant, increase in proportion of CD56$^+$ (NK) cells Enhanced NK activity (target cell lysis of PBMC against labeled K562 cells)
L. rhamnosus	Comparison of pre- and	5×10^{10}	54	44–80	Increased PMN phagocytosis

Probiotic	Study design	Dose	n	Age	Results
HN001	postintervention in LFM or lactose-hydrolyzed LFM				Increased NK activity No significant differences between LFM and lactose-hydrolyzed LFM groups
S. thermophilus + L. johnsonii La1	Comparison of pre- and postintervention	1.5×10^9 or 1.5×10^8 of L. johnsonii La1*	42	21–57	S. thermophilus alone weakly enhanced respiratoryburst, but not phagocytosis Higher dose of L. johnsonii La1 significantly enhanced both; lower dose showed the same trend, but the difference was not statistically significant
L. acidophilus La1) now: L. johnsonii La1 or B. bifidum Bb12	Comparison of pre- and postintervention	La 1: 7×10^{10} Bb 12: 10^{10}	28	23–62	Significantly enhanced phagocytosis by monocytes and PMN with both L. johnsonii La1 and B. bifidum Bb12 No significant changes in lymphocyte subsets or cells expressing T cell activation markers
L. casei strain Shirota	Placebo-controlled with subjects on a controlled diet	3×10^{11} 55.8 ± 7.5	20	mean age 55.8 ± 7.5	No significant differences in: lymphocyte subsets, NK activity, phagocytosis or oxidative burst, mitogen-stimulated production of IL-1β, IL-2, or IFN-γ

*Lower dose was obtained by storing the product for 21–28 d, which may have resulted in changes other than reduction of viable bacterial count.

229

In developed countries, allergic diseases have increased dramatically over the last decades. The hygiene hypothesis attributes this a to lack of microbial stimuli owing to increased hygiene resulting in an imbalance between Th1- and Th2-type immune responses that favors the development of IgE-mediated allergies. The earliest and largest exposure to microbial antigens occurs during intestinal colonization starting at birth. Thus, the intestinal microflora may provide a major stimulus in shifting the immune responses of neonates and infants from the initial Th2-type to the Th1-type response that predominates in nonatopic adults.

The above is supported by the findings that the balance of supposedly beneficial and potentially harmful bacteria in the large intestine of allergic infants is altered (20). Compared with infants who remained healthy, fewer of those who later developed allergy were colonized with enterococci during the first month of life and with bifidobacteria during the first year of life, whereas colonization with *Staphylococcus aureus* was higher at 6 mo. In addition, allergic infants had greater numbers of clostridia at 3 mo of age, but lower *Bacteroides* counts at 12 mo. Somewhat conflicting results have been obtained regarding lactobacilli. A cross-sectional analysis showed a lower prevalence of lactobacilli in allergic compared with nonallergic children, whereas a prospective study detected lactobacilli in a higher proportion of allergic infants throughout the first year of life, although the difference was significant only at 1 wk of age.

A group of Finnish researchers have conducted a series of randomized placebo-controlled trials to examine whether probiotic supplementation during the perinatal period can affect the development of atopic disease. In the first study, 31 infants with atopic eczema and a history of atopic disease or food allergy were put on a cow's milk elimination diet and received extensively hydrolyzed whey formula with or without LGG (5×10^8 CFU/g formula) for 1 mo and were evaluated after a further month during which all infants received unsupplemented formula (21). Supplementation with LGG resulted in significant improvements in atopic dermatitis. Tumor necrosis factor (TNF)–α and α1-antitrypsin were elevated compared with healthy controls at baseline, but both markers of inflammation decreased significantly in the group supplemented with LGG, whereas no significant change was observed in the control group. These results suggest that LGG ingestion can alleviate intestinal inflammation.

In a subsequent study, 27 infants who experienced onset of atopic disease while still being exclusively breastfed were weaned to extensively hydrolyzed whey formulae with or without LGG or *B. lactis* Bb-12 (22). After two months, atopic eczema in both probiotic-supplemented groups had improved significantly, whereas no improvement was observed in the unsupplemented group.

Serum soluble CD4 and urinary eosinophilic protein X, both markers of inflammation, were significantly reduced in both supplemented groups. Supplementation did not affect the serum concentrations of TNF-α, a variety of chemokines (GM-CSF, RANTES and MCP-1a), or of soluble ICAM and IL-1ra. In contrast, serum transforming growth factor (TGF)-β concentrations significantly decreased from baseline to 2 mo in the *B. lactis* group, but tended to increase in the LGG group, while remaining unchanged in the non-supplemented controls. The latter findings underscore that the immunomodulatory effects of probiotics can be highly strain-specific.

Two further studies addressed the question of whether there was a correlation between TGF-β concentrations in breast milk and the incidence of atopic eczema in the infants, and investigated the effect of LGG ingestion in this context. TGF-β is a pleiotropic immunoregulatory cytokine that can be produced by and act on every type of leukocyte and a variety of other cell types. The actions of its three isoforms, TGF-β 1, 2, and 3, can be both immunostimulatory or immunosuppressive, with the nature of the ultimate effect depending on the context provided by the state of differentiation and activation of their target cells and the total milieu of cytokines present. TGF-β is a key regulator in the establishment of immunologic tolerance both at the level of deletion of self-reactive cells and at the level of anergy induction for peripheral tolerance. In addition, it induces isotype switching to IgA production in B-cells.

Human breast milk contains TGF-β in latent form, which is thought to be activated in the intestine of the neonate or infant. By antagonizing IFN-γ and TNF-α, it may prevent induction of MHC class II by these two cytokines on intestinal epithelial cells thereby preventing premature stimulation of the immature immune system of the neonate and subsequent sensitization. In addition, by inducing isotype switching to IgA, it may reduce intestinal inflammation.

The concentration of TGF-β1 and TGF-β2 was found to be higher in colostrum of mothers whose infants developed atopic disease only after weaning compared with the colostrum of mothers with infants in whom atopic disease manifested itself in the preweaning period (23). Three-mo-old infants with IgA-secreating cells specific to at least one of the four dietary antigens tested had received colostrum with significantly higher TGF-β2 concentration and marginally higher TGF-β1 levels. It was thought that TGF-β in early milk may have stimulated the neonate's own intestinal production of this cytokine, thereby enhancing mucosal IgA secretion.

A subgroup of 62 of the 159 infants enrolled in the LGG supplementation trial (24) was exclusively breastfed for 3 mo, and the mothers ingested either LGG or placebo during that period. Fifty-seven of these infants were followed for 24 mo, and the effect of LGG supplementation on the concentration of

TGF-β in colostrum and breast milk at 3 mo was assessed. Both parameters were correlated with the incidence of atopic eczema in these infants (25). The incidence of chronic relapsing atopic eczema was significantly lower in children whose mothers had received LGG (15% vs 47%). A significantly higher concentration of TGF-β2 was detected in the breast milk of mothers receiving LGG than in that of mothers taking placebo, while the concentration of TGF-β1 was similar in both groups.

The results from some of the previously discussed clinical trials and studies in experimental animals conducted by the same laboratories suggest that the anti-inflammatory effects of LGG ingestion are not attributable to modulation of the intestinal microflora towards a more beneficial bacterial composition. Instead, normalization of intestinal permeability and modification of the degradation, permeation, and targeting of food antigens to Peyer's patches, as well as direct anti-inflammatory activities, all appear to be mechanisms contributing to the beneficial effects of LGG in allergies.

Dose-Response

It appears to be widely accepted that most bacterial strains have to be used at a minimum dose of 10^9 CFU to produce some sort of health benefit, but the existing data are limited and in some cases methodologically flawed. There are indications that the tested doses have to differ by at least a factor of 10 in order to allow the detection of significant differences in the magnitude of the response. One of the most clear-cut demonstrations of a dose response comes from a study comparing two concentrations of L. reuteri that differed by three orders of magnitude (10^{10} or 10^7 CFU/d) in children with rotavirus-induced diarrhea. There was a significant correlation between the ingested dose and the number of bacteria colonizing the GI tract, the shortening of the duration of diarrhea, and the percentage of children in whom watery diarrhea persisted on the second day of treatment. In another instance, a lower dose of B. lactis HN019 (5×10^9 organisms/d) was associated with greater increases in PMN and mononuclear cell phagocytosis and NK cell activity than the 10-fold higher dose. Although none of the differences between the two doses reached statistical significance, this nonetheless suggests that there may be a maximum dose beyond which no further increases in response are observed.

Probiotics for Normalizing the Vaginal Microflora

Lactobacillus is the predominant bacterial genus in the normal vaginal microbial flora of women in their reproductive years, but in peri- and postmenopausal women lactobacilli are frequently absent. Whereas earlier studies had suggested that L. acidophilus and L. fermentum were the dominant species, recent investigations using molecular approaches have identified L. crispatus,

L. gasseri and/or *L. jensenii* as the most prevalent strains in women from numerous different areas of the world. In contrast, the dominant species of microorganisms in a group of women from Ontario, Canada (in 42%) was the newly identified *L. iners*.

The vaginal microflora is a dynamic ecosystem undergoing frequent changes in at least some women, with 66 to 75% of women either acquiring or losing vaginal lactobacilli during extended observation periods. A variety of factors have been reported to influence the vaginal lactobacillus composition, but apart from estrogen-dependent variables—such as menstrual cycle, peri- and post-menopausal status, and hormone replacement therapy—and the use of antibiotics and spermicides, there is little consensus concerning the nature of these factors.

A lactobacillus-dominated vaginal flora is considered normal; progressively greater disturbances of this ecosystem manifest themselves as decreasing lactobacillus and increasing gram-negative and gram-variable organisms, with bacterial vaginosis (BV) constituting the most severe form of abnormality. BV is a condition characterized by decreased lactobacilli, particularly H_2O_2-producing lactobacilli, and increased concentrations of anaerobic bacteria, such as *Gardnerella* species and *Mobiluncus*. It is diagnosed by the presence of three of the four following criteria: a vaginal pH > 4.5, presence of clue cells in the vaginal fluid, a milky homogeneous vaginal discharge, and the release of an amine (fishy) odor upon addition of potassium hydroxide. The 10-point Nugent scoring method based on gram staining of vaginal fluid is frequently used not only for the confirmation of BV, but also for scoring the status of the vaginal flora as normal, intermediate, or BV.

It should be noted that BV is not an inevitable consequence of the absence of lactobacilli. Conversely, lactobacilli can still be detected in some women with BV. Nonetheless, both cross-sectional and longitudinal studies have shown that the acquisition of BV is associated with the lack or loss of H_2O_2-producing lactobacilli. There are indications that some species of H_2O_2-generating lactobacilli are among the most persistent lactobacilli in the vagina of nonpregnant women, and that women colonized with these strains are significantly more likely to remain colonized.

A variety of probiotics administered as vaginal suppositories exhibit some effectiveness in normalizing the vaginal microflora and treating urogenital infections *(26)*. Recently, a randomized placebo-controlled trial demonstrated that oral administration of probiotics could have similar effects *(27)*. A daily dose of 10^9 viable *L. rhamnosus* GR-1 and 10^9 *L. fermentum* RC-14 was chosen because a dose-response study by the same group of researchers had shown that a dose of $> 8 \times 10^8$ viable organisms was required in order to achieve a significant effect. For a period of 60 d, 64 healthy women consumed one capsule containing this combination or placebo daily. Within 4 weeks, a significant increase in vaginal lactobacilli and concomitant decrease in yeasts and coliforms was observed in women receiving lactobacilli compared with those taking placebo. Some of these changes persisted for up to 30 d after cessation of supplementation. Among the subgroup of women with asymptomatic BV at baseline, 59% of the lactobacillus-treated women improved compared with only 31% of the placebo-treated women. The same group of researchers had previously reported similar findings from two open trials.

Vaginal Microflora and HIV-1 Infection

A system consisting of peroxidase (present in vaginal fluid) and H_2O_2-producing lactobacilli, particularly in the presence of halide, has been reported to exert in vitro antimicrobial effects against the BV-associated microorganisms, *Gardnerella vaginalis*, *Bacteroides bivus*, and also against HIV. Of note, however, an H_2O_2- and lactobacillus-dependent mechanism has also been implicated in the activation of the HIV-1 long terminal repeat, and this activation can result in increased production of intact virions by latently HIV-1-infected cells in vitro. This suggests that H_2O_2-producing lactobacilli have the potential to influence HIV-1 infection in two opposing ways, namely by exhibiting a viricidal effect on the one hand and enhancing virus replication on the other hand.

The evidence to date, however, suggests that the presence of H_2O_2-generating lactobacilli provides some protection against HIV infection. A positive association was observed between abnormal vaginal flora and seropositivity for HIV-1 in several cross-sectional studies in rural Ugandan women, female sex workers in Thailand, two different cohorts of pregnant women in urban Malawi, and also a group of pregnant women in North Carolina. Two prospective studies, one in 1196 pregnant Malawi women *(28)* and one in 657 Kenyan sex workers *(29)*, confirmed the significant increase in the risk of seroconversion with increasing severity of vaginal disturbance. In the Kenyan study the risk of gonorrhea and Trichomonas infection was also higher in women with abnormal vaginal flora on Gram stain *(29)*. The authors of this and other studies urged that treatment of BV and promotion of vaginal colonization with lactobacilli should be evaluated as potential interventions to reduce a woman's risk of acquiring HIV-1 and other sexually transmitted diseases.

Prebiotics and Synbiotics

A review published as part of the European project on non-digestible oligosaccharides (ENDO) concluded that the evidence from clinical trials that inulin-type fructans or $\beta(2{\rightarrow}1)$ fructans are prebiotics is strong *(30)*. The evidence for transgalactosylated oligosaccharides is equivocal and limited for other NDOs such as lactulose, soybean oligosaccharides, xylo-oligosaccharides, and pyrodextrins. In experimental animals, intake of inulin-type fructans and other NDOs enhances the absorption and bioavailability of minerals, such as calcium, magnesium, zinc, and iron. In humans, however, only the absorption of calcium, but not that of other minerals, has been found to be enhanced during consumption of NDOs in some studies, but not in others. The discrepancies are most likely due to methodological differences. Other beneficial effects of NDO supplementation include regulation of bowel habit and possibly reduction of cholesterol levels.

The effect of prebiotics on immune parameters has not been investigated in humans. In experimental animals, supplementation with oligofructose is associated with a variety of imunomodulating activities, including changes in lymphocyte subset, increased phagocytic activity, and enhanced IgA secretion *(31)*. It appears that many of these effects are observed in GALT, but not in peripheral blood immune cells. Since PBMC are the most easily accessible and most frequently sampled compartment of the human immune system, it may be difficult to demonstrate similar immunomodulatory effects of prebiotics in humans.

Two studies have investigated the influence of combined administration of a potential prebiotic, lactose-hydrolyzed milk, and a probiotic on immune parameters in healthy human volunteers *(32,33)*. Lactose-hydrolyzed milk contains galacto-oligosaccharides, a type of nondigestible oligosaccharide that is considered to have prebiotic potential, although studies to date have yielded conflicting results concerning its bifidogenic effects *(30)*. Subjects consuming *B. lactis* HN019 in lactose-hydrolyzed low-fat milk achieved greater increases in PMN phagocytic activity and NK cell activity than subjects consuming the same amount of microbes in low-fat milk *(32)*. Although both of these activities were also greater in a group of volunteers consuming *L. rhamnosus* HN001 in lactose-hydrolyzed milk compared with a group consuming the same probiotic in non-hydrolyzed milk, the difference was not statistically significant *(33)*. Given the similarity in study protocol and age range of the volunteers, the difference in bacterial strains is the most likely explanation for the observed difference. Unfortunately, fecal bacterial composition was not monitored in either of these studies.

Safety

Lactic acid bacteria have been used for the production of fermented dairy products and a variety of other fermented foods and beverages for thousands of years, and this is generally accepted as a demonstration of their overall safety. Nonetheless, because of the enormous variability in the activities not only of bacterial species, but even of strains of the same species, it has repeatedly been urged that each strain be assessed separately and on its own merit. In evaluating the probiotic potential of a bacterial strain, its safety is the most important consideration. Whereas GRAS (generally recognized as safe) status is commonly conferred on lactobacilli, lactococci, and some bifidobacteria, the genera *Streptococcus* and *Enterococcus* contain some opportunistic pathogens *(34)*. A few cases of fungemia during treatment with *Saccharomyces boulardii* have been reported, all in patients with a catheter, and all resolved with standard antifungal therapy. There have also been isolated cases of bacteremia because of lactic acid bacteria, mostly in immunocompromised hosts, but to date none of the isolates from blood cultures of these patients corresponded to a strain used in dairy, other commercial foods, or pharmaceutica. Furthermore, although many lactic acid bacteria are naturally resistant to some antibiotics, there still are safe antibiotics to which they are sensitive. To date, there have been no reports of adverse events from lactobacillus supplementation in AIDS patients or patients with Crohn's disease, although digestive lesions and/or immunodeficiency might be expected to favor bacterial translocation and systemic infections. Nonetheless, special precautions and close monitoring are probably warranted during probiotic supplementation in these and other high-risk groups.

Plasmid-linked antibiotic resistances, although rare, are known to occur in lactic acid bacteria and need to be assessed in potential probiotics. This is of particular importance in the case of entercococci, many of which contain conjugative antibiotic resistance plasmids. In vitro transfer of vancomycin resistance has been shown to be possible not only between enterococcal strains but also between enterococci and other gram-positive bacteria, such as *Listeria* and *Staphylococcus aureus*. This is cause for serious concern because vancomycin is one of the few remaining antibiotics for the treatment of certain multidrug-resistant pathogens.

A further safety issue arises from the fact that good manufacturing practices are not followed by all providers of commercially available probiotic preparations. Several recent analyses indicate that such products (1) do not always contain all of the species declared on the label; (2) often have lower bacterial counts than stated on the label; and (3) sometimes contain species not listed on the label. In addition, the available evidence does not always support the health benefit claims printed on the label.

Applicability in Developing Countries

Studies in Peru, Pakistan, and India have shown that supplementation with probiotics is a feasible approach to reducing the incidence or shortening the duration of acute diarrhea in developing countries. Difficulties arise, however,

Table 6
Examples of Lactic Acid-Fermented Cereals (85,97)

Raw material*	Product name	Country/region	Lactic acid bacteria	Other microorganisms
Maize, also sorghum or millet	Ogi	Nigeria/West Africa	L. plantarum L. fermentum L. delbrueckii	Saccharomyces busae
Maize	Banku	Ghana	lactic acid bacteria unidentified	Moulds
Maize, also rice or sorghum	Kenkey	Ghana	lactobacilli related to L. fermentum and L. reuteri	Candida, Saccharomyces, Penicillum, Aspergillus, Fusarium species
Maize, sorghum, or millet	Mawe	South Africa	L. fermentum, L. cellobiosis, L. brevis	Candida krusei Saccharomyces cerevisiae
Maize	Pozol	Southeastern Mexico	L. plantarum L. confusus Lactococcus lactis Lactococcus raffinolactis Leuconostoc mesenteroides	Aerobic mesophiles Enterobacteriacea Yeast Moulds
Sorghum	Abreh	Sudan	Lactobacillus spp L. mesenteroides L. plantarum	
Sorghum, millet, maize or cassava	Uji	Kenya/East Africa	L. plantarum Leuconostoc mesenteroides	
Millet, wheat	Mahewou/Magou	South Africa	L. delbrueckii L. bulgaricus L. acidophilus Streptococcus lactis	

*Note that different sources list different raw materials for most of the products. Because each grain is associated with its own characteristic lactic acid bacteria, the choice of grain also determines which bacterial strains are involved in fermentation.

237

from the short shelf life and the need for refrigeration of many of the commercially available products.

Nonviable microorganisms offer a more stable alternative. Heat-inactivated
LGG or *L. acidophilus* LB were shown to be effective in shortening the duration of acute rotavirus-induced diarrhea and diarrhea of unknown etiology
(11,35). Apart from one of these studies *(11)*, there are few other examples of
direct comparisons of the in vivo activities of viable and nonviable bacteria. In
several studies, however, fermented products containing heat (or otherwise)
inactivated bacteria have been used as controls. These studies indicate that
nonviable bacteria or products containing them can exert some, but clearly not
all, of the same effects as live bacteria *(36)*. It appears, however, that live bacteria have considerably greater immunomodulatory activities than their nonviable counterparts. This could be attributable to the demonstrated ability of
viable bacteria to gain direct access to immune cells by translocating from the
intestinal tract into mesenteric lymph nodes and other extraintestinal sites. That
hypothesis is consistent with the observation that, upon parenteral administration, viable and nonviable bacteria activate the immune system to a similar
extent. This suggests that, for the purpose of modulating the immune system,
live bacteria are preferable.

In many African, Asian, and South American countries, there is a long tradi-
tion of using lactic acid-fermented preparations as weaning and therapeutic
foods (*see* Table 6 for examples of cereal-based fermented foods). There is
some interest in designing starter cultures for some of these products to ensure
that their nutrient content is preserved and their safety (absence of pathogenic
microorganisms) enhanced *(37)*. It may be desirable to make probiotic status
one of the criteria in choosing bacterial strains for such starter cultures.

References

1. Fuller R. (1989) Probiotics in man and animals. *J. Appl. Bacteriol.* **66**, 365–378.
2. Gibson, G.R. and Roberfroid, M.B. (1995) Dietary modulation of the human colonic microbiota: introducing the concept of prebiotics. *J. Nutr.* **125**, 1401–1412.
3. Cebra, J.J. (1999) Influences of microbiota on intestinal immune system develop-ment. *Am. J. Clin. Nutr.* **69**, 1046S–1051S.
4. Claeson, M. and Merson, M.H. (1990) Global progress in the control of diarrheal diseases. *Pediatr. Infect. Dis. J.* **9**, 345–355.
5. Elmer, G.W. and McFarland, L.V. (2001) Biotherapeutic agents in the treatment of infectious diarrhea. *Gastroenterol. Clin. North Am.* **30**, 837–854.
6. Szajewska, H. and Mrukowicz, J.Z. (2001) Probiotics in the treatment and pre-vention of acute infectious diarrhea in infants and children: a systematic review of published randomized, double-blind, placebo-controlled trials. *J. Pediatr. Gastroenterol. Nutr.* **33**, S17–S25.

7. D'Souza, A.L., Rajkumar, C., Cooke, J., and Bulpitt, C.J. (2002) Probiotics in prevention of antibiotic associated diarrhoea: meta- analysis. *Brit. Med. J* **324**, 1361.
8. Elmer, G.W., McFarland, L.V., Surawicz, C.M., Danko, L., and Greenberg, R.N. (1999) Behaviour of *Saccharomyces boulardii* in recurrent *Clostridium difficile* disease patients. *Aliment. Pharm. Ther.* **13**, 1663–1668.
9. Isolauri, E., Kaila, M., Mykkänen, H., Ling, W.H., and Salminen, S. (1994) Oral bacteriotherapy for viral gastroenteritis. *Dig. Dis. Sci.* **39**, 2595–2600.
10. Shornikova, A.V., Casas, I.A., Mykkänen, H., Salo, E., and Vesikari, T. (1997) Bacteriotherapy with *Lactobacillus reuteri* in rotavirus gastroenteritis. *Pediatr. Infect. Dis. J.* **16**, 1103–1107.
11. Kaila, M., Isolauri, E., Saxelin, M., Arvilommi, H., and Vesikari, T. (1995) Viable versus inactivated lactobacillus strain GG in acute rotavirus diarrhoea. *Arch. Dis. Child.* **72**, 51–53.
12. Majamaa, H., Isolauri, E., Saxelin, M., and Vesikari, T. (1995) Lactic acid bacteria in the treatment of acute rotavirus gastroenteritis. *J. Pediatr. Gastroenterol. Nutr.* **20**, 333–338.
13. Isolauri, E., Joensuu, J., Suomalainen, H., Luomala, M., and Vesikari, T. (1995) Improved immunogenicity of oral D x RRV reassortant rotavirus vaccine by *Lactobacillus casei* GG. *Vaccine* **13**, 310–312.
14. Fang, H., Elina, T., Heikki, A., and Seppo, S. (2000) Modulation of humoral immune response through probiotic intake. *FEMS Immunol. Med. Microbiol.* **29**, 47–52.
15. Link-Amster, H., Rochat, F., Saudan, K.Y., Mignot, O., and Aeschlimann, J.M. (1994) Modulation of a specific humoral immune response and changes in intestinal flora mediated through fermented milk intake. *FEMS Immunol. Med. Microbiol.* **10**, 55–63.
16. Kimura, K., McCartney, A.L., McConnell, M.A., and Tannock, G.W. (1997) Analysis of fecal populations of bifidobacteria and lactobacilli and investigation of the immunological responses of their human hosts to the predominant strains. *Appl. Environ. Microbiol.* **63**, 3394–3398.
17. Spanhaak, S., Havenaar, R., and Schaafsma, G. (1998) The effect of consumption of milk fermented by *Lactobacillus casei* strain Shirota on the intestinal microflora and immune parameters in humans. *Eur. J. Clin. Nutr.* **52**, 899–907.
18. Gill, H.S., Rutherfurd, K.J., Cross, M.L., and Gopal, P.K. (2001) Enhancement of immunity in the elderly by dietary supplementation with the probiotic *Bifidobacterium lactis* HN019. *Am. J. Clin. Nutr.* **74**, 833–839.
19. Pelto, L., Isolauri, E., Lilius, E.M., Nuutila, J., and Salminen, S. (1998) Probiotic bacteria down-regulate the milk-induced inflammatory response in milk-hypersensitive subjects but have an immunostimulatory effect in healthy subjects. *Clin. Exp. Allergy* **28**, 1474–1479.
20. Kirjavainen, P.V., Arvola, T., Salminen, S.J., and Isolauri, E. (2002) Aberrant composition of gut microbiota of allergic infants: a target of bifidobacterial therapy at weaning? *Gut* **51**, 51–55.

21. Majamaa, H. and Isolauri, E. (1997) Probiotics: a novel approach in the management of food allergy. *J. Allergy Clin. Immunol.* **99**, 179–185.
22. Isolauri, E., Arvola, T., Sütas, Y., Moilanen, E., and Salminen, S. (2000) Probiotics in the management of atopic eczema. *Clin. Exp. Allergy* **30**, 1604–1610.
23. Kalliomäki, M., Ouwehand, A., Arvilommi, H., Kero, P., and Isolauri, E. (1999) Transforming growth factor-β in breast milk: a potential regulator of atopic disease at an early age. *J. Allergy Clin. Immunol.* **104**, 1251–1257.
24. Kalliomäki, M., Salminen, S., Arvilommi, H., Kero, P., Koskinen, P., and Isolauri, E. (2001) Probiotics in primary prevention of atopic disease: a randomised placebo-controlled trial. *Lancet* **357**, 1076–1079.
25. Rautava, S., Kalliomäki, M., and Isolauri, E. (2002) Probiotics during pregnancy and breast-feeding might confer immunomodulatory protection against atopic disease in the infant. *J. Allergy Clin. Immunol.* **109**, 119–121.
26. Reid, G. and Burton, J. (2002) Use of *Lactobacillus* to prevent infection by pathogenic bacteria. *Microbes. Infect.* **4**, 319–324.
27. Reid, G., Charbonneau, D., Erb, J., et al. (2003) Oral use of *Lactobacillus rhamnosus* GR-1 and *L. fermentum* RC-14 significantly alters vaginal flora: randomized, placebo-controlled trial in 64 healthy women. *FEMS Immunol. Med. Microbiol.* **35**, 131–134.
28. Taha, T.E., Hoover, D.R., Dallabetta, G.A., et al. (1998) Bacterial vaginosis and disturbances of vaginal flora: association with increased acquisition of HIV. *AIDS* **12**, 1699–1706.
29. Martin, H.L., Richardson, B.A., Nyange, P.M., et al. (1999) Vaginal lactobacilli, microbial flora, and risk of human immunodeficiency virus type 1 and sexually transmitted disease acquisition. *J. Infect. Dis.* **180**, 1863–1868.
30. Van Loo, J., Cummings, J., Delzenne, N., et al. (1999) Functional food properties of non-digestible oligosaccharides: a consensus report from the ENDO project (DGXII AIRII-CT94-1095). *Br. J. Nutr.* **81**, 121–132.
31. Schley, P.D. and Field, C.J. (2002) The immune-enhancing effects of dietary fibres and prebiotics. *Br. J. Nutr.* **87(suppl 2)**, S221–S230.
32. Chiang, B.L., Sheih, Y.H., Wang, L.H., Liao, C.K., and Gill, H.S. (2000) Enhancing immunity by dietary consumption of a probiotic lactic acid bacterium (*Bifidobacterium lactis* HN019): optimization and definition of cellular immune responses. *Eur. J. Clin. Nutr.* **54**, 849–855.
33. Sheih, Y.H., Chiang, B.L., Wang, L.H., Liao, C.K., and Gill, H.S. (2001) Systemic immunity-enhancing effects in healthy subjects following dietary consumption of the lactic acid bacterium *Lactobacillus rhamnosus* HN001. *J. Am. Coll. Nutr.* **20**, 149–156.
34. Salminen, S., von Wright, A., Morelli, L., et al. (1998) Demonstration of safety of probiotics-a review. *Int. J. Food. Microbiol.* **44**, 93–106.
35. Simakachorn, N., Pichaipat, V., Rithipornpaisarn, P., Kongkaew, C., Tongpradit, P., and Varavithya, W. (2000) Clinical evaluation of the addition of lyophilized, heat-killed *Lactobacillus acidophilus* LB to oral rehydration therapy in the treatment of acute diarrhea in children. *J. Pediatr. Gastroenterol. Nutr.* **30**, 68–72.

36. Ouwehand, A.C. and Salminen, S.J. (1998) The health effects of cultured milk products with viable and non-viable bacteria. *Int. Dairy J.* **8**, 749–758.

37. Mensah, P., Harrison, D.T.J., and Tomkins, A.M. Fermented cereal gruels: Towards a solution of the weanling's dilemma [electronic version]. Food and Nutrition Bulletin 1991; 13:retrieved from http://www.unu.edu/unupress/food/8F131e/8F131E08.htm.

38. Havenaar, R., Ten Brink, B., Huis in't Veld, J.H.J. (1992) Selection of strains for probiotic use, in *Probiotics: The Scientific Basis.* (Fuller, R., ed.) Chapman & Hall, London, U.K., pp. 209–224.

39. Guarner, F. and Schaafsma, G.J. (1998) Probiotics. *Int. J. Food. Microbiol.* **39**, 237–238.

40. Food and Agriculture Organization of the United Nations, World Health Organization. Health and Nutrition Properties of Probiotics in Food including Powder Milk with Live Lactic Acid Bacteria. Córdoba, Argentina, 2001:http://www/fao.org/es/ESN/Probio/probio.htm.

41. Salminen, E., Ouwehand, A., Benno Y., and Lee Y.K. (1999) Probiotics: how should they be defined? *Trends Food. Sci. Technol.* **10**, 107–110.

42. Saavedra, J. (2000) Probiotics and infectious diarrhea. *Am. J. Gastroenterol.* **95**, S16–S18.

11 Malaria And Immunity

CLARA MENÉNDEZ AND CARLOTA DOBAÑO

CONTENTS

KEY POINTS

- A considerable number of children under 5 yr of age in sub-Saharan Africa are sick or die from infection with *Plasmodium falciparum*.
- Heavy uninterrupted exposure to *P. falciparum* leads to the development of naturally acquired immunity (NAI) that protects first against death or severe malaria, then against mild malaria (antidisease immunity), and finally, against parasite infection (antiparasite immunity).
- The onset of NAI may be governed by parasitic factors (poor immunogenicity or antigenic diversity, exposure-dependent), or by intrinsic host factors (age, exposure-independent).
- Interventions to control malaria that reduce exposure to *P. falciparum* (for example, insecticide-impregnated bednets) diminish parasitemia and related morbidity and mortality, but some exposure may be needed to sustain NAI.
- NAI is primarily directed against the parasite in its asexual erythrocytic stage.

From: *Handbook of Nutrition and Immunity*
Edited by: M. E. Gershwin, P. Nestel, and C. L. Keen © Humana Press, Totowa, NJ

- Passive transfer of immune immunolglobin (Ig)G has demonstrated a role for antibodies in protection, particularly cytophilic isotypes (IgG1 and IgG3).
- Agglutinating antibodies recognizing antigens on the surface of the infected erythrocyte may contribute to NAI.
- Further research is required on the role of cell-mediated immunity and cytokines in NAI in humans.
- Susceptibility to malaria is increased during pregnancy.
- Malaria during pregnancy causes anemia in the mother and low birth weight in the baby.
- HIV infection increases the risk to malaria during pregnancy.
- Pregnant women in malaria endemic areas need to be protected with insecticide-treated nets and prophylactic antimalarial drugs.
- Nutritional status is adversely affected by malaria.
- Undernutrition is associated with higher malaria-related morbidity and mortality.
- Oral iron supplementation in prophylactic doses to infants in malaria endemic areas is safe and efficacious, but it increases the risk of developing diarrhea.

Introduction

People living in malaria-affected areas are more likely to be undernourished than those in nonmalarial areas. Because both conditions generally coexist, they interact. That is, malaria can adversely affect nutritional status and nutritional status can modulate susceptibility to malaria, creating a vicious circle in which it is not always clear what is the cause and what is the consequence. Relatively few studies have examined the nature of this interaction with an adequate number of patients and some of the findings remain controversial. Recent studies showed that nutrition strongly influences the disease burden of malaria (1,2), but earlier ones suggested that undernourished children may be protected from malaria (3). The groups at highest risk of being adversely affected by malaria are children and pregnant women, who are also most vulnerable to undernutrition. Understanding the association between these two populations is a priority. To better understand how nutrition and the immune system can be altered by malarial infection and disease, this chapter first reviews general aspects of immunity to malaria before discussing the particularities of malaria immunity in children and pregnant women and the association between nutritional status and malaria.

Malaria: The Parasite and the Disease

Malaria is an infectious disease caused by protozoan parasites of the genus *Plasmodium* that is transmitted by female Anopheline mosquitoes throughout the tropical world. The World Health Organization (WHO) estimates that 4 billion people in approx 90 countries are at risk of becoming infected, and 300–500 million cases and 1–3 million deaths occur each year *(4)*. Moreover, these estimates have increased over the last three decades. Most of the disease and deaths can be attributed to a single species—*P. falciparum*, although *P. vivax* is important in Asia and Latin America. The highest morbidity and mortality occur in sub-Saharan African children under the age of 5 yr, but a significant number of adults including pregnant women are also affected.

Controlling the disease has proven to be very difficult because of the complex life cycle of the parasite. *Plasmodium* requires a vertebrate and an invertebrate host to complete its development, with a changing morphology and antigenic composition in each life stage. A blood-feeding mosquito takes up parasites in the form of male and female gametocytes contained within red blood cells (RBC) that develop into gametes in the mosquito's gut. Fertilization produces zygotes that develop into motile ookinetes that burrow into the gut wall to form oocysts. Immature sporozoites divide within the oocyst, and then migrate to the salivary glands where they mature, ready to be inoculated into the next host. After the bite, sporozoites spend less than 30 min in the blood circulation before invading hepatocytes or being cleared by other tissues of the body. In a hepatocyte, depending on the species of Plasmodia, a single sporozoite develops into 30,000–40,000 merozoites (exoerythrocytic or preerythrocytic stage), over 5–8 d or longer. Each merozoite, when released, can invade a RBC. During the asexual or blood cycle, the parasite develops inside the RBC over 2 (*P. falciparum*, *P. vivax*, and *P. ovale*) or 3 d (*P. malariae*). The parasite changes its morphology from ring to trophozoite and finally schizont. Six to thirty-two merozoites develop inside each schizont and, following its rupture, each merozoite can continue the asexual cycle by invading a fresh RBC. The blood phase includes a period of exponential growth in the number of parasites within the host, but it takes several cycles of multiplication before parasite numbers increase to levels detectable by microscopy. Finally, some parasites undergo sexual differentiation into male and female gametocytes (sexual stage) ready to make the transition from a vertebrate host to the next blood-feeding mosquito.

In addition to the complexity of the life cycle, the diversity of the malaria parasite is a significant problem for vaccine development. Within a single species of *Plasmodium*, allelic polymorphisms originate the coexistence of different genotypes, clones or so-called "strains." Allelic polymorphisms give rise to structurally distinct forms of particular proteins in different parasite clones. In particular, genetic polymorphisms in certain protein loci are thought to lead to the expression of antigenically distinct forms of the proteins *(5)*. An alternative concept is phenotypic antigenic variation *(6)*. Broadly, this refers to changes in antigenic phenotype by regulated expression of different genes of a clonal population of parasites over the natural course of an infection. Life-cycle-related antigenic changes are an example of this biochemical and antigenic phenotypic variation. Antigenic variation in several species of *Plasmodium* has been shown to be a feature of antigens expressed on the surface of parasitized RBC (PRBC) *(7)*.

Pathology of Malarial Disease

In malaria endemic areas, probably only a small proportion of people who become infected with *P. falciparum* develop clinical disease. The reasons why many infections remain asymptomatic or why a few symptomatic infections evolve into severe illness are not understood. Clinical symptoms of malaria often commence at about the same time or just before parasites are diagnosed in blood by microscopy; more-sensitive detection by polymerase chain reaction (PCR) can detect parasites up to 1 wk before they can be detected in slides *(8)*. In Africa, the majority of symptomatic infections occur between 6 mo and 5 yr of age *(9)*. The most common clinical presentation of all malarias is acute febrile illness. Other frequent symptoms are headache, anorexia and nausea, myalgia, arthralgia, and general prostration. Typical signs are splenomegaly and hepatomegaly. These are features of mild or uncomplicated malaria (UM).

The manifestations of severe malaria (SM), as defined by WHO criteria, are highly variable and associated almost exclusively with *P. falciparum* infections *(10)*. The spectrum of severe *P. falciparum* disease includes severe malarial anemia (SMA), cerebral malaria (CM), acidosis, respiratory distress, shock, apparent disseminated intravascular coagulation, renal failure, and pulmonary edema. Some manifestations are more common in particular age groups and/or geographical areas. CM is widespread in sub-Saharan Africa and Southeast Asia, and can occur in South America. In Africa, about 2% of malaria cases between 6 mo and 5 yr of age are classified as severe, mainly involving CM. A few CM cases also occur in the 5–10 yr old age group, and are only occasionally reported in adults. In contrast, in Southeast Asia CM typically occurs in adults as well as children. Anemia is common mainly in African children and pregnant women. Organ failure mainly affects adults in Asia and South America. Malaria mortality in African children, where the heaviest burden of disease falls, is attributed mostly to CM and SMA. Other life-threatening conditions include pulmonary, kidney, and liver complications, and malaria-induced metabolic acidosis.

Cerebral malaria is defined clinically as both the presence of coma and malaria parasites *(10)*. The mortality rate for CM is between 15 and 30% in Africa. In addition, a consistent minority of survivors (5–20%) are discharged with neurological sequelae *(11)*, although one-half of these recover fully within 4–6 wk. Two phenomena have been considered in CM pathogenesis. First, adherence of PRBC to host cells, either endothelial cells in the post capillary venules of the brain (cytoadherence) or circulating noninfected RBC (rosetting). Second, induction of host cytokines and their effects on brain tissues via induction of secondary mediators, for example, nitric oxide (NO) and free oxygen radicals. These phenomena are not mutually exclusive as suspected causes of CM.

Severe malarial anemia is defined as a hemoglobin (Hb) concentration below 50 g/L, or a hematocrit (or packed cell volume) below 16%, in a patient with a parasitemia above 10,000 trophozoites/mL of blood, although SMA can develop at lower parasitemias *(10)*. In most cases, blood transfusions improve the clinical findings. Overall, mortality rates for children admitted with SMA in hospitals with blood transfusion facilities range from 4.7 to 14–16% *(12)*. Regarding the pathophysiology of SMA, it is generally thought that the destruction of RBCs is more than can be accounted for by the number of RBCs infected and directly destroyed by parasites. In addition to RBCs lost by lysis when schizonts rupture, various immunopathological mechanisms may contribute to SMA. Parasite antigens, immune complexes containing them, or autoantibodies could bind to unparasitized RBCs and accelerate their clearance by cells of the macrophage/monocyte lineage in the spleen and liver, or by complement-mediated lysis. Non-infected RBCs could also be damaged by disease-induced free-oxygen radicals leading to rigidification of the RBC membrane and thus their increased clearance by a hyperactive spleen. At the same time, chronic release of tumor necrosis factor (TNF)-α or other cytokines in response to the infection could inhibit RBC development from bone marrow stem cells (dyserythropoiesis) and alter the kinetics of RBC turnover. Alternatively, blocking of bone marrow sinusoids with PRBC could also cause dyserythropoiesis, which has been described both morphologically and functionally in SMA patients. These findings have led to the idea that SMA may be caused by a chronic process as well as by acute events *(13)*. However, the question of whether presentations with SMA are essentially acute episodes related primarily to uncontrolled exponential parasite growth, or whether they are cases of chronically progressive anemia that finally crosses some critical threshold, remains unsolved.

Naturally Acquired Immunity (NAI)

People living in malaria endemic areas who are exposed to repeated *P. falciparum* infections from infancy develop immunity to the disease later in life. Children are more susceptible to clinical malaria and also to the more severe life-threatening forms of the disease, and have the highest mortality rates. Adults in endemic areas, although often harboring low, but detectable, numbers of parasites in the blood, rarely develop clinical symptoms or die as a result of the infection. This form of NAI to the disease, also referred to as "premunition," "clinical tolerance," or "antitoxic/antidisease immunity," develops slowly over years and is never complete. There is, generally, also a substantial decrease in the parasite load in infected adults, indicating an "antiparasite immunity" component malaria in protection that develops with age. Parasite density is linked to disease, and diminished parasite counts almost certainly contribute to diminished risk of disease. The dominant factor driving protection from disease may be specific to effectors that diminish parasite numbers, but the activity of other effectors, for example, responses that diminish proinflammatory cytokines, remain possible as well.

In naïve individuals of any age acutely infected with malaria, clinical disease almost always appears with relatively low densities of parasitemia, even when subpatent. However, in highly endemic areas, the patterns of disease are sometimes distinct from parasitemia, and both are age-dependent. Among very heavily exposed children, high-density parasitemia may occur in the absence of obvious clinical symptoms. The greatest disease risk for these children is SMA rather than CM. Adults in such areas rarely have high-density parasitemia, but their risk of disease is higher when they do.

In holoendemic Africa, onset of clinical immunity requires 10–15 yr of roughly five infections per year. The seemingly long period required to achieve protection is probably dependent on age and exposure, but the prevailing component has not been conclusively explained. On one hand, the malaria parasite may be poorly immunogenic at inducing protective responses. On the other hand, if immunity is essentially strain-specific, a long period could be required to be exposed to a large repertoire of diverse strains *(14)*. An alternative hypothesis, based largely on the observations of malaria-naïve Javanese transmigrants in Indonesian Papua, attributes the onset of clinical immunity to recent heavy exposure and development of a strain-transcending immune response governed predominantly by the stage of physiological development of the human host independent of lifelong exposure *(15)*. Thus, a mature immune system could allow an adult to acquire immunity more rapidly than a child under the same level of exposure. In the context of modeling NAI for vaccine development, it is crucial to distinguish between these hypotheses in order to understand the molecular and cellular events that drive the onset of clinical immunity.

Epidemiological Considerations: The Effect of Exposure

The intensity of exposure to biting infectious mosquitoes, measured by the entomological inoculation rate (EIR), influences the distribution of malaria morbidity and mortality within communities. In general, the more intense the transmission, the earlier and more confined the age range of susceptibility to disease. Thus, in high endemic areas, risk of SM is limited to visitors, infants, small children, and pregnant women, whereas in low endemic areas almost all exposed people are at risk of debilitating or severe disease.

EIR is associated with parasitemia density: increased exposure to infected mosquitoes can lead to more sporozoites reaching the liver, and consequently, more parasites developing to mature liver-stage schizonts, which then rupture resulting in more PRBCs. A high density of *P. falciparum* asexual parasitemia correlates with SM *(10)*, which is linked to risk of death. Therefore, interventions that reduce *P. falciparum* transmission intensity can reduce high-density parasitemia and related morbidity and mortality. Indeed, insecticide-impregnated bednets reduce the prevalence or incidence of parasitemia and provide protection against morbidity and mortality attributable to malaria *(16)*. The intensity of transmission also influences the risk of SM: the risk of CM or SMA is lowest among children with the highest transmission intensities, and highest among those exposed to low to moderate intensities of transmission *(17)*. To avoid the possibility that interventions to diminish risk of infection could increase the risk of poor clinical outcomes, these interventions would have to push the attack rate below the threshold of risk of SM without crossing the threshold of exposure needed to sustain NAI.

Epidemiological Considerations: The Effect of Age

The prevalence and density, but not incidence, of infection decrease with age. This is mainly caused by the development of antiparasite immunity that restricts the density of asexual parasitemia. In children less than 1 yr of age, the prevalence and density of *P. falciparum* infection, and the incidence of overall fevers and of malaria-associated fevers, increase with age for the first 6 mo of life and then gradually decline. In highly endemic areas, parasitemia peaks in children under 5 yr old and subsequently declines in an age-dependent manner.

Innate age-related distinctions, about which very little is known in the context of malaria, may have a dominant effect on the clinical course of disease. Studies of transmigrants in Indonesian Papua have suggested that age-dependent immunity occurs in both acute and chronic exposure to infection, with apparently critical effects on the course of infection that differ sharply between children and adults *(15)*. The adult immune system apparently develops clinical immunity more rapidly and completely than in children under chronic heavy exposure. However, the adult immune response to acute heavy exposure seems to put them at much greater susceptibility to SM. A relatively exaggerated production of proinflammatory cytokines by adult humans in response to a primary infection by *P. falciparum* that wanes with continued exposure could explain these differences.

Epidemiological Considerations: Patterns of Severe Disease

The incidence of CM and SMA differ with age and vary with endemicity. In African children, the peak of SMA occurs within the first 2 yr of life, whereas CM occurs later, between 3 and 4 yr of age. Different levels of NAI could influence the different age patterns of disease severity, for example, children who develop CM may have "less" immunity than children who develop UM, but there is no evidence to support this possibility. Alternatively, the gap of several years before an increased probability that a *P. falciparum* infection gives rise to CM is compatible with the idea that a degree of immunological sensitization by prior malaria infections could predispose an individual to developing CM. Another possibility is that particular *P. falciparum* strains may differentially predispose to CM, SMA, or UM *(18)* by exhibiting phenotypes associated with varying degrees of "virulence," for example, the ability to invade RBCs, to adhere to endothelial cells, or to stimulate TNF-α.

Naturally Acquired Immunity in Children

An estimated 2% of African children succumb to death caused by malaria before the age of 5 yr *(19)*. The protection afforded by NAI manifests first against death or SM, followed by a gradually diminishing risk of even mild attacks that mostly plateaus during or soon after puberty. After birth, the prevalence of parasitemia increases sharply with age. For the first few months of life, children may be resistant to SM. Although almost always challenged and infected, mortality among infants less than 3 mo of age rarely occurs in holoendemic areas. This protection is thought to be associated with the presence of maternal antibodies (Ab). Immunoglobin (Ig) G is acquired by the fetus *in utero*, mainly during the third trimester of pregnancy, and IgG levels decrease from birth until about 4 mo of age. Inhibitory factors against in vitro growth of *P. falciparum* such as lactoferrin and secretory IgA have been demonstrated in breastmilk and maternal and infant sera *(20)*. Begining at 3–4 mo of age, young children become susceptible to SM and death. Between 4 and 6 mo of age, almost all infants are seronegative. Consequently, the risk of clinical disease increases from birth to about 6 mo of age, depending on the transmission rate. At about 2–5 yr of age, the frequency of clinical disease begins to diminish and risk of mortality sharply decreases. The age of onset of this protection is somewhat earlier with heavier transmission, but rarely occurs before the age of 2 yr. In holoendemic areas, the presence and density of parasites at any given time does not correlate well with clinical disease. Children may have high parasite loads but no symptoms, or disease with low parasitemias. At the age of peak parasite prevalence, the number of clinical attacks of malaria per year and the risk of mortality dramatically declines. From adolescence onwards SM very rarely occurs.

Mechanisms of Protective Immunity

Parasites can be killed by effector mechanisms from both the innate and the adaptive immune system, but the relative contributions of each have not been established. Effector cells of innate immunity such as tissue macrophages, monocytes, and granulocytes may have an intrinsic antiparasitic activity, for example, phagocytosis of sporozoites when they enter the body. Cytokines such as TNF-α induced by parasite products released by rupturing schizonts (exoantigens) in monocytes and macrophages and interferon (TFN)-γ secreted by T-cells or natural killer (NK) cells may act by activating macrophages and neutrophils to kill parasites via reactive oxygen or nitrogen intermediates, primarily L-arginine-derived NO *(21)*. TNF-α and NO can have both harmful and beneficial effects in the infected host, depending on the amount produced. Soluble malaria antigens containing phosphatidylinositol moieties, for example, glycosylphosphatidyl-inositol anchors on plasmodial proteins, can be responsible for the toxic overproduction of TNF-α implicated in disease severity. Other mechanisms proposed for high concentrations of TNF-α are IgE elevation *(22)* or low interleukin (IL)-10 concentrations *(23)*. Periodic fever, produced when large numbers of PRBC rupture, is the most characteristic feature of malaria, and infected individuals have elevated levels of the endogenous pyrogens, TNF-α, IL-1, and IL-6. Febrile temperatures may be acting as density-dependent regulators of the growth of intraerythrocytic *P. falciparum (24)*.

Little is known about the protective underlying mechanisms for acquired immunity. Both humoral and cellular mechanisms have been implicated: Ab target extracellular parasites and block their capacity to invade new cells, and cell-mediated responses prevent the development of intracellular forms. The widespread persistence of patent parasitemia in asymptomatic individuals resident in malaria-endemic areas suggests that NAI is primarily directed against the parasite in its asexual erythrocytic stage and does not effectively block sporozoite invasion or intrahepatic development.

Mechanisms of Asexual Erythrocytic Stage Immunity–Antibody Responses

Evidence suggests that circulating extracellular merozoites are the primary targets of the protective immunity conferred by the passive transfer of immune serum. The reduction in parasitemia occurs following schizogony, and the serum does not appear to be effective against trophozoites or gametocytes *(25)*. Considerable evidence has accumulated which supports a role for Ab in the protective immunity directed against the asexual erythrocytic stage of *Plasmodia*. Classical passive transfers of immune Ab demonstrated that IgG protect against malarial infection. Transfer of pooled γ-globulin from West African immune adults into West African *(25)*, East African *(26)*, or Thai *(27)* children acutely infected with *P. falciparum* caused a marked reduction in parasitemia and clinical symptoms. Some evidence shows that this protective immunity is mediated by cytophilic Ab of the IgG1 and IgG3 isotypes, in association with monocytes. These Ab had no direct effect on the invasion or intraerythrocytic development of *P. falciparum*, as assessed by the in vitro growth inhibition assay, but induced a marked specific inhibition of parasite growth in the presence of monocytes in an Ab-dependent cellular inhibition assay *(28)*. Cytophilic Ab cooperated with monocytes in vitro via Fc receptor to produce TNF-α. In West Africa, analysis of the Ab isotype predominating in individuals with defined clinical states of resistance or susceptibility to malaria revealed that cytophilic IgG1 and IgG3 isotypes predominated in immune individuals, compared with individuals experiencing a primary clinical attack *(29)*. The data supporting the relevance of IgG1 and IgG3, but not IgG2 or IgG4, subclasses in NAI against *P. falciparum*, have led to hypothesizing that during childhood nonprotective Ab isotypes may block the activity of protective isotypes, and thus explain the age-related acquisition of immunity *(29)*.

Ab agglutinating PBRC have also been associated with reduced episodes of clinical disease *(30)*. Such Ab could agglutinate the merozoite at rupture of mature schizonts, and block merozoite invasion of new RBC. Apart from the above, other putative effector mechanisms involving Ab can be envisaged: (i) direct damage to free parasites, either by themselves or by activating the complement system; (ii) neutralization of a parasite function, for example, block its adherence and/or subsequent invasion to a host cell; (iii) neutralization of harmful toxins released from PBRC; and (iv) enhancement of phagocytosis by macrophages, which could be increased further by the presence of complement.

Given the complexity of the parasite and the multitude of immune responses that can be involved, it is unlikely that a single immune response directed against a single antigen expressed during one stage of the parasite's life cycle is responsible for the NAI against malaria. The publication of the *P. falciparum* genome will hopefully lead to the discovery of the targets of protective immunity. Possible targets antigens of erythrocytic stage immunity characterized thus far include: (i) merozoite surface proteins (MSP1, MSP2, other MSPs); (ii) soluble proteins associated with the merozoite surface or exported to the parasitophorous vacuole during the later stages of parasite intracellular development (SERA; Exp-1, HRP-2, MSP-3, GLURP, ABRA, S-antigen); (iii) proteins in the apical organelles (AMA-1, RAP-1, RAP-2, EBA-175); and (iv) proteins in the surface of PRBC (PfEMP-1, rifins) *(31)*.

Mechanisms of Asexual Erythrocytic Stage Immunity–Cellular Immunity

Most of the research on cell-mediated immunity in malaria has been done in rodent models, and the understanding of cellular mechanisms in humans is limited. CD4$^+$ T-cells are thought to regulate the immune response to erythrocytic stage antigens *(32)*. In vitro stimulation with parasite extracts or antigens induce T-cell proliferation and/or cytokine secretion (for example, IFN-γ, IL-4), which not always correlate with antigen-specific Ab levels. In addition, CD4$^+$ T-cells may provide T-cell help for Ab production.

T-cells from malaria-naïve individuals may also proliferate and/or release cytokines in response to in vitro stimulation with parasite extracts *(33)*, presumably as a consequence of crossreactive stimulation with other pathogens. Additionally, in endemic areas, asymptomatic falciparum infections have been associated with spontaneous apoptosis of the host lymphocytes in vitro that could be modulated by different cytokines *(34)*.

Lymphopenia, which is a lower numbers of T-cells in the peripheral circulation, is a feature of acute falciparum malaria, presumably because of sequestration in lymphoid organs in response to the infection *(35)*. Another feature of malaria is a transient inability of peripheral T-cells to respond to antigenic stimulation in vitro that could be explained by the reallocation hypothesis or, alternatively, by some immunosuppressive mechanisms *(35)*. Finally, increased levels of circulating soluble markers of T-cell activation in acute malaria, for example, IL-2 receptor, CD4, and CD8 have suggested a systemic T-cell activation that correlates with disease severity *(36)*.

Malaria During Pregnancy
Epidemiology (37)

Pregnant women are at increased risk of falciparum malaria compared with nonpregnant women, male adults, or the same women before pregnancy. These observations are consistent across all malaria-endemic areas in Asia, Latin America, and Africa.

The negative effects of malaria in the woman and her fetus depends on the level of prepregnancy immunity against malaria, which in general reflects the level of exposure to the infection. In areas of low and unstable endemicity, malaria may be a common cause of maternal and perinatal mortality, whereas it is rarely a direct cause of death in settings of stable transmission, where pregnant women can be considered semiimmune. In the latter situation, however, malaria may indirectly contribute to maternal, perinatal, and infant death through the development of severe anemia in the mother and low birth weight in the fetus.

Another important epidemiological aspect is the effect of parity on the susceptibility and severity of malaria infection. Parity influences vulnerability to the infection with lower risk with increasing parity. This is especially marked in areas of stable transmission. Younger age, independent of parity, has been associated with increased risk. The prevalence of infection and parasite density is highest in the first half of pregnancy and decreases progressively until delivery. Usually, the prevalence of infection in the postpartum period is similar to that before pregnancy.

In general, pregnant women with the Hb genotype AS, whose prevalence may be up to 40% of the adult population in some sub-Saharan countries have been found to have similar parasite prevalence and risk of infection compared with those with the Hb genotype AA.

Effects of Malaria During Pregnancy (see Table 1)

On the Mother

The consequences of maternal malaria vary depending on the level of NAI against the infection and parity. In general, severe complications of *P. falciparum* infection, such as CM, affect mainly nonimmune women of all parities. Semiimmune primigravidae suffer mild clinical episodes, whereas multigravidae are relatively symptom-free *(38)*. However, this classical clinical pattern is changing in some malaria endemic areas because of the AIDS epidemic. HIV$^+$ pregnant women are more likely to suffer severe malaria infection and disease regardless of their parity *(39)*.

In all areas, malaria infection during pregnancy causes anemia, being more frequent in lower parity groups. Anemia contributes indirectly to maternal mortality. Up to one-third of maternal deaths are related to SMA in malaria endemic areas (Bernard Brabin, personal communciation).

On the Fetus

Abortion and stillbirth rates can be high during malaria epidemics and in nonimmune women *(40)*. These consequences are more difficult to establish in stable endemic regions. In all areas, maternal malaria may be associated with reduced birth weight, being most marked in first-born children. This may result from intrauterine growth restriction (IUGR), premature delivery, or both *(41)*. Congenital malaria may occur in all endemic areas, although it is said to be more common during malaria epidemics *(42)*.

On the Infant

Data are lacking for the effects of malaria during pregnancy on subsequent mortality and morbidity in the infant. Maternal anemia is a risk factor for peri-

Table 1
Effects of Malaria During Pregnancy

Effects of malaria	Malarial endemicity	
	Low or unstable	High or stable
On the mother		
Severe disease, including death[a]	(++)[b]	(+) (indirectly through anemia ?)[c]
Acute disease/anemia	(+++) (everyone)	(+++) (mainly primigravidae)[c]
Placental infection	(−)	(+++) (mainly primigravidae)[c]
On the fetus		
Abortion/perinatal death	(++)	(+++) (mainly primigravidae)[c]
Intra uterine growth retardation	(+++) (everyone)	(++) (mainly primigravidae)[c]
Prematurity	(++)	(+)?
Congenital infection	(++)	?
On the infant		
Increased risk of death	?	?
Increased/decreased susceptibility to malaria	?	

[a]probably more frequent in HIV+ women
[b](−), rare; (+), infrequent; (++), not infrequent; (+++), frequent; ?, not known
[c]also frequent in HIV+ multigravidae

natal mortality, and may also influence the infant's morbidity and mortality by reducing the baby's birth weight. Malaria infection during pregnancy may also influence the risk of death and disease during the first year of life by directly inducing growth retardation and/or prematurity. Infants born with IUGR frequently show impaired cell-mediated immunity, which may adversely affect their chances of survival by increasing the susceptibility of infections including malaria. Finally, as for other infections, the influence of in utero exposure to malaria antigens on the postnatal response to the infection remains to be established. It could be either beneficial or harmful depending on the intensity of the infection and the gestational time at which the first exposure occurs *(37)*.

The Placenta in Malaria Infection

The placenta is a preferential site for parasite invasion during malaria infection, especially in primigravidae semiimmune women. Parasite densities may be several times higher in the placenta than in peripheral blood. The infection is accompanied by an intense inflammatory reaction in the placental intervillous spaces *(43)*.

Mechanisms for the Increased Risk

During pregnancy, there is a physiological immune adaptation that develops to prevent the rejection of the immunologically different fetus.

Immunological Mechanisms

HUMORAL IMMUNITY

Although mean IgG titers fall progressively as pregnancy advances, this seems to be a relative rather than absolute decrease, probably explained by the hemodilution in the second half of pregnancy *(37)*. Humoral responses to vaccination are intact in pregnant women and do not differ by parity group, which suggests that an impaired humoral immunity does not explain the increased susceptibility to malaria infection observed in pregnant women *(37)*.

CELL-MEDIATED IMMUNITY

Cell-mediated immunity is depressed transiently during pregnancy owing to the increased production of hormones and proteins that occur as part of the adaptive process essential to maintaining gestation. Among the hormones, cortisol and oestrogens have been primarily associated with in vitro suppression of cell-mediated responses *(37)*. Although cortisol levels are increased in pregnant women, especially primigravidae, the general immunodepression they induce does not adequately explain the consistent preference for placental infection. Oestrogens are found in higher titers in the placental intervillous spaces than in peripheral plasma and are also higher in primigravidae compared with other parities. Thus, they might better explain the epidemiological observations (37). However, more information is needed to establish their exact role in parasite invasion.

Parasite Factors

In vitro studies have shown cytoadherence of a particular subpopulation of *P. falciparum* parasites to adhesion molecules present on the trophoblastic tissue (Condroitin sulphate A), which may also explain the mechanism for placental infection during pregnancy (44).

Mechanical Factors

Another explanation is the accumulation of maternal PRBCs in the intervillous spaces giving rise to mechanical sequestration.

Entomological Factors

Higher exposure to mosquitoes of the pregnant woman related to behavioral and physical changes are also through to contribute to the increased risk of malaria during pregnancy (45).

Malaria Control During Pregnancy

The current WHO recommendation for malaria control during pregnancy (46) rely on the combination of the following strategies.

- Adequate case management of the clinical episode with effective and safe antimalarial drugs.
- Use of insecticide treated nets and other materials.
- Chemoprophylaxis through intermittent preventive treatment (IPT) in areas of stable endemicity, which is the administration of an antimalarial at specified intervals during pregnancy. At present, the only recommended antimalarial to be used in IPT is sulfadoxine-pyrimethamin; one dose to be administered at the beginning of the second trimester and the second during the third trimester.

Malaria and Nutrition

The association between malaria infection and nutrition is complex and the exact mechanisms have not been fully elucidated. Early observational studies noted that malaria episodes were associated with loss of weight in children (3). Another report suggested that undernourished children were protected against malaria infection and disease including CM (47). Two recent studies, however, showed that undernutrition was associated with increased malaria mortality *(48)* and more severe malaria-associated anemia *(1)*.

The causal association between malaria infection and nutrition can only be established through malaria control intervention studies, in which the nutritional status of protected and unprotected individuals is compared. Results from these studies suggest that protection against malaria infection is followed by an improvement in anthropometric parameters mainly observed in children *(2)*. Undernutrition may increase malaria severity and malaria infection may negatively affect nutritional status by reducing appetite *(49)* and increasing metabolic demands *(50)* among other factors.

Malaria and Iron

The safety of administering iron to individuals exposed to malaria has long been questioned. The discussion is based on the findings of a report showing an increased risk of malaria infections or episodes in individuals receiving iron therapy *(51)*. However, a meta-analysis of iron intervention studies concluded that iron supplementation did not significantly increase the incidence of infections (incidence rate ratio and incidence rate difference), irrespective of the quality of survey methods, methods of surveillance, route of iron supplementation, duration of supplementation, geographic location of the study population, or the baseline Hb concentration of the iron-supplemented group *(52)*.

Several practical conclusions can be drawn from the scientific evidence in relation to iron supplementation and malaria.

- Parenteral iron should be avoided because it increases the risk of malaria in pregnant women and infants and Gram-negative sepsis in neonates.
- Oral therapeutic iron should be administered concurrently with or preceded by effective antimalarial therapy.
- Prophylactic iron can be given to pregnant women exposed to malaria. An exception is women with Hb genotype AS because administration of iron in prophylactic doses is associated with no hematological improvement and with an increased risk of placental malaria infection.
- Prophylatic iron can be safely administered in low doses during the first year of life.

Malaria and Vitamin A

Vitamin A deficiency is prevalent in many developing countries including those where malaria is also endemic. Vitamin A supplementation reduces overall child mortality and the WHO recommends it as part of routine primary health care in developing countries. Plasma retinol has been negatively correlated with falciparum parasitemia *(53)*, but this could reflect an acute phase response rather than liver depletion *(54)*. Vitamin A supplementation to malaria exposed children reduced the risk of malaria episodes in an intervention study in Papua New Guinea *(55)*, but this finding was not confirmed in Ghana *(56)*. No conclusions can be drawn about the effect of vitamin A on malaria risk.

Malaria and Zinc

A study among Malawian children and pregnant women exposed to malaria reported inverse associations between zinc status and falciparum parasitemia *(57)*. An intervention study of zinc supplementation to children in Papua New Guinea found a reduction in the risk of malaria episodes in children receiving the supplements *(58)*, but this was not confirmed in a similar study in Burkina Faso, West Africa *(59)*. As with vitamin A, the interaction between zinc and malaria infection is not fully understood and more studies are needed before recommendations of zinc supplementation can be made.

Malaria and Folic Acid

Low infection rates were reported in pregnant women consuming a diet high in folates, and greater infection rates were reported in those with megaloblastic anemia *(60)*. However, malaria itself may induce folate deficiency. Some folic acid supplementation trials found no effect on malaria anemia *(61)*. In contrast, children experiencing malaria episodes who were treated concurrently with pyrimethamine-sulfadoxine, an antimalarial with antifolate properties, and high-dose folate supplements had increased frequencies of malaria parasitemias *(62)*. Whether this happens when folic acid is administered at the lower WHO-recommended dosage is unknown.

Malaria and Riboflavin (Vitamin B₂)

Riboflavin-deficient children and adults are less likely to be infected with malaria parasites *(63)*. However, studies in animals found that high-doses of riboflavin suppress parasite growth, suggesting that high-dose riboflavin therapy may be beneficial for malaria patients. This potential use of riboflavin remains to be studied in humans.

Conclusion

Adults living in malaria hyper- and holoendemic areas develop an immunity that is effective against severe disease and death. Children in sub-Saharan Africa suffer the greatest malaria morbidity and mortality. Apart from good empirical evidence that IgG is involved, there is no consensus on what constitutes the key determinants of protection or the mechanism(s) of immunity. Vaccine strategies aimed at inducing an adult-like immune status and duplicating the protection achieved by NAI in endemic areas would greatly diminish disease and death caused by *P. falciparum* in young children.

Pregnant women are vulnerable to both malaria infection and undernutrition. In stable malaria endemic areas, primigravidae and adolescent pregnant women are particularly susceptible to the infection owing to factors not yet well understood. In general, pregnant women require special attention by nutritional and malaria control programs.

The interaction between malaria infection and nutrition is complex. Malaria control intervention studies have consistently shown improvements in nutritional status in the protected groups, suggesting that the adverse effects of malaria on nutritional status are probably caused by the combined effects of decreased appetite and increased metabolic demands. Undernutrition is associated with poor outcome in infected individuals, but the mechanisms remain unclear. It is speculated that the immunomodulatory properties of different micronutrients are likely to be relevant in this interaction, but little is known about their metabolism in malaria infection. Despite the lack of definitive knowledge, the implementation of programs both to improve the overall nutritional status of populations exposed to malaria, especially the most at-risk young children and pregnant women, and to control malaria is essential to reduce the burden of malaria mortality and morbidity.

References

1. Verhoef, H., West, C.E., Veneemans, J., Beguin, Y., and Kok, F.J. (2002) Stunting may determine the severity of malaria-associated anemia in African children. *Pediatrics* **110**, 48–52.
2. Bradley-Moore, A.M., Greenwood, B.M., and Bradley, A.K. (1985) Malaria chemoprophylaxis with chloroquine in young Nigerian children. III. Its effect on nutrition. *Ann. Trop. Med. Parasitol.* **79**, 575–584.
3. Hendrickse, R.G., Hasan, A.H., Olumide, L.O., and Akinkunmi, A. (1971) Malaria in early childhood. An investigation of five hundred seriously ill children in whom a "clinical" diagnosis of malaria was made on admission to the children's emergency room at University College Hospital, Ibadan. *Ann. Trop. Med. Parasitol.* **65**, 1–20.
4. World Health Organization Expert Committee on Malaria. (2000) Twentieth Report, WHO Tech. Rep. Ser. 892, WHO, Geneva.
5. Borst, P., Bitter, W., Mcculloch, R., Vanleeuwen, F., and Rudenko, G. (1985) Antigen variation in malaria. *Cell* **82**, 1–4.
6. Bickle, A., Anders, R.F., Day, K., and Coppel, R.L. (1993) The S-antigen of *Plasmodium falciparum*: repertoire and origin of diversity. *Mol. Biochem. Parasitol.* **61**, 189–196.

7. Brown, K. and Brown, N. (1965) Immunity to malaria: antigenic variation in chronic infections of Plasmodium knowlesi. *Nature* **208**, 1286–1288.

8. Cheng Q, Lawrence G, Reed C, et al. (1997) Measurement of Plasmodium falciparum growth rate in vivo: a test of malaria vaccines. *Am. J. Trop. Med. Hyg.* **57**, 495–500.

9. Murphy, S.C. and Breman, J.G. (2001) Gaps in the childhood malaria burden in Africa: cerebral malaria, neurological sequelae, anemia, respiratory distress, hypoglycemia, and complications of pregnancy. *Am. J. Trop. Med. Hyg.* **64(1–2 Suppl)**, 57–67.

10. Warrell, D.A., Molyneux, M.E., and Beales, P.F. (1990) Severe and complicated malaria. *Trans. R. Soc. Trop. Med. Hyg.* **84(Suppl 2)**, 1–65.

11. Holding, P.A. and Snow, R.W. (2001) Impact of Plasmodium falciparum malaria on performance and learning: review of the evidence. *Am. J. Trop. Med. Hyg.* **64(1–2 Suppl)**, 68–75.

12. Newton, C.R.J.N., Taylor, T.E., and Whitten, R.O. (1998) Pathophisiology of fatal falciparum malaria in African children *Am. J. Trop. Med. Hyg.* **58**, 673–683.

13. Menendez, C., Fleming, A.F., and Alonso, P.L. (2000) Malaria-related anaemia. *Parasitol. Today* **16**, 469–476.

14. Day, K.P. and Marsh, K. (1991) Naturally acquired-immunity to *Plasmodium falciparum*. *Immunoparasitol. Today* **12**, A68–A71.

15. Baird, J.K. (1995) Host age as a determinant of naturally acquired immunity to *Plasmodium falciparum*. *Parasitol. Today* **11**, 105–111.

16. Alonso, P.L., Lindsay, S.W., Armstrong, J.R., et al. (1991) The effect of insecticide-treated bed nets on mortality of Gambian children. *Lancet* **337**, 1499–1502.

17. Snow, R.W., Omumbo, J.A., Lowe, B., et al. (1997) Relation between severe malaria morbidity in children and level of Plasmodium falciparum transmission in Africa. *Lancet* **349**, 1650–1654.

18. Gupta, S., Hill, A.V.S., Kwiatkowski, D., Greenwood, A.M., Greenwood, B.M., and Day, K.P. (1994) Parasite virulence and disease patterns in *Plasmodium falciparum* malaria. *Proc. Nat. Acad. Sci. USA* **91**, 3715–3719.

19. Marsh, K. (1992) Malaria—a neglected disease? *Parasitol.* **104(Suppl)**, S53–S69.

20. Kassim, O.O., Ako-Anai, K.A., Torimiro, S.E., Hollowell, G.P., Okoye, V.C., and Martin, S.K. (2000) Inhibitory factors in breastmilk, maternal and infant sera against in vitro growth of *Plasmodium falciparum* malaria parasite. *J. Trop. Pediatr.* **46**, 92–96.

21. Clark, I.A., Rockett, K.A., and Cowden, W.B. (1991) Proposed link between cytokines, nitric oxide and human cerebral malaria. *Parasitol. Today* **7**, 205–207.

22. Perlmann, H., Helmby, H., Hagstedt, M., et al. (1994) IgE elevation and IgE antimalarial antibodies in *Plasmodium falciparum* malaria: association of high IgE levels with cerebral malaria. *Clin. Exp. Immunol.* **97**, 284–292.

23. Kurtzhals, J.A.L., Adabayeri, V., Goka, B.Q., et al. (1998) Low plasma concentrations of interleukin 10 in severe malarial anaemia compared with cerebral and uncomplicated malaria. *Lancet* **351**, 1768–1772.

24. Kwiatkowski, D. (1990) Tumor necrosis factor, fever and fatality in falciparum malaria. *Immunol. Letters* **25**, 213–216.
25. Cohen, S., McGregor, I.A., and Carrington, S. (1961) Gamma globulin and acquired immunity to human malaria. *Nature* **192**, 733 737.
26. McGregor, I.A. and Carrington, S. (1963) Treatment of East African *P. falciparum* malaria with West African human gammaglobulin. *Trans. R. Soc. Trop. Med. Hyg.* **57**, 170–175.
27. Sabchareon, A., Burnouf, T., Ouattara, D., et al. (1991) Parasitologic and clinical human response to immunoglobulin administration in falciparum malaria. *Am. J. Trop. Med. Hyg.* **45**, 297–308.
28. Bouharoun-Tayoun, H., Oeuvray C., Lunel F., and Druilhe P. (1995) Mechanisms underlying the monocyte-mediated antibody-dependent killing of *Plasmodium falciparum* asexual blood stages. *J. Exp. Med.* **182**, 409–418.
29. Bouharoun-Tayoun, H. and Druilhe, P. (1992) *Plasmodium falciparum* malaria: evidence for an isotype imbalance which may be responsible for delayed acquisition of protective immunity. *Infect. Immun.* **60**, 1473–1481.
30. Marsh, K., Otoo, L., Hayes, R.J., Carson, D.C., and Greenwood, B.M. (1989) Antibodies to blood stage antigens of *Plasmodium falciparum* in rural Gambians and their relation to protection against infection. *Trans. R. Soc. Trop. Med. Hyg.* **83**, 293–303.
31. Moore, S.A., Surgey, E.G., and Cadwgan, A.M. (2002) Malaria vaccines: where are we and where are we going? *Lancet Infect. Dis.* **2**, 737–743.
32. Taylor-Robinson, A.W., and Smith, E.C. (1999) A role for cytokines in potentiation of malaria vaccines through immunological modulation of blood stage infection. *Immunol. Rev.* **171**, 105–123.
33. Good, M.F., Quakyi, I.A., Saul, A., Berzofsky, J.A., Carter, R., and Miller, L.H. Human T clones reactive to the sexual stages of *Plasmodium falciparum* malaria. High frequency of gamete-reactive T cells in peripheral blood from nonexposed donors. *J. Immunol.* **138**, 306–311.
34. Balde, A.T., Aribot, G., Tall, A., Spiegel, A., and Roussilhon, C. (2000) Apoptosis modulation in mononuclear cells recovered from individuals exposed to *Plasmodium falciparum* infection. *Parasite Immunol.* **22**, 307–318.
35. Hviid, L., Kurtzhals, J.A., Goka, B.Q., et al. (1997) Rapid reemergence of T cells into peripheral circulation following treatment of severe and uncomplicated *Plasmodium falciparum* malaria. *Infect. Immun.* **65**, 4090–4093.
36. Jakobsen, P.H., Hviid, L., Theander, T.G., et al. (1993) Specific T-cell recognition of the merozoite proteins rhoptry-associated protein 1 and erythrocyte-binding antigen 1 of *Plasmodium falciparum*. *Infect. Immun.* **6**, 268–273.
37. Menendez, C. (1995) Malaria during pregnancy: a priority area of malaria research and control. *Parasitol. Today* **11**, 178–183.
38. MacGregor, I.A. (1987) Thoughts on malaria in pregnancy with consideration of some factors which influence remedial strategies. *Parassitologia* **29(2–3)**, 153–163.
39. Verhoeff, F.H., Brabin, B.J., Hart, C.A., Chimsuku, L., Kazembe, P., and Broadhead, R.L. (1999) Increased prevalence of malaria in HIV infected pregnant women and its implications for malaria control. *Trop. Med. Int. Hlth.* **4**, 5–12.

40. Wickramasuriya GAW. (1937) *Malaria and Ankylostomiasis in the Pregnant Woman. Their more serious complications and sequelae.* Oxford University Press, UK, pp. 52,57.
41. Menendez, C., Ordi, J., Ismail, M.R., et al. (2000) The impact of placental malaria on gestational age and birth weight. *J. Infect. Dis.* **181**, 1740–1745.
42. Giglioli, G. (1972) Changes in the pattern of mortality following the eradication of hyperendemic malaria from a highly susceptible community. *Bull. WHO* **46**, 181–202.
43. Ordi, J., Menendez, C., Ismail, M.R., et al. (1998) Massive chronic intervillositis associated with malaria infection. *Am. J. Surg. Pathol.* **22**, 1006–1010.
44. Fried, M. and Duffy, P.E. (1996) Adherence of Plasmodium falciparum to chondroitin sulfate A in the human placenta. *Science* **272**, 1502–1504.
45. Lindsay, S., Ansell, J., Selman, C., Cox, V., Hamilton, K., and Walraven, G. (2000) Effect of pregnancy on exposure to malaria mosquitoes. *Lancet* **55**, 1972.
46. World Health Organisation. (2000) The African Summit on Roll Back Malaria. WHO, Geneva.
47. Edington, G.M. (1954) Cerebral malaria in the Gold Coast African: four autopsy reports. *Ann. Trop. Med. Parasitol.* **48**, 300–306.
48. Schellenberg, D., Menendez, C., Kahigwa, E., et al. (1999) African children with malaria in an area of intense *Plasmodium falciparum* transmission: features on admission to the hospital and risk factors for death. *Am. J. Trop. Med. Hyg.* **61**, 431–438.
49. Bruce-Chwatt, L.J. (1952) Malaria in African infants and children in Southern Nigeria. *Ann. Trop. Med. Parasitol.* **79**, 549–562.
50. Frood, J.D.L., Whitehead, R.G., and Coward, W.A. (1971) Relationship between pattern of infection and development of hypoalbuminaemia and hypo-beta-lipoproteinaemia in rural Ugandan children. *Lancet* **ii**, 1047–1049.
51. Murray, M.J., Murray, A.B., Murray, M.B., and Murray, C.J. (1978) The adverse effect of iron repletion on the course of certain infections. *Brit. Med. J.* **2**, 1113–1115.
52. Gera, T. and Sachdev, H.P.S. (2002) Effect of iron supplementation on incidence of infectious illness in children: systematic review. *Brit. Med. J.* **325**, 1142–1152.
53. Hautvast, J.L., Tolboom, J.J., West, C.E., Kafwembe, E.M., Sauerwein, R.W., and van Staveren, W.A. (1998) Malaria is associated with reduced serum retinol levels in rural Zambian children. *Int. J. Vitam. Nutr. Res.* **68**, 384–388.
54. Filteau, S.M., Morris, S.S., Abbott, R.A., Tomkins, A.M., Kirkwood, B.R., Arthur, P., et al. (1993) Influence of morbidity on serum retinol of children in a community-based study in northern Ghana. *Am. J. Clin. Nutr.* **58**, 192–197.
55. Shankar, A.H., Genton, B., Semba, R.D., et al. (1999) Effect of vitamin A supplementation on morbidity due to *Plasmodium falciparum* in young children in Papua New Guinea: a randomised trial. *Lancet* **354**, 203–209.
56. Binka, F.N., Ross, D.A., Morris, S.S., et al. (1995) Vitamin A supplementation and childhood malaria in northern Ghana. *Am. J. Clin. Nutr.* **61**, 853–859.

57. Gibson, R.S. and Huddle, J.M. (1998) Suboptimal zinc status in pregnant Malawian women: its association with low intakes of poorly available zinc, frequent reproductive cycling, and malaria. *Am. J. Clin. Nutr.* **67**, 702–709.

58. Shankar, A.H., Genton, B., Baisor, M., et al. (2000) The influence of zinc supplementation on morbidity due to *Plasmodium falciparum*: a randomized trial in preschool children in Papua New Guinea. *Am. J. Trop. Med. Hyg.* **62**, 663–669.

59. Muller, O., Becher, H., van Zweeden, A.B., et al. (2001) Effect of zinc supplementation on malaria and other causes of morbidity in west African children: randomised double blind placebo controlled trial. *Brit. Med. J.* **322**, 1–6.

60. Fleming, A.F. (1989) Tropical obstetrics and gynaecology. 1. Anaemia in pregnancy in tropical Africa. *Trans. R. Soc. Trop. Med. Hyg.* **83**, 441–448.

61. Fleming, A.F., Ghatoura, G.B., Harrison, K.A., Briggs, N.D., Dunn, D.T. (1986) The prevention of anaemia in pregnancy in primigravidae in the guinea savanna of Nigeria. *Ann. Trop. Med. Parasitol.* **80**, 211–233.

62. van Hensbroek, M.B., Morris-Jones, S., Meisner, S., et al. (1995) Iron, but not folic acid, combined with effective antimalarial therapy promotes haematological recovery in African children after acute falciparum malaria. *Trans. R. Soc. Trop. Med. Hyg.* **89**, 672–676.

63. Bates, C.J., Powers, H.J., Lamb, W.H., Anderson, B.B., Perry, G.M., and Vullo, C. (1986) Antimalarial effects of riboflavin deficiency. *Lancet* **1**, 329–330.

12 Acute Respiratory Infections

Ian Douglas Riley

Contents

Key Points

- Acute respiratory infections (ARI) cause more than 25% of all deaths in children under the age of 5 worldwide. Two-thirds of these deaths are as a result from pneumonia.
- Severe disease is an outcome of frequent exposure to pathogenic organisms, virulence, and host susceptibility.
- High acquisition rates of *Streptococcus pneumoniae* and *Haemophilus influenzae* by the upper respiratory tract predispose to pulmonary invasion.
- *S. pneumoniae* and *H. influenzae* capsular polysaccharide determines invasiveness and immunogenicity of these organisms. Polysaccharide is a weak immunogen in infants.

From: *Handbook of Nutrition and Immunity*
Edited by: M. E. Gershwin, P. Nestel, and C. L. Keen © Humana Press, Totowa, NJ

- The lungs are protected by an integrated set of biologic, mechanical, phagocytic, and immunologic defenses with built-in redundancies.
- The major risk factors for severe ARI are poor nutrition, indoor smoke pollution, and substandard living conditions.
- Undernourished children, very young infants, and HIV-infected children are susceptible to invasion by many different opportunistic pathogens. Nevertheless, *S. pneumoniae* and *H. influenzae* are the most important pathogens.
- Conjugate polysaccharide vaccines are effective in preventing pneumonia from *S. pneumoniae* and *H. influenzae*, but are too expensive for use in developing countries.
- Reduction of mortality from ARI depends on an integrated approach including promoting good nutrition, immunizing infants, controlling HIV transmission, and standardizing case management with selective treatment of pneumonia with antibiotics.

Introduction *(1)*

Acute respiratory infections (ARI) are the leading cause of death in children worldwide. Most ARI deaths are caused by pneumonia. The most recent data relate to 1998 when ARI caused 1.9 million child deaths, but a further 1.1 million ARI deaths were caused by specific diseases including 67% of all measles deaths, 83% of all pertussis deaths, and 25% of AIDS deaths in children. A further 10% of perinatal deaths were a result of pneumonia. All told, 28% of the estimated 10.8 million deaths in children under the age of 5 yr were caused by ARI and almost all of them occurred in developing countries.

ARI range in severity from the common cold to life-threatening pneumonia and are the most common cause for attendance at health services. Children in both developing and developed countries experience four to eight "coughs and colds" each year, but the incidence of severe ARI is 10–30 times higher in developing countries. Two bacteria–*Streptococcus pneumoniae* (pneumococcus) and *Haemophilus influenzae*—are responsible for two-thirds of all severe ARI cases.

A public health approach to ARI was slow to develop. In the early 1980s, the World Health Organization (WHO) sponsored research that defined the causative agents of severe disease in developing countries to standardize case management. The results showed that selective antibiotic treatment of severe ARI could reduce population mortality by 20–35%. A systematic review of risk factors identified interventions most likely to reduce severe disease and death. New vaccines were evaluated. In the early 1990s, ARI, along with diarrhea, malaria, measles, and undernutrition, were included in the WHO strategy for the integrated management of childhood illness (IMCI) that shifted the emphasis of case management from specific diseases to the sick child.

This chapter describes the interventions to control ARI as well as the reasons for the high morbidity and mortality rates found in developing countries. Severe ARI is the outcome of three sets of interacting factors. First, the frequency of exposure to pathogenic organisms. Second, virulence, which is the relative ability of organisms to cause severe disease. Third, host susceptibility.

Anatomical Classification and Pathology *(2–4)*

Official reports of morbidity and mortality are based on the International Classification of Disease. ARI are grouped into three categories, namely, acute upper respiratory infections, influenza and pneumonia, and other acute lower respiratory infections. Specific infections are grouped separately as are perinatal conditions.

It is standard clinical practice to classify ARI first by the anatomical site of maximum inflammation and second by causative agent (*see* Table 1). Inflammation of the respiratory system is a threat to life at three levels: at or about the larynx or glottis, in the bronchioles, and within the alveoli. Inflammation of the first two leads to obstruction of the airways, and of the third to diminished capacity to exchange gases. The work of respiration is increased either because of obstruction or of increased stiffness of the lungs.

In infancy, the airways are most narrow just below the larynx. Inflammatory swelling, typically from a viral laryngo-tracheo-bronchitis (croup) causes stridor—a harsh inspiratory sound. The effort of respiration brings accessory muscles of respiration into play and the child is seen to be in extreme distress. The whoop, heard in about one-third of cases of pertussis, is the sound of inhalation through an obstructed glottis following a paroxysm of coughing.

Bronchiolitis, commonly associated with respiratory syncytial virus (RSV) infection, leads to trapping of air, hyperinflation, and an expiratory noise or wheeze: respiratory effort is directed at the act of expiration.

S. pneumoniae and *H. influenzae* stimulate an outpouring of exudate into the alveoli, in which it is spread throughout the lungs. This results in a segmental or lobar pneumonia. At autopsy, pneumonic lung is solid and airless, and is described as being consolidated. Bronchopneumonia is caused by invasion of alveoli from the airways by bacteria frequently less virulent than those causing lobar pneumonia. Bacterial pneumonias cause dense opacities in chest radiographs. Infection with staphylococcus and Gram-negative bacteria may cause abscesses or empyema (pus in the pleural cavity).

Viral pneumonia causes lymphocytic infiltration of the interstitium and has a cytopathic effect in alveolar and bronchial cells. Typically, viral pneumonias

Table 1
Anatomical Classification of ARI by Site of Maximum Inflammation

Acute upper respiratory infections
- Nasopharyngitis (common cold, coryza)
- Otitis media
- Pharyngitis (sore throat)
- Tonsillitis
- Sinusitis (especially of the faciomaxillary sinuses)

Acute lower respiratory infections
- Epiglottitis
- Laryngitis
- Bronchitis
- Bronchiolitis
- Pneumonia

cause nodular or reticular opacities in chest radiographs. The radiographic appearances of bacterial and viral pneumonia overlap, however, and neither pattern is absolutely diagnostic.

WHO Clinical Classification *(2)*

Clinical Decision-Making

The WHO clinical classification is a severity-based classification that was developed for health workers untrained in auscultation and without access to radiography or laboratory support. It is used to make decisions about whether a child requires antibiotics and whether a child should be admitted to the hospital. It sets the criteria for referral between different level health facilities.

A history of cough or difficult breathing suggests that a child may be suffering from pneumonia. Fast breathing is the single most specific sign of pneumonia. Cut-off points are 60 breaths/min in infants under 2 mo old, 50 breaths/min in infants 2–11 mo old, and 40 breaths/min in children 1–4 yr old. Chest indrawing indicates severe pneumonia. It is a paradoxical movement of the lower part of the chest wall, flexible in infancy, which is drawn inward during inspiration. It is caused by increased work of respiration resulting in increased negative intrapleural pressure. It is to be distinguished from, but often associated with, indrawing of supracostal and intercostal soft tissues. The presence of these signs increases the specificity of the diagnosis.

Stridor in the calm child and central cyanosis are indications for immediate admission. A neonate with fast breathing or chest indrawing requires admission. A child over 2 mo old with chest indrawing also requires admission. A

Table 2
Summary of the Clinical Classification and Management
at the Periphery of the Child 2–59 mo With a History of Cough or Difficult Breathing

Clinical Signs	Classification	Management
Danger signs:		
• Convulsions this illness	Very severe disease	Admit to hospital for treatment and investigation
• Lethargic or unconscious		
• Unable to drink or breastfeed		
• Vomits everything		
Respiratory signs:		
• Chest indrawing	Severe pneumonia	Admit to hospital for antibiotics
• Cyanosis		
• Stridor in the calm child		
Fast breathing	Pneumonia	Treat with antibiotics at home
None of the above	Cough or Cold	Symptomatic treatment

child over 2 mo old with fast breathing, but not chest indrawing, has pneumonia and can be treated with antibiotics at home. Children with a history of cough or difficult breathing, but with none of these signs, have a "cough or cold" and should be treated symptomatically.

The IMCI also identifies certain danger signs that may be associated with pneumonia or with a nonrespiratory bacterial infection. Classification and management of children 2–59 mo old and of infants under 2 mo old are summarized in Tables 2 and 3.

Epidemiological Studies

The clinical classification is used increasingly as an outcome measure for epidemiological studies. In this classification, pneumonia refers to a mix of conditions including laryngeal obstruction, bronchitis, bronchiolitis, and pneumonia. Many such cases will not have radiographic signs of pneumonia. Acute lower respiratory tract infection (ALRI) is a more appropriate term.

The global estimates of mortality referred to at the beginning of the chapter depend heavily on the use of verbal autopsies (3). In general, the higher the mortality rate in a country, the more likely it is that a child will die without making contact with the health services. Verbal autopsy diagnoses are based

Table 3
Summary of the Clinical Classification and Management of Severe
Bacterial Infection and ARI at the Periphery for the Infant Under 2 mo of Age

Clinical Signs	Classification	Management
Danger signs:		
• Convulsions this illness	Possible severe bacterial infection	Admit to hospital for treatment and investigation
• Lethargic or unconscious		
• Less than normal movement		
• Unable to feed		
• Bulging fontanelle		
• Pus draining from ear		
• Fever or hypothermia		
Respiratory signs:		
• Severe chest indrawing	Severe pneumonia	Admit to hospital for antibiotics
• Nasal flaring		
• Grunting		
• Fast breathing		
• Stridor in the calm child		
Local signs:		
• Red umbilicus or draining pus	Local bacterial infection	Admit to hospital for antibiotics
• Skin pustules		
No fast breathing; no signs of pneumonia	Cough or cold	Symptomatic treatment

on field surveys and retrospective histories taken from mothers. Essentially, the diagnosis of ALRI depends on a history of cough and difficult breathing. The coexistence of malaria and measles reduces the specificity of the diagnosis. The tendency is to over diagnose if a study focuses on ALRI to the exclusion of other conditions.

Etiologic Agents of Respiratory Disease

Known Etiologic Agents

An extraordinary number of organisms are capable of invading the respiratory tract (*see* Table 4). Although some pathogens are strongly associated with particular diseases, no single pathogen is known to cause only the one disease, and no disease is caused by a single pathogen.

The principal causes of population mortality are *S. pneumoniae*, *H. influenzae*, influenza A virus, measles virus, RSV, and *Bordetella pertussis* (1,4,5). Each can cause severe disease in previously healthy persons. Recently described infective agents include the variant coronavirus that is thought to be responsible for the severe acute respiratory distress syndrome (SARS) and metapneumovirus, which appears to be responsible for a spectrum of disease similar to that of RSV (6,7).

Pathways of Spread and of Transmission (8)

Organisms enter the lungs by inhalation, aspiration, invasion from the upper respiratory tract, or from the blood stream. They exit the respiratory tract in secretions. Coughing and sneezing create aerosols and droplets. Microbial aerosols can be inhaled directly into the alveoli. Droplets and other large particles settle out quickly; organisms are transmitted directly through kissing and fondling or from contaminated objects (fomites). The fetus is susceptible to vertical transmission in the birth canal. Poor management of a birth delivery exposes the fetus to organisms from the mother's bowel, or from the hands of the mother or midwife. Organisms from the skin, such as *S. aureus* and *S. pyogenes*, can invade the lungs by way of the blood stream as do *Salmonella* from bowel.

An opportunistic pathogen as distinct from a true pathogen is an organism that is not capable of invading the body and causing disease in a healthy person, but able to do so in a person with weakened immunity. Although useful conceptually, the distinction between opportunistic and true pathogens is not clear cut. Virulence and its correlate invasiveness are relative rather than absolute properties of microorganisms. Opportunistic pathogens are less virulent and less invasive than true pathogens.

Activation of latent infections, for example, *M. tuberculosis* or cytomegalovirus, is also more likely in persons with weakened immunity.

S. pneumoniae and H. influenzae (9–11)

S. pneumoniae and *H. influenzae* are upper respiratory commensals and extracellular pathogens. They possess a polysaccharide capsule that appears to swell in the presence of specific antibody. On the basis of this reaction, more than 80 distinct serotypes of pneumococcus and seven serotypes of *H.*

Table 4
Respiratory Pathogens
and the Diseases They Cause

Coryza (common cold)
- Rhinoviruses
- Respiratory syncytial virus (RSV)
- Influenza viruses
- Parainfluenza viruses
- Coronavirus

Pharyngitis and tonsillitis
- Respiratory viruses as above
- Adenoviruses
- Coxsackie viruses
- Herpes simplex virus
- Measles virus
- *Corynebacterium diphtheriae*
- β-haemolytic *Streptococcus pyogenes*

Acute otitis media, acute sinusitis
- Respiratory viruses
- *H. influenzae*
- *S. pneumoniae*

Acute epiglottitis
- *Haemophilus influenzae* type b

Acute laryngo-tracheo-bronchitis (croup)
- Parainfluenza virus
- RSV
- Rhinoviruses
- Measles virus
- *Corynebacterium diphtheriae*

Acute bronchitis
- Respiratory viruses as above

Whooping cough
- *Bordetella pertussis*
- Adenoviruses

Acute bronchiolitis
- RSV
- Other respiratory viruses
- *Chlamydia trachomatis*

continued

Table 4 (*Continued*)
Respiratory Pathogens
and the Diseases They Cause

Pneumonia

- Respiratory cyncitial virus
- Parainfluenza 3 virus
- Influenza virus
- Adenoviruses
- Measles virus
- Cytomegalovirus (CMV)
- *S. pneumoniae*
- *H. influenzae*
- *Staphylococcus aureus*
- Gram negative bacilli
- *Mycobacterium tuberculosis*
- *Chlamydia trachomatis*
- *Mycoplasma pneumoniae*
- *Legionella pneumophila*

influenzae have been described. The capsule enables resistance to phagocytosis and determines the organism's immunogenicity and invasiveness. There are also non capsulated strains. Virulence factors include cell wall adhesins and a toxic protein, pneumolysin, which contributes to the inflammatory response.

Some serotypes and all non capsulated strains invade only rarely and can be regarded as opportunistic pathogens; noncapsulated strains fall into this category. Other serotypes are true pathogens. They are highly invasive, are rarely found as carriage organisms, and multiply in large numbers in the alveolar exudate that they provoke *(12)*. Immune competence against capsular polysaccharide is acquired serotype by serotype as a child grows older *(13)*. It is generally poor in children less than 2 yr of age, but competence against some serotypes is not attained until after the age of 5 yr.

Children in developing countries encounter these organisms at a much younger age and have much higher carriage rates than do children in developed countries. A study of neonates in the Papuan New Guinean highlands showed the mean age of acquisition of *S. pneumoniae* to be 17 d and of *H. influenzae* to be 31 d *(14)*. In contrast, the mean age of acquisition in a US series was 6 mo *(15)*. In the US series, acquisition was associated with subsequent disease in 15% of cases. Preschool children introduced pneumococcus into households. Day care has increased the prevalence of upper respiratory colonization of infants in the United States.

Case fatality rates correlate with the degree of invasion. In the preantibiotic era, case fatality in adults was shown to increase with the extent of pulmonary involvement, and again with bacteraemia. In the 1920s, less than 20% of adult patients with bacteremic pneumococcal pneumonia survived *(16)*. Today, in developing countries, bacteremia occurs in between 5 and 20% of children who have not received prior antibiotics. Case fatality is increased fivefold in these cases.

Respiratory Viruses

Coinfection with bacteria and viruses is common. Viral nasopharyngitis spreads bacteria through sneezing and coughing. Viruses damage respiratory epithelium and upregulate epithelial receptors for bacterial attachment. Only three respiratory viruses—influenza A, measles, and RSV—are independently associated with high mortality. These are enveloped RNA viruses that attach to respiratory epithelial cell membranes.

Influenza A Virus (17)

In temperate climate countries influenza A virus causes winter epidemics associated with high mortality in the very young and the old, but is not associated with a specific respiratory syndrome. It is frequently isolated from children with pneumonia in developing countries. Epidemics are associated with "drift" and pandemics with "shift" in the molecular structure of the haemagglutinin (HA) and neuraminadase (NA) glycoproteins that are required for attachment and exit from epithelial cells. Virulence is associated with the number of points on an HA precursor that can be cleaved by proteases. The more points at which this can take place, and the greater the number of host proteases that can cleave the virus, the greater the extent of its cell tropism and hence of its virulence. Bacteria, too, produce proteases that cleave the precursor and extend cell tropism.

The primary site of attachment is usually the epithelial cells of the tracheobronchus. Primary influenzal pneumonia is rare, but can be extremely severe. Secondary pneumonia due to *S. pneumoniae* or *H. influenzae* is comparatively common. Influenza vaccine is considered to be 60–90% effective providing it contains HA and NA antigens from current epidemic strains.

Measles (18)

Measles is a disease of epithelial surfaces, and is particularly severe in undernourished children. It causes immunosuppression and vitamin A depletion. Despite mass immunization and the elimination of measles from many industrialized countries, measles was still responsible for nearly 800,000 deaths in 2000. Vaccine coverage over 95% is required to eliminate measles from a population. Even with 80% coverage, the disease remains a major public health problem. Young infants experience very severe disease probably because they are exposed to a higher infective dose when an older sibling introduces the disease into a household.

An HA glycoprotein enables measles attachment to respiratory epithelium. Subsequent spread through the lymphatic system is followed by a secondary viremia and widespread infection of epithelium. The typical rash is caused by T-cell damage to virus-infected epithelial cells. Viral pneumonia early in the infection causes high case fatality. Later in the course of illness, secondary infection with *S. pneumoniae*, *H. influenzae*, *S. aureus*, or Gram-negative bacteria may develop. Coinfection with other respiratory viruses is also common.

Respiratory Syncytial Virus (RSV) (19)

RSV causes seasonal epidemics that often occur during the rainy season in tropical countries. Most bronchiolitis occurs in children under 12 mo old with the peak incidence at 2–6 mo of age. Immunity is not protective and reinfection occurs throughout life. The available evidence is that it is a leading cause of mortality from ARI worldwide—certainly the most important viral pathogen after measles *(7,20)*.

RSV infects upper respiratory mucosa. An asymptomatic period of 4–5 d is followed by nasopharyngitis with profuse discharge of secretions. Cough develops on about the seventh day and a wheeze about the eighth day. In cases of bronchiolitis, RSV infects bronchiolar epithelium producing edema and mucus secretion. The lumen contains thick plugs of necrotic debris. Virulence factors are not well understood. Trials of an inactivated virus vaccine in the 1960s did not protect against subsequent infection; 80% of the recipients were admitted to hospital and two died. These deaths appeared to be caused by a virus-induced cell-mediated immune process. Subunit vaccines are currently under development but routine immunization is thought to be 5–10 yr away.

HIV-Associated Respiratory Infection (21,22)

A vicious cycle involving HIV, tuberculosis, and undernutrition is now common in sub-Saharan Africa. Active tuberculosis hastens the onset of HIV. HIV and protein-energy deficiency suppress Th1 and macrophage functions and result in the reactivation of latent tuberculosis. HIV-1 and tuberculosis worsen nutritional status.

Bacterial pneumonia caused by the usual pathogens is common in HIV-1 infected individuals and is frequently associated with bacteremia, abscess formation, and empyema. *Pneumocystis carinii*, an airborne fungus, is an opportunistic pathogen of low virulence. It was first described as a cause of pneumonia in undernourished African children. *P. carinii* pneumonia is the most common cause of death in HIV-infected children in Africa.

Respiratory Defenses Against Bacterial Invasion of the Lungs *(23,24)*

The lungs are protected by an integrated set of biologic, mechanical, phagocytic, and immunologic defenses. Because the system contains redundancies, invasion is only likely to occur when more than one level of defense has been compromised. Commensal bacteria of the upper respiratory tract inhibit colonization by pathogenic bacteria including enteric Gram-negative bacteria. Colonization is also regulated by the availability of adherence sites, and secretory immunoglobulin (Ig) A. Undernutrition, passive smoking, abnormalities of mucociliary clearance, and antibiotics all increase colonization.

Branching of the airways and the consequent sudden alterations in the direction of airflow lead to the deposition of foreign particles onto epithelial mucosa. The mucus layer covering ciliated epithelial cells carries trapped particles upward to where they trigger the cough reflex and are expelled. Particles less than 10 mm diameter (PM_{10}) are sufficiently small not to be affected by turbulent airflow and can penetrate into alveoli where they are either deposited on alveolar walls or exhaled. Respiratory mucosa also secretes surfactant (that has antibacterial activity), immunoglobulins, and complement.

Successful eradication of bacteria depends principally on phagocytosis. Experiments on mice using a bolus of *S. aureus*, an extracellular pathogen, emphasize that inoculum size as well as bacterial virulence and the state of host defenses determine whether bacteria will be eradicated or not. At the lowest dose, 10^5 bacteria were completely cleared by alveolar macrophages. At the next level, 10^6 bacteria were cleared slowly but completely; this required a granulocyte response. 10^7 *S. aureus* evoked a marked granulocytic response, but the number of organisms remained constant. After the greatest inoculum of 10^8 *S. aureus*, the organisms proliferated; most of the mice died from pneumonia despite an even greater granulocytic response *(25)*.

Secretory IgA is the predominant immunoglobulin of the upper airways. IgA does not activate complement but neutralizes viruses and agglutinates bacteria. Mucosal immunity to bacterial polysaccharide matures much earlier than does systemic immunity. IgG enters the airways from the circulation, but is also produced in the lung. Deficiencies of immunoglobulin lead to infection by encapsulated extracellular bacteria.

Risk Factors

Poor nutrition, environmental pollution, and substandard living conditions all contribute to the high burden of disease and death from ARI. Increasingly, population-based descriptive and intervention studies that depend on household monitoring of disease events are using the WHO clinical definition of ALRI as their principal morbidity outcome. Verbal autopsies are used to measure disease-specific mortality. A WHO systematic review of interventions for the prevention of childhood pneumonia included a meta-analysis of potential risk factors. The more important of these are described below *(26)*.

The contribution of the major risk factors to the global burden of disease has also been assessed recently *(27)*. Low weight-for-age (below −1 standard deviation [SD]) was responsible for 9.5% of the total burden; vitamin A deficiency for 1.8%; zinc deficiency for 1.9%; and indoor smoke from solid fuels for 2.6%. Principal outcomes of poor nutrition were pneumonia, measles, diarrhea, and malaria. For indoor smoke they were ALRI and chronic lung disease. The effects of these risk factors are thus substantially mediated through ARI.

Nutrition

With the exception of measles, there is little theory and less evidence relating particular nutritional deficiencies to specific respiratory infections. Interactions and confounding among nutritional and other risk factors, the extent of the deficiency, the complexities of immunological deficits, and the multiplicity of opportunistic pathogens and respiratory syndromes make prediction difficult. Variation between populations in the effectiveness of nutritional interventions can be difficult to explain.

The association between vitamin A deficiency and measles is well established. Vitamin A deficiency causes squamous metaplasia and impairs the integrity of respiratory epithelium. Squamous metaplasia of the thymus was observed at autopsy in Filipino children who had died from pneumonia *(4)*. A meta analysis showed that the administration of massive doses of vitamin A to patients hospitalized with measles reduced case fatality by approx 60%; deaths related to respiratory infections accounted for 80% of mortality in these studies *(28)*. Furthermore, the administration of vitamin A to children older than 6 mo as part of a community-based prevention study reduced all-cause mortality by about 30%. This was associated with a reduction of diarrheal and measles mortality but not of pneumonia mortality. In community-based studies, vitamin A affected neither the incidence nor the severity of pneumonia *(29)*. No consistent effect of vitamin A supplements on the course of nonmeasles pneumonia has been shown in hospitalized children. Indeed, under certain circumstances, most notably in children who are not undernourished, vitamin A may increase the severity of respiratory infections. This may be because of a pharmacologic effect of the supplement on the inflammatory response. Vitamin A supplements are indicated for children with clinical evidence of vitamin A deficiency and for measles. They are not indicated for children with nonmeasles pneumonia *(29,30)*.

An important unifying hypothesis is that as deficiency of zinc or protein energy becomes limiting, the myeloid series of cells is maintained but lymphopoiesis is severely limited. In other words, macrophages and neutrophils are spared at the expense of humoral- and cell-mediated immunity *(31)*. Supplementation with zinc reduced the incidence of pneumonia by more than 40%. Zinc was effective whether serum levels were normal or low, whether the child was wasted or not wasted, or whether vitamins were administered concurrently *(32)*. The effect on mortality from ALRI is still not known.

The risk of dying from ALRI increases as weight-for-age decreases. The risk of dying from ALRI is four times higher in a child with a z-score below –2 SD than in a child with a z-score above 0. The incidence of pneumonia is higher in low weight-for-age children. Those with pneumonia and z-scores below –2 SD experienced case fatality rates about double those of children with normal weight-for-age *(33)*.

Breastfeeding reduces the frequency of infection with encapsulated organisms, even though breast milk has little effect on rates of upper respiratory colonization *(27)*. Breastfeeding reduces mortality from ALRI by about 50%, the effect being relatively constant during the first year of life *(34)*.

Indoor Air Pollution (35)

Because of poverty, more than 2 billion people rely on biomass fuels. Dung, crop residues, and wood are burned indoors in open fires or poorly functioning stoves. Industrial and vehicle emissions and tobacco smoke are other sources of indoor pollution.

Exposure to indoor air pollution varies greatly through the day and is greatest when a household member is closest to the fire—lighting the stove, adding fuel, stirring the cooking pot, and so forth. Women are more likely to be exposed than men. An infant may be carried on its mother's back or suspended in a cradle from the wall where the height, and hence the exposure, may vary.

The US standard for 24-h average PM_{10} is less than 150 mg/m^3. An intervention study in Kenya found PM_{10} in one house to be in excess of 7000 mg/m^3. Improvements to wood stoves reduced the incidence of ALRI by more than 50% in houses where PM_{10} was initially more than 1000 mg/m^3 *(36)*. Switching to charcoal as fuel would have been even more effective.

Upper Respiratory Carriage of Pathogenic Bacteria

Crowding and poor hygiene increase the transmission and acquisition of upper respiratory pathogens. A post-World War II longitudinal study of 1000 children in Newcastle-upon-Tyne, England, identified chronic upper respiratory infection as a significant precursor of ALRI *(37)*. A chronic nasal discharge is common in children living under conditions of poverty. Little attention has been paid to this phenomenon, which must necessarily increase the size of bacterial inocula to the lungs during sleep.

Interpretation of Etiologic Studies

Proving that a particular organism isolated from a patient with pneumonia has actually caused the disease is difficult. Because respiratory secretions may contaminate the lower respiratory tract, even organisms isolated from bronchoscopic aspirate may have been derived from the upper respiratory tract and not be invasive. Isolation from lung aspirate or blood culture is regarded as definite proof of invasion. However, now that the etiology of community-acquired pneumonia in developing countries has been established as the basis for the first line of treatment, it is no longer considered ethical to take lung aspirates for research purposes only. Vaccine trials, for example, now depend on blood culture as the only specific outcome measure available. Blood culture, however, is quite insensitive. An assay such as polymerase chain reaction (PCR) is sensitive, but its specificity is low because of its propensity to detect commensals, particularly if their total mass has been increased because of upper respiratory infection.

When more than one organism has been isolated from the same site, the known virulence of these isolates is the only guide to their pathogenicity. For example, in the 1980s, an influential study from Papua New Guinea confirmed *S. pneumoniae* and *H. influenzae* as significant pathogens *(38)*. The two organisms were isolated alone or in combination from more than 50% of patients with severe pneumonia. However, in 28% of cases, commensals of lesser virulence were isolated from lung or blood. These included non typable and non b serotypes of *H. influenzae*, *Moraxella catarrhalis*, *Staphylococcus epidermidis*, *Streptococcus viridans*, and *Acinetobacter*. It was concluded that even though the infants were likely to have poor immunity these organisms were not pathogenic. The most likely explanation of their presence in the lungs was that the child had inhaled a bolus of secretions and opportunistic pathogens had multiplied in the exudate stimulated by true pathogens. Even so, the question of whether vaccines should be developed against non b serotypes of *H. influenzae* remains open to debate *(38)*.

S. pneumoniae and *H. influenzae* have fastidious growth requirements. Also, they are more sensitive to antibiotics administered before admission to the hospital than *S. aureus* and the Gram-negative bacteria. Because of poor laboratory techniques, early studies underestimated the significance of these organisms. This problem still affects many hospital service laboratories today.

Patterns of Disease in Developing Countries

The significance of *S. pneumoniae* and *H. influenzae* as major pathogens was established during the 1980s. First-line antibiotic treatment guidelines were based on their susceptibility and resistance patterns. It needed to be known, however, whether the guidelines were valid for special groups such as undernourished children, very young infants, and children with associated HIV infection. Recent etiologic studies have focused on these susceptible groups. It must be remembered that hospital series reflect the pattern of pulmonary invasion and the relative importance of pathogens but, without a baseline population, do not indicate the true incidence of disease.

Clinical Undernutrition and ARI

Very few studies have examined the association between clinical undernutrition and ARI. A study in The Gambia in the early 1990s compared commensal organisms and pathogens in undernourished and well-nourished children with and without radiographic pneumonia. Children were enrolled if their weight-for-age was below 70% of the United States National Center for Health Statistics median or if they were edematous. One-half of the sample were undernourished, severely undernourished, or had edematous malnutrition (*see* Chapter 4). Measles and HIV infection were uncommon *(40)*. Carriage rates of *S. pneumoniae* and *H. influenzae* were high (more than 70%) in all children. These were also the most common invasive bacteria to be isolated. Gram-negative carriage and bacteremia, *Salmonella* bacteremia, and pulmonary *M. tuberculosis* infection were all more common in undernourished children. RSV infection was more common in well-nourished children. The undernourished children were susceptible to invasion by a wide spectrum of bacteria and viruses which, overall, were less virulent than the organisms causing pneumonia in the well-nourished group. These included both extracellular and intracellular pathogens, upper respiratory commensals, and blood borne organisms suggesting impairment of defenses at all levels. That undernourished children were less able to localize infection was suggested by radiographic consolidation being less well defined. The authors saw no justification for changing recommendations for first line therapy.

Serious Infections in Young Infants

Etiologically, pneumonia, meningitis, and sepsis in the neonate are part of a single problem of exposure and susceptibility. Because of their naïve, immature immune systems, very young infants have difficulty in localizing infection; clinical signs are not well expressed. Clinically, it is difficult to distinguish between these diseases. Case management strategies, therefore, tend to refer to the seriously ill infant rather than to anatomically classified diseases. Although the demographic definition of a neonate is an infant less than 1 mo of age, the boundary between the susceptible, very young infant and the older infant is not well demarcated.

In the 1990s, WHO coordinated a multicenter study in Ethiopia, Papua New Guinea, The Philippines, and The Gambia of serious infections in infants under 3 mo old *(41)*. Overall case fatality was 5.4%, being highest in the youngest infants: 63% of deaths occurred in children less than 1 mo of age, and 51% occurred in children less than 1 wk old. Case fatality of infants with clinical signs suggestive of serious bacterial infection and a positive blood culture was 30%. Between 4 and 11% of the children were bacteremic. Three organisms, *S. pneumoniae*, *S. aureus*, and *S. pyogenes*, accounted for nearly 60% of blood culture isolates. *S. pneumoniae* was the cause of more than 40% of cases of bacterial meningitis. Many different Gram-negative bacteria including *Acinetobacter* spp., *Klebsiella* spp., *E. coli*, and *Salmonella* spp. caused invasive disease. *Chlamydia trachomatis*, a sexually transmitted infection, was strongly associated with severe pneumonia in Papua New Guinea. These results are consistent with early and intense upper respiratory colonization by *S. pneumoniae* and *H. influenzae*. Most of the Gram-negative bacteremia was probably a consequence of poor birth delivery techniques. Guidelines for first-line antibiotics for neonatal pneumonia were revised to take into account the frequency of *Salmonella*.

HIV and Respiratory Infections (42,43)

The number of HIV-infected children, particularly in sub-Saharan Africa is continuing to increase. The countries that had contributed most to the disease burden from ARI in childhood are the same as those where HIV infection is now endemic. The clinical features of tuberculosis, bacterial sepsis, and *P. carinii* pneumonia overlap, but treatment guidelines have been slow to reflect this.

The prevalence of HIV in children in a South African population was below 5%, but HIV-infected children comprised 45% of hospital admissions for pneumonia and 85% of those who died. An HIV-infected child in the community was more than 40 times more likely to develop pneumococcal bacteremia, 20 times more likely to develop *H. influenzae* bacteremia, and 20 times more likely to develop tuberculosis than were non-HIV-infected children. HIV-infected children who were undernourished experienced even higher rates of bacteremia. *P. carinii* pneumonia was extremely common. These observations suggest global immune defects.

Conjugate Polysaccharide Vaccines

Conjugation of the polysaccharide to a carrier protein alters the immune response that becomes T-cell dependent. A conjugated polysaccharide vaccine is effective in young infants and stimulates immune memory. Hib conjugate vaccines, which were introduced into industrialized countries in the late 1980s, have been shown to prevent more than 90% of cases of invasive disease, principally meningitis. They prevent *H. influenzae* type b carriage so that in addition to a direct effect they have an indirect effect through "herd immunity." In randomized, controlled trials, Hib vaccines were shown to prevent more than 20% of radiographic pneumonia in Chile and The Gambia *(44,45)*.

Because of the larger number of potentially invasive serotypes, pneumococcal conjugate vaccines are more complex and more expensive to produce than the Hib vaccine. In the United States, a 7-valent vaccine was shown to prevent nearly 90% of invasive pneumococcal disease in children and more than 20% of radiographic pneumonia *(46)*. This vaccine was licensed in the United States in 2000. Since then, the incidence of invasive pneumococcal disease has not only declined by nearly 70% in children under 5 yr old, it has also declined markedly in adults *(47)*. In the absence of other causes, this suggests a herd effect. Currently, vaccine trials are underway in The Gambia and the Philippines. A South African trial should be reported shortly.

Although conjugate vaccines could be expected to have major impact on the burden of ARI, the Hib conjugate has not been introduced into a national immunization program in any country in Africa or Asia. The problem is one of cost. Even if the price were reduced to $US 1.50 per dose, vaccine cost per child for routine immunization in the poorer countries of Asia, including India and China, would rise from $4.50 to $6 *(48)*. This increase would represent between 1 and 3% of GNP in those countries where treatment costs are low. Paradoxically, high income countries with a lesser burden of disease have far greater financial incentive to introduce Hib conjugate vaccine because of comparatively high treatment costs. Pneumococcal conjugate vaccines are expected to be even more expensive.

Management of ARI by Peripheral Health Services in Developing Countries

International research and program development focus on cost-effective interventions. Peripheral health services are concerned with cost-efficiency, that is, with providing the highest possible levels of population coverage of interventions within the limits of a restricted health budget. Devolution of health services gives greater responsibility to local government and greater budgetary control to local politicians. Advocacy is needed to get the right mix of resources allocated to curative and outreach services, staff training, health promotion, transport, and logistics. Prepackaging of interventions, as with IMCI, should make advocacy and planning easier *(49)*.

A program based on case management raises questions about the equitable distribution of health resources. The health manager may need to advocate cost-effective treatment to both public and private sector physicians. In the event of life-threatening disease, families deserve the right of access to potentially life-saving drugs for their children at a cost that will not cripple them economically. Far too often, physicians prescribe a cocktail of drugs of which only one or two are likely to be effective. Drug costs, especially when drugs are purchased retail, tend to reflect international and not domestic cost structures. It is not unusual for a family to have to draw on their capital by selling farm animals, for example, because of a child's illness.

The incidence of severe ARI will reflect the socioeconomic status of the population as well as the adequacy of immunization, nutrition, and HIV control programs. Diagnosis and treatment require community health workers to have high levels of skill. High quality supervision is necessary. Drug supplies must be maintained. Management practices need to be integrated in primary, secondary, and tertiary facilities so that referral systems function efficiently.

The effectiveness of case management depends on the mother accessing services as soon as possible after the onset of fast breathing. Her decisions will depend on traditional beliefs, the severity of the infection, and her expectation of cost. Reduction of mortality from ARI still depends on selective treatment with highly effective antimicrobial agents.

References

1. Rasmussen, Z., Pio, A., and Enarson, P. (2000) Case management of childhood pneumonia in developing countries: recent relevant research and current initiatives. *Int. J. Lung Dis.* **4**, 807–826.
2. Rasmussen, Z., Pio, A., and Enarson, P. (2000) Case management of childhood pneumonia in developing countries: recent relevant research and current initiatives. *Int. J. Lung Dis.* **4**, 807–826.
3. World Health Organization. (1992) ICD10: inernational statistical classification of diseases and related health problems. 10th revision. WHO, Geneva.
4. Phelan, P.D., Olinsky, A., and Robertson, C.F. (1994) *Respiratory Illness in Children*. Oxford, England: Blackwell Scientific.
5. World Health Organization. (2001) IMCI: Integrated Management of Childhood Illneses. Model Chapter for Textbooks. WHO/FCH/CAH/00.40. Geneva: WHO.
6. Williams, B.G., Gouws, E., Boschi-Pinto, C., Bryce, J., and Dye, C. (2002) Estimates of world-wide distribution of child deaths from acute respiratory infections. *Lancet Infect. Dis.* **2**, 25–32.
7. World Health Organization. (2001) The World Health Report 2001. Mental Health: New understanding, new hope. Geneva: WHO. Accessed May 14, 2002, at http://www.who.int/whr/annex/en.

8. Stensballe, L.G., Devasundaram, J.K., and Simoes, E.A.F. (2003) Respiratory syncytial virus epidemics: the ups and the downs of a seasonal virus. *Pediatr. Infect. Dis. J.* **22**, S21–S32.
9. Peiris, J.S.M., Lai, S.T., Poon, L.L.M., et al. (2003) Coronavirus as a possible cause of severe acute respiratory syndrome. *Lancet* **361**, 1319–1325
10. den Hoogen, B., Garofalo, R.P., Osterhaus, A., and Ruuskanen, O. (2002) Metapneumovirus and acute wheezing in children. *Lancet* **360**, 1393–1394.
11. Evans, A.S. (1991) Epidemiological concepts, in *Bacterial Infections of Humans: Epidemiology and Control.* (Evans, A.S. and Brachman, P.S., eds.), 2nd ed. Plenum, New York.
12. Baltimore, R.S. and Shapiro, E.D. (1991) Pneumococcal infections, in *Bacterial Infections of Humans: Epidemiology and Control.* (Evans, A.S. and Brachman, P.S., eds.), 2nd ed. Plenum, New York.
13. Cochi, S.L. and Ward, J.L. (1991) Haemophilus influenzae Type b, in *Bacterial Infections of Humans: Epidemiology and Control.* (Evans, A.S. and Brachman, P.S., eds.), 2nd ed. Plenum, New York.
14. Salyers, A.A. and Whitt, D.D. (2002) *Bacterial pathogenesis: A molecular approach.* ASM, Washington, DC.
15. Smith, T., Lehmann, D., Montgomery, J., Gratten, M., Riley, I.D., and Alpers, M.P. (1993) Acquisition and invasiveness of different serotypes of *Streptococcus pneumoniae* in young children. *Epidemiol. Infect.* **111**, 27–39.
16. Douglas, R.M., Paton, J.C., Duncan, S.J., and Hansman, D.J. (1983) Antibody response to pneumococcal vaccination in children younger than five years of age. *J. Infect. Dis.* **148**, 131–137.
17. Gratten, M., Gratten, H., Poli, A., Carrad, E., Raymer, M., and Koki, G. (1986) Colonisation of *Haemophilus influenzae* and *Streptococcus pneumoniae* in the upper respiratory tract of neonates in Papua New Guinea: primary acquisition, duration of carriage, and relationship to carriage in mothers. *Biol. Neonate.* **50**, 114–120.
18. Gray, B.M., Converse, G.M., and Dillon, H.C. (1980) Epidemiologic studies of *Streptococcus pneumoniae* in infants: acquisition carriage, and infection during the first 24 months of life. *J. Infect. Dis.* **142**, 923–933.
19. Austrian, R. and Gold, J. (1964) Pneumococcal bacteremia with especial reference to bacteremic pneumococcal pneumonia. *Ann. Intern. Med.* **60**, 759–776.
20. Hilleman, M.R. (2002) Realities and enigmas of human viral influenza: pathogenesis, epidemiology and control. *Vaccine* **20**, 3068–3087
21. Duke, T. and Mgone, C.S. (2003) Measles: not just another viral exanthem. *Lancet* **361**, 763–773.
22. McIntosh, K. (1999) Pathogenesis of severe acute respiratory infections in the developing world: respiratory syncytial virus and parainfluenza virus. *Rev. Infect. Dis.* **13(Suppl 6)**, S492–S500.
23. Bustamente-Calvillo, M.A., Velszquez, F.R., Cabrera-Munoz, L., et al. (2001) Molecular detection of respiratory syncytial virus in postmortem lung tissue

samples from Mexican children deceased with pneumonia. *Pediatr. Infect. Dis.* **20**, 495–501.

24. Jartti, J. and van Miller, R. (1996) HIV-associated respiratory disease. *Lancet* **348**, 307–312.

25. Boelaert, .JR. and Gordeuk, V.R. (2002) Protein energy malnutrition and risk of tuberculosis infection. *Lancet* **360**, 1102.

26. Busse, W.W. (1991) Pathogenesis and sequelae of respiratory infections. *Rev. Infect. Dis.* **13(Suppl 6)**, S477–S485.

27. Ghaffar, F., Friedland, I., and McCracken, G. (1999) Dynamics of nasopharyngeal colonization by *Streptococcus pneumoniae*. *Pediatr. Infect. Dis. J.* **18**, 638–646.

28. Onofrio, J.M., Toews, G.B., Lipscomb, M.F., and Pierce, A.K. (1983) Granulocyte-alveolar-macrophage interaction in the pulmonary clearance of *Staphylococcus aureus*. *Am. Rev. Resp. Dis.* **127**, 335–341.

29. Kirkwood, B.R., Gove, S., Rogers, S., Lob-Levyt, J., Arthur, P., and Campbell, H. (1995) Potential interventions for the prevention of childhood pneumonia in developing countries: a systematic review. *Bull. WHO* **73**, 793–798.

30. Ezzati, M., Lopez, A.D., Rodgers, A., et al. (2002) Selected major risk factors and global and regional burden of disease. *Lancet* **360**, 1347–1360.

31. Fawzi, W.W., Chalmers, T.C., Herrera, M.G., and Mosteller, F. (1993) Vitamin A supplementation and child mortality: A meta-analysis. *J. Am. Med. Assoc.* **269**, 898–903.

32. Villamor, E. and Fawzi, W.W. (2000) Vitamin A supplementation: Implications for morbidity and mortality in children. *J. Infect. Dis.* **182(Suppl 1)**, S122–S133.

33. Ramakrishnan, U. and Martorell, R. (1998) The role of vitamin A in reducing child mortality and morbidity and improving growth. *Salud. Publica. Mex.* **40**, 189–198.

34. Fraker, P. (2000) Impact of nutritional status on immune integrity, in, *Nutrition and Immunology: Principles and Practice*. (Gershwin, M.E., German, J.B., Keen, C.L., eds.) Humana, Totowa, NJ, pp. 147–156.

35. Zinc Investigators' Collaborative Group. Prevention of diarrhea and pneumonia by zinc supplementation in children in developing countries: pooled analysis of randomized controlled trials. *J. Pediatr.* 135,689–697.

36. Victora, C.G., Kirkwood, B.R., Ashworth, A., et al. Potential interventions for the prevention of childhood pneumonia in developing countries: improving nutrition. *Am. J. Clin. Nutr.* **70**, 309–320.

37. WHO Collaborative Study Team on the role of breastfeeding on the prevention of infant mortality. (2000) *Lancet* **355**, 451–455.

38. Bruce, N., Perez-Padilla, R., and Albalak R. (2000) Indoor air pollution in developing countries: a major environmental and public health challenge. *Bull. WHO* **78**, 1078–1092.

39. Ezzati, M. Kammen, D.M. (2001) Indoor air pollution from biomass combustion and acute respiratory infections in Kenya: an exposure response study. *Lancet* **358**, 619–624.

40. Miller, F.J.W., Court, S.D., Walton, N.S., and Knox, E.G. (1960) Growing up in Newcastle upon Tyne: a continuing study of health and illness in young children within their families. Oxford University Press, London.
41. Shann, F., Germer, S., Hazlett, D., Gratten, M., Linneman, V., and Payne, R. (1984) Aetiology of pneumonia in children in Goroka Hospital, Papua New Guinea. *Lancet* **ii**, 537–541.
42. Shann F. (1999) *Haemophilus influenzae* pneumonia: type b or non-type b? *Lancet* **354**, 1488–1490.
43. Adegbola, R.A., Falade, A.G., Sam, B.E., et al. (1984) The etiology of pneumonia in malnourished and well-nourished Gambian children. *Pediatr. Infect. Dis. J.* **13**, 975–982.
44. WHO Young Infants Study Group. (1999) Serious infections in young infants in developing countries: rationale for a multicenter study. *Pediatr. Infect. Dis. J.* S4–S7.
45. Madhi, S.A., Petersen, K., Madhi, A., Khoosal, M., and Klugman, K.P. (2000) Increased disease burden and anitbiotic resistance of bacteria causing severe community acquired lower respiratory tract infections in children in human immunodeficiency virus type 1-infected children. *Clin. Infect. Dis.* **31**, 170–176.
46. Chintu, C., Mudenda, V., Lucas, S., et al. (2002) Lung disease at necropsy in African children dying from respiratory illnesses: a descriptive necropsy study. *Lancet* **360**, 985–990.
47. Levine, O.S., Lagos, R., Munoz, A., et al. (1999) Defining the burden of pneumonia in children preventable by vaccination against *Haemophilus influenzae* type b. *Pediatr. Infect. Dis.* **18**, 1060–1064.
48. Mulholland, E.K., Hilton, S., Adegbola, R., et al. (1997) Randomised trial of *Haemophilus influenzae* type-b tetanus protein conjugate vaccine for prevention of pneumonia and meningitis in Gambian infants. *Lancet* **349**, 1191–1197.
49. Black, S.B., Shinefield, H.R., and Ling, S. (2002) Effectiveness of heptavalent pneumococcal conjugate vaccine in children younger than five years of age for prevention of pneumonia. *Pediatr. Infect. Dis.* **21**, 810–815.
50. Whitney, C.G., Farley, M.M., Hadler, J., et al. (2003) Decline in invasive pneumococcal disease after the introduction of protein-polysaccharide conjugate vaccine. *N. Engl. J. Med.* **348**, 1737–1746.
51. Miller, M. (1998) An assessment of the value of *Haemophilus influenzae* type b conjugate vaccine in Asia. *Pediatr. Infect. Dis.* **17**, S152–S159.
52. World Health Organization. (1994) Health Facility Survey Manual: case management of acute respiratory infections. WHO, Geneva.

13 Diarrhea and Other Gastrointestinal Diseases

Douglas L. Taren

Contents

Key Points

- Diarrheas and gastrointestinal infections are a leading cause of childhood morbidity and mortality in developing countries.
- Undernutrition increases diarrheal morbidity by increasing the incidence, severity, and duration of infections.
- Increased diarrheal morbidity occurs with undernutrition primarily caused by impaired cellular immunity.
- The pathophysiology of diarrheal episodes is dependent on the infectious agent.
- Micronutrient supplementation, especially zinc and vitamin A, can have an important role in providing adjuvant therapy for diarrhea.
- Infectious gastrointestinal diseases may not cause diarrhea, but can continue to affect the immune system and, therefore, indirectly increase the onset of acute diarrhea.

From: *Handbook of Nutrition and Immunity*
Edited by: M. E. Gershwin, P. Nestel, and C. L. Keen © Humana Press, Totowa, NJ

- Impaired immune status, particularly cellular immunity, is a major risk factor for persistent diarrhea.
- Probiotics have an important role in the prevention and treatment of diarrheal diseases.
- Only a limited number of vaccines are available against agents that cause infectious diarrhea.

Introduction

Infectious diarrheas and gastrointestinal diseases are leading causes of childhood morbidity and mortality in developing countries. More than 1.4 billion cases of diarrhea occur each year leading to about 3 million deaths, most in children under 2 yr of age living in developing countries. A greater severity of diarrhea is often associated with reduced nutritional status and an impaired immune response. Persistent diarrhea can occur in 3–23% of all diarrheal episodes and accounts for about 40% of diarrheal-related deaths.

This chapter discusses the bidirectional interaction between nutritional status and gastrointestinal infections and the accompanying immune system response. Many intestinal infections are causative agents for diarrhea. However, many of the organisms that infect the intestinal tract do not overtly cause diarrhea, but their presence affects the body's immune system leading to comorbid conditions. The associations between nutritional status and the immune status presented in this chapter relate to those found among children living in developing countries, although they do reflect the physiological responses in all children.

Diarrhea and Gastrointestinal Infections

Various definitions can be used for diarrhea (1). The quantitative definition is a stool volume greater than 10 mL/kg/d. The clinical definition for acute diarrhea is a report of three or more loose or watery stools within a 24-h period. In both cases, the consistency of the stools is not firm. The severity of diarrhea can be determined by an increase in the total volume of stool produced or the number of stool movements in a 24-h period. The presence of steatorrehea (fatty stools), mucus, dysentery (blood), and the degree of dehydration are additional criteria for defining the severity of diarrheas. A diarrheal episode ends when the symptoms have stopped for at least 24 h.

Persistent diarrhea is defined as diarrhea that had an acute start, occurs for 14 or more consecutive days, is presumed to be caused by an infectious agent, and is not responsive to appropriate treatment. Undernutrition, including micronutrient deficiency, particularly zinc and vitamin A, impaired cell-mediated immunity, and not exclusively breastfeeding during the first 4 mo of life are risk factors for developing persistent diarrhea (2). The organisms associated with persistent diarrhea are usually different to those that started the initial

Table 1
Leading Causes of Diarrhea and Gastrointestinal Infections

Viruses	Protozoa
Rotavirus	*Entomoeba histolytica*
Adenovirus	*Giardia lamblia*
Astrovirus	Cryptosporidium
Calicivirus	*Isospora belli*
Cytomegalovirus	*Balantidium coli*
Torovirus	Cryptosporidium
Enteric Coronavirus	Microsporidium
Picobirnaviruses	
	Helminthes
Bacteria	*Ascaris lumbricoides*
Escherichia coli	*Trichuris trichuria*
Salomonella typhi	Hookworms
Shigella spp	*Stronglyloides stercoralis*
Clostridium difficle	
Vibrio cholerae	
Campylobacter	
Yersinia	
Aeromonas	
Plesiomonas	
Edwardsiella	

episode of acute diarrhea. This strongly suggests that children whose immune status is compromised during the initial episode of acute diarrhea are vulnerable to other infectious agents becoming established in the gastrointestinal tract. Once this happens, trauma to the intestinal epithelial tissues continues. Nutritional status and the cellular immune response deteriorate further, and persistent diarrhea becomes established.

Many different infections cause diarrhea. The most common include viral, bacterial, and protozoan infections that are normally present in the gastrointestinal tract (*see* Table 1). However, diarrhea can also be caused by infectious agents that are not usually associated with the gastrointestinal tract, such as malaria, and by noninfectious states such as celiac disease, allergic enteropathies, tropical sprue, and hereditary disorders. The epidemiology of infectious agents that cause diarrheas varies throughout the world. Rotavirus is the major viral agent and responsible for about 140 million diarrheal cases and 900,000 deaths/yr (1). The incidence of rotavirus infections peaks between 6 and 24 mo of age. However, other viruses also contribute significantly to diarrheal episodes and these include Norwalk-like viruses, adenoviruses, caliciviruses, retroviruses, and astroviruses. The toxins produced as a result of viral infections can have a direct effect on the enteric nervous system that control peristalsis and stimulate epithelial cells to secrete more water *(3)*, and it is hypothesized that this mechanism may also occur with bacterial infections such as cholera and infections with *Escherichia coli* (*E. coli*). If so, it may be possible to direct interventions at the enteric nervous system to decrease the amount of water lost in the increased volume of stools that is produced in many diarrheas.

The most common bacterial causes of diarrheas include *Shigella* bacteria and the intestinal toxin producing *E. coli*. Five strains of *E. coli* cause diarrhea: enterotoxigenic *E. coli*, enteroinvasive *E. coli*, enterohemorrhagic *E. coli*, enteropathogenic *E. coli*, and enteroaggregative *E. coli*. Each *E. coli* has its own mechanism of damaging epithelial tissue. The combined infections from *Shigella* and *E. coli* account for nearly 1 billion cases of diarrhea and 1.4 million deaths each year. *Vibrio cholerae* is also a leading cause of diarrhea accounting for 7 million cases and more than 100,000 deaths/yr *(4)*. Although there are often large outbreaks of cholera, the case mortality rates for cholera have decreased during the last decade *(4)*. *Clostridium difficile* is a spore-forming toxigenic bacterium that also causes diarrhea, but the proportion of diarrheas in the world caused by its occurrence is unknown as it most often occurs after a course of broad-spectrum antibiotics.

Protozoa and helminthes are the major intestinal parasitic infections associated with diarrhea. Protozoa are more commonly associated with diarrhea, but helminthes independently affect nutritional status and alter the anatomy and physiology of the gastrointestinal tract, making them important comorbid infections that increase the risk for diarrhea. Other parasitic infections that do not harbor in the gastrointestinal tract can also cause diarrhea, such as visceral leishmaniasis. The modes of action of intestinal parasitic infections are very different to those of viruses and bacteria, and they can also differ among each other. For example, *Entomoeba histolytic*, the infectious agent for amebic dysentery, is more likely to invade the intestinal epithelium causing traumatic damage to the intestinal lining and disrupting intestinal functions. In contrast, the protozoan *Giardia lamblia* is less invasive although it too can cause trauma to the intestinal lining. Diarrhea associated with *G. lamblia* leads to poor absorption and steatorrhea because the protozoa can attach themselves to the intestinal epithelial and, in sufficiently large numbers, they decrease the area available for digestion and absorption. Electron micrographs showed that *G. lamblia* can also change the microflora of the gastrointestinal track and create an environment that is favorable for more pathologic organisms *(5,6)*. Other diarrheal causing protozoa, such as cryptosporidium and microsporidium, are usually only present in children who have a reduced immune status.

Intestinal helminthes, such as hookworm and trichuriasis, can damage the epithelial wall without causing acute diarrhea. However, the ensuing blood loss lowers the body's immune response to infection as a result of the loss of iron and other nutrients and may be one of the reasons that helminthes may increase the risk for diarrhea (7,8). Similarly, infections with *Ascaris lumbricoides* (roundworm) may affect nutritional status notably vitamin A by shortening transit time and decreasing the absorption of fat and fat-soluble vitamins possibly as a result of damage to the gut wall (9,10). Intestinal helminthes are important comorbid infections along with other diarrheal causing agents.

The parasitic disease–diarrhea–nutritional status triad is a good example of the different ways that infections can alter nutritional status. Parasitic infections can decrease nutritional status, and thus the cellular immune response, through at least four distinct mechanisms (11): They can cause anorexia thereby reducing the availability of nutrients; increase the utilization and excretion of nutrients; several can effectively compete and sequester essential nutrients from their host; and, in adults, the infections can affect an individual's work capacity or productivity which, in turn, can limit their purchasing power thereby lowering the availability of nutrients for consumption by both the individual and their families.

Immune Response to Persistent Diarrhea

A cell-mediated immune response involving T-helper (Th) cells is responsible for providing the primary resistance against viral, bacterial, and protozoan and intracellular parasites. However, cell-mediated antibody-dependent immunity through a second type of Th cell is the primary immune response to extracellular parasites such as helminthes (12). In helminth infections, the Th2 cells secrete a series of interleukins (IL) that promote the production of IgE and IgG1. However, the cell-mediated Th cells produce interferon (IFN)-γ and IL-2 to promote macrophage activity and the production of IgG2a, IgG2b, and IgG3. Both systems can be affected by nutritional status and it is important to recognize that the gastrointestinal tract is the body's first level of defense against invasive organisms. Therefore, studying the response of the intestinal immunity against infectious agents with changes in nutritional status provide a model for understanding nutrition-immunity interactions.

Studies on helminth infections have indicated that undernutrition is associated with a decrease in Th2 cell responses including IgE, and parasite-specific IgG (12). Furthermore, a deficit in zinc and energy intakes may suppress specific cellular responses (13,14). More importantly, studies on nematodes have shown that in laboratory animals each nutrient may have its own role in modifying immune responses and is dependent on the nutrient, the infectious agent, and the location of the infection *(12)*.

Early exposure to infections may play an important role in decreasing a healthy child's risk of future diarrheal episodes. Lymphocyte subsets in children with greater exposure to gastroenteritis have peripheral blood lymphocyte profiles that are more similar to adults than children who have fewer episodes of gastroenteritis. In particular, several studies have indicated that early exposure increase the proportion of CD4 cells that display a memory phenotype *(15)*. The increased number of memory T-cells was similar to adult levels in these children who ranged from 6 mo to 3 yr of age. Furthermore, the increased number of memory CD4$^+$ T-cells occurred in children with acute diarrhea and not in children with upper respiratory infections, but this difference disappeared as children become older (closer to 3 yr of age). It may be possible that children who are undernourished early in life are not able to rapidly develop the memory cells and this places them at risk for future infections. Thus, early and controlled exposure to potential infectious agents is important when a very young child has a good nutritional status and responsive immune system. Early undernutrition in the first year of life may increase the risk for diarrheal mortality over a period of time.

Persistent diarrhea is associated with severe morphological changes in the microvilli as well as the permeability of the small intestine. Several studies in the Gambia showed that children with persistent diarrhea had chronic cell-mediated enteropathy, a high number of intraepithelial lymphocytes and an increased number of activated T cells, and a decreased number of B-cells *(16)*. Studies in Bangladesh have looked at the immune response of children who developed persistent diarrhea following acute diarrhea caused by rotavirus infection *(17)*. Among all the observed parameters for the cellular immune response, only an elevated IFN-γ level was associated with the development of persistent diarrhea compared with acute diarrhea. However, only 29 of the 149 children with an initial diarrhea were diagnosed with rotavirus and only 10 of these children developed persistent diarrhea. More studies are needed to determine which immune reactions play the major roles in the development of persistent diarrhea.

Expanding the Undernutrition-Diarrhea Interaction Paradigm

The association between undernutrition and diarrhea can be a vicious cycle. Simply stated, poor nutritional status increases a child's susceptibility to infection and infection decreases a child's nutritional status. This cycle continues until there is a successful intervention. The use of appropriate nutrition interventions can be an important adjuvant to conventional therapies during diar-

Table 2
Nutrition Interventions As an Adjuvant to Diarrhea Prevention and Treatment

Nutrition Intervention	Results
Zinc	Decrease duration and severity of acute and persistent diarrhea with doses of 20 mg/d
Iron	Parenteral administration is life-threatening. Iron supplement in nonmalarial areas may be beneficial for lowering the risk of diarrhea in nonbreastfed infants. However, nondiscretionary iron supplementation may slightly increase the risk of diarrhea. Breastmilk has greater advantages compared with iron-fortified formula for preventing diarrhea
Vitamin A	Supplements decrease the severity of diarrheal episodes and diarrhea case-fatality rates. However, equivocal results exist regarding vitamin A supplementation on the incidence of diarrhea
Protein and Energy	Decreased wasting and stunting associated with lower incidence, severity, and duration of diarrhea primarily through improved cellular immunity
Probiotics	Consumption of specific lactic acid producing organisms reduces the incidence of diarrheal infections by as much as 50%

rheal episodes. Thus, nutrition interventions need to be included in the current undernutrition-diarrhea paradigm (*see* Fig. 1). A variety of interventions have now been studied (*see* Table 2) including the use of micronutrients and probiotics.

Poor nutritional status is not only related to the onset of an initial diarrheal episode, but also to the severity of the episodes and the duration of the diarrheal episode including the development of persistent diarrhea (*18–20*). This suggests the existence of a specific undernutrition-diarrhea cycle that is mediated by the lack of a proper immune response. Infectious diarrheas induce undernutrition by inducing catabolic cytokines such as tumor necrosis factor (TNF) and IL-1, IL-6, and IL-8 (*17,21,22*). Undernutrition, usually defined as wasting or underweight, inhibits the repair of intestinal tissue because of a slower production of mature epithelial cells resulting in immature crypts. Trauma to the gastrointestinal epithelium causes a flattening of the microvilli

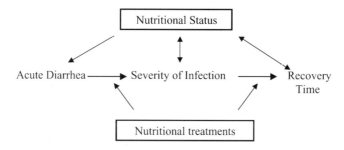

Fig. 1. Expansion of the two-way interaction between nutritional status and infection.

Table 3
The Nine Pillars of Good Treatment of Acute Gastroenteritis

1. Use of oral rehydration therapy
2. Hypotonic solution (Na 60mmol/L, glucose 74–11 mmol/L (industrialized countries only)
3. Fast oral rehydration, over 3–4 h
4. Rapid realimentation with normal feeding (including solids) thereafter.
5. Use of special formula is unjustified
6. Use of diluted formula is unjustified
7. Continuation of breast feeding at all times
8. Supplementation with oral rehydration solution for ongoing losses
9. No unnecessary medication

Source: Ref. 23.

and significantly decreases the absorptive surface of the small intestines. This leads to malabsorption and poor electrolyte balance and thus changes the intestinal environment, which makes it possible for opportunistic pathogens to colonize and continue the cycle of diarrhea.

The nine pillars of good treatment of acute gastroenteritis developed by the European Society of Pediatric Gastroenterology, Hepatology, and Nutrition (ESPHGHN) are based on the oral rehydration therapy, feeding the sick child, continuous breastfeeding, and limiting unnecessary interventions (see Table 3) (23). These pillars are appropriate for children in developing countries with one exception. The World Health Organization (WHO) recommends a greater sodium content for oral rehydration solution compared with the hypotonic solution recommended by the ESPHGHN (24). Other treatment strategies for diarrhea still need to be scrutinized including the use of smectite (unabsorbable clay) that is popular in some areas because it increases the appearance of formed stools, but it may be masking the loss of liquid (25).

Although a child's initial nutritional status has been the focus of increased risk for diarrheal morbidity and mortality, nutrition interventions during acute infections are being tested as an adjuvant to traditional interventions. Zinc supplementation during an acute diarrheal episode reduces both the duration and severity of acute and persistent diarrhea within a certain set of define parameters *(26)*. About 20 mg/d of zinc, or twice the recommended daily allowance (RDA), is needed. Zinc supplementation resulted in a 15% lower probability that acute diarrhea would continue on any given day and it decreased the probability of having an acute diarrheal episode for at least 7 d by 27%. The results for acute diarrhea did not vary by child age, gender, or nutritional status as measured by weight-for-age. Zinc supplementation also reduced the risk of continuing diarrhea by 24% in children who entered treatment with persistent diarrhea. However, in contrast to the results for acute diarrhea, the effect of zinc supplementation on persistent diarrhea was only significant for male children below 12 mo of age who were wasted at the start of treatment.

Vitamin A supplementation decreases the risk of mortality in infants and young children. Much of the decrease in case mortality is associated with lower case-fatality rates from diarrhea *(27,28)*. A meta-analysis on the affect of vitamin A supplementation on the incidence of diarrheal episodes provided equivocal results. The same analysis indicated that vitamin A supplementation reduces the severity and duration of diarrheal diseases *(29)*. This suggests that vitamin A is able to prevent the death of children who may have the pathology, but it has little affect in children whose diarrhea is not severe and who would not die without the supplement. The mechanism for the lower case-fatality rates in children with severe diarrhea may be by upregulating the cellular immune systems of the weakest children during diarrheal episodes *(29)*.

Although zinc and vitamin A supplementation are beneficial for managing diarrheal disease, the situation with iron is different—particularly in malaria endemic areas. Treating iron deficiency reverses impaired immune responses, but no studies have looked at its effect as an adjuvant to diarrheal treatments. A meta-analysis of the effect of iron supplementation on infectious disease found children supplemented with iron are at 11% greater risk of developing diarrhea, but this translated to only 0.05 episodes per child year *(30)*. In a comprehensive review on the association between iron and immunity and infection, Oppenheimer *(31)* concluded "that breast milk confers greater advantages than powdered milk, iron fortified or otherwise" for reducing the risk of diarrhea.

Probiotics, the use of live microorganisms of human origin to improve health, have been shown to be a successful strategy to prevent diarrheal infections *(32)*. The major probiotics studied in conjunction with diarrhea are *Lactobacillus GG, Bifidobacterium, Streptococcus thermophilous*, and

Saccharomyces boulardii (nonhuman origin). Studies with *Lactobacillus GG* reduced the incidence in diarrheal episodes in formula-fed infants. *Lactobacillus GG* also reduced non-*Clostridium difficile* antibiotic induced diarrhea by 66% when children weighing less than 12 kg were given two capsules containing $\geq 10^{10}$ organism. *Lactobacillus GG* also reduced the risk of traveler's diarrhea by 25–50%. The mechanism for these outcomes may be a direct competition to the colonization of the gastrointestinal tract. However, it is also known that these lactic acid bacteria may be improving immune function by enhancing phagocytosis, cellular immune response, and the humoral immune response.

Infant Feeding Patterns

The most important nutritional prevention of infant diarrheas is breast-feeding along with the introduction of liquids and solids at the appropriate age. Thus, infant feeding practices have a strong effect on the likelihood of a child developing diarrhea, as well as being an antecedent for undernutrition.

Studies on the pattern of infant feeding in Lima, Peru, described an environment that led to a high incident of diarrhea (33). In this community, formula milk was introduced at an early age along with other liquid foods and, by 4 mo of age, more than 80% of infants were consuming a liquid other than breast milk. Close monitoring of infant feeding and diarrheal episodes, through home visits every third day, showed that the relative risk for both the number and the duration of diarrheas was significantly greater in children not exclusively breastfed. Infants fully weaned before 6 mo of age who were receiving formula milk were three times more likely to get diarrhea than those who were exclusively breastfed: The incidence rate for diarrhea increased from 7.6 to 26.1 per 100 d of observation. The trend continued for infants who were both breastfed and receiving complementary food. Furthermore, formula-fed infants were at five times-greater risk of being ill for more days. This study illustrates both the clear benefit of exclusively breastfeeding to limit diarrheal morbidity to a minimum and also the detrimental affect of introducing complementary food too early.

Exclusive breastfeeding can also prevent acute diarrhea from becoming persistent diarrhea (34). The continuation of breastfeeding during diarrheal episodes provides children with a number of substances that protect against infections. Both specific and nonspecific immune substances such as lymphocytes, macrophages, and secretary IgA assist infected hosts with combating infectious agents. At the same time, breast milk promotes the repair of damaged epithelial tissues (35,36). The naturally low pH in the intestinal tract, along with exclusive breastfeeding, promotes the growth of probiotics, especially bifidobacterium. An effective treatment for persistent diarrhea in the

Table 4
WHO Recommendations for Treating Persistent Diarrhea

Continue breastfeeding
Provide a nutritious age-appropriate diet
Limit the content of lactose from animal milk
Provide at least 110 kcal/kg/d of energy
Include supplementary vitamins and minerals
Feed small amounts of food at one time, at least six times/d

Source: Ref. *25.*

young child includes breast milk along with age-appropriate feeding practices (*see* Table 4).

Most children can be treated at home for persistent diarrhea if proper nutrition can be provided and action is taken to prevent dehydration. However, some children may need to be hospitalized. The criteria for hospitalization include cases with moderate or severe dehydration in children who are not candidates for enteral feeds or with stool outputs that can exceed 30 g/kg/d. Nonetheless, any partial parental nutrition is only feasible in specialized hospitals in developing countries *(7)*. Children with serious systemic infectious such as pneumonia or sepsis also need to be admitted and observed. Special care must also be given to younger infants. Infants less than 4-mo-old should be cared for in a clinic or hospital setting.

Diarrheal Vaccines

The development of vaccines to prevent and treat diarrheas is underway. Vaccines to provide both active and passive immunity are being developed (*see* Table 5). The most promising progress has been made for rotavirus and cholera *(4,37)*, but studies are ongoing for *Shigella* and *E. coli* vaccines *(38)*. Vaccines for larger parasites such as *Entomoeba histolytica*, *Giardia lamblia*, and helminthes have required different approaches. For helminthes, the goal of an effective vaccine is to reduce the worm burden to a nonpathologic level rather than to provide sterilizing immunity or to focus on reducing the pathologic properties of the helminthes *(39)*. The approach being followed in the development of nematode vaccines is also to target parasite molecules that are required for nutrition or survival *(40)*. Hyperimmune milk has been investigated for cryptosporidium and other small protozoa and may provide some protection for at-risk individuals *(17)*. A hyperimmune bovine colostrum product is also available for rotavirus and is licensed in Australia *(41)*.

Data on the efficacy of diarrhea preventing vaccines are limited. At most, only data on basic protection are available for the viral and bacterial vaccines. Few trials have determined how much protection the vaccines provide when

Table 5
Immunological Approaches to Preventing Selected Diarrheal Diseases

Active Immunity (Vaccinations)	Passive Immunity (Hyperimmune Colostrum)	Targeted Immunity (Harm Reduction)
	Rotavirus	Hookworm
Rotavirus	Cryptosporidium	
Cholera	Enterotoxic *E. coli*	
Shigella	*Clostridium difficile*	
Campylobacter	Campylobactor	
Enterotoxic *E. coli*		
Salomenella typhi		

Source: Refs. *1, 39, 40.*

given to children with different nutritional status or concomitant infections. This is an important consideration because there is some evidence that polio vaccine is not completely protective when given to infants who have diarrhea *(42)*. This is clearly an important concern and may be specific to an oral vaccine compared with intramuscular injections.

Three oral cholera vaccines are currently available and licensed in some countries *(4)*. The development of these vaccines took different routes. One vaccine comprises killed whole-cell *V. cholerae* O1 with a purified subunit of the cholera toxin (WC/rBS). The vaccine provides 85–95% protection for at least 6 mo after two administrations 1 wk apart. Booster doses can be given every 6 mo. Protection remains high at about 60% 6 mo later, but may decline rapidly after this. A similar vaccine has been developed with the purified subunit and field trials suggest it has 66% protection at 8 mo. The third vaccine is an attenuated live oral genetically modified *V. cholerae* O1 strain that provides 95% protection after one dose for *V. cholerae* and 65% protection against *V. cholerae* El Tor for at least 3 mo. Given these results, the WHO has recommended giving the WC/rBS to populations that are at risk for a cholera outbreak within 6 mo *(4)*.

A tetravalent rhesus rotavirus vaccine has been developed and tested in several field trials. Vaccine effectiveness varied between developed and developing countries. Under more ideal conditions, the vaccine is able to prevent 50–70% of all rotavirus cases and 70–90% of severe rotavirus cases. However, reports from in Brazil and Peru suggested that the effectiveness of the vaccine was 35–66% *(37)*. The vaccine schedule indicates it is to be given in three doses at ages 2, 3, and 6 mo. Adverse effects have been reported, including fever after the first dose and the risk of adverse effects increase with age. The most serious adverse effect reported was intussusception (bowel obstruction) among infants during the first 1–2 wk following vaccination. Fifteen cases were reported from September 1998 to July 1999. Based on these findings, the Advisory Committee on Immunization Practices for the US Centers for Disease Control and Prevention recommended the suspension of the rotavirus vaccine until further studies could be conducted *(43,44)*.

Conclusion

Undernutrition is a major causal factor for persistent diarrhea because it depresses the cell-mediated response and delays repair of the intestinal epithelium. Acute diarrheal episodes elicit an immune response that exacerbates undernutrition by inducing anorexia and increased catabolism. The mechanisms underlying the interaction between diarrhea and undernutrition continue to be elucidated in order to develop appropriate prevention and treatment protocols. The issues that have to be identified when examining this association include the specific pathogenic agents involved, the energy/nutrients (macronutrients and/or micronutrients) required for prevention and treatment, and the temporal sequence between nutritional status and infection. Prevention and treatment protocols for diarrheas, in most cases, will be similar and include preventing dehydration, breastfeeding, and providing an age-appropriate diet. Other nutrition interventions, such as zinc supplementation, are being recognized as additional adjuvant to the treatment of diarrhea. In measuring the outcome of interventions, public health professionals and clinicians must focus not only on the incidence of diseases, but also the severity and duration of diarrheal episodes including the development of persistent diarrhea.

Nutritional interventions must also be accompanied by other preventive behaviors to decrease a child's exposure to infectious agents. Good access to safe water and sanitation facilities is critical for decreasing exposure to pathogens. Improved hygiene from hand washing at home and in child- or day-care centers will also prevent infections and epidemics of infectious diarrheas. Personal hygiene and public health interventions need to work hand in hand to decrease the incidence of diarrhea and the devastating outcomes associated with it. The morbidity and mortality associated with diarrhea is a priority for improving the health of children worldwide. Millions of childhood deaths can only be averted by improved nutrition and hygiene. Public health and clinical approaches to preventing and treating diarrhea need to incorporate proven nutritional strategies. These strategies include micronutrient supplementation, food-based programs, and community education programs. The general public and health care professionals need to be aware of the effect that nutrition interventions can have on decreasing diarrheal morbidity and mortality. Thus, the new knowledge that is rapidly being accumulated on how nutrition and infant feeding practices improve the lives of children need to be incorporated into daily practice.

References

1. Davidson, G., Barnes, G., Bass, D., et al. (2002) Infectious diarrhea in children: working group report of the first world congress of pediatric gastroenterology, hepatology, and nutrition. *J. Pediatr. Gastroenterol. Nutr.* **35**, S143–S150.
2. Bhutta, Z.A. and Hendricks, K.M. (1996) Nutritional management of persistent diarrhea in childhood: a perspective from the developing world. *J. Pediatr. Gastroenterol. Nutr.* **22**, 17–37.
3. Lundgren, O., Peregrin, A.T., Persson, K., Kordasti, S., Uhnoo, I., and Svensson, L. (2000) Role of the enteric nervous system in the fluid and electrolyte secretion of rotavirus diarrhea. *Science* **287**, 491–495.
4. World Health Organization. (2002) Cholera 2001. *Weekly epidemiological record.* **31**, 257–268.
5. Tandon, B.N., Puri, B.K., Gandhi, P.C., et al. (1974) Mucosal surface injury of jejunal mucosa in patients with giardiasis an electron microscope study. *Ind. J. Med. Res.* **62**, 1838–1842
6. Tandon, B.N., Tandon, R.K., Sapathy, B.K., et al. (1971) Mechanism of malabsorption in giardiasis: a study of bacterial flora and bile salt deconjugation in upper jejunum. *Gut* **18**, 176–181.
7. Ighogboja, I.S. and Ikeh, E.I. (1997) Parasitic agents in childhood diarrhoea and malnutrition. *West Afr. J. Med.* **16**, 36–39.
8. Nwabuisi, C. (2001) Childhood cryptosporidiosis and intestinal parasitosis in association with diarrhoea in Kwara State, Nigeria. *West Afr. J. Med.* **20**, 165–168.
9. Taren, D.L., Nesheim, M.C., Crompton, D.W.T., et al. (1987) Contributions of ascariasis to poor nutritional status of children from chiriqui province, Republic of Panama. *Parasitol.* **95**, 603–613.
10. Brown, J.H., Gilman, R.H., Khatun, M., et al. (1980) Absorption of macronutrients from a rice-vegetable diet before and after treatment of ascariasis in children. *Am. J. Clin. Nutr.* **33**, 1875–1882.
11. Taren, D.L. and Crompton, D.W.T. (1990) Mechanisms for interactions between parasitism and nutritional status. *Clin. Nutr.* **8**, 227–238.
12. Koski, K.G. and Scott, M.E. (2001) Gastrointestinal nematodes, nutrition and immunity: breaking the negative spiral. *Ann. Rev. Nutr.* **21**, 297–321.
13. Sazawal, S., Jalla, S., Mazumder, S., Sinha, A., et al. (1997) Effect of zinc supplementation on cell-mediated immunity and lymphocyte subsets in preschool children. *Ind. Pediatr.* **34**, 589–597.
14. McMurray, D.N., Watson, R.R., and Reyes, M.A. (1981) Effect of renutrition on humoral and cell-mediated immunity in severely malnourished children. *Am. J. Clin. Nutr.* **34**, 2117–2126.
15. Granot, E., Rabinowitz, R., and Schlesinger, M. (1999) Lymphocyte subset profile of young healthy children residing in a rural area: possible role of recurrent gastrointestinal infections. *J. Pediatr. Gastroenetrol. Nutr.* **28**, 147–151.

16. Sullivan, P.B. (2002) Studies of the small intestines in persistent diarrhea and malnutrition: the gambian experience. *J. Pediatr. Gastroenetrol. Nutr.* **34**, S11–S13.
17. Azim, T., Ahmed, S., Sefat-E-Khuda, et al. (1999) Immune response of children who develop persistent diarrhea following rotavirus infection. *Clin. Diagn. Lab. Immunol.* **6**, 690–695.
18. Food and Nutrition Board. (1992) Relation between nutrition and diarrhea, in *Nutrition Issues in Developing Countries*. National Academy of Sciences, Washington, DC, pp. 21–41.
19. Bhandari, N., Bhan, M.K., Sazawal, S., et al. (1989) Association of antecedent malnutrition with persistent diarrhea-a case control study. *Brit. Med. J.* **298**, 1284–1297.
20. Deivanayagam, N., Mala, N., Ashok, T.P., et al. (1992) Risk factors for persistent-diarrhea among children under 2 years of age: case control study. *Ind. J. Pediatr.* **30**, 177–185.
21. Kutukeuler, N., Caglayan. (1997) Tumor necrosis factor-a and interleukin-6 in stools of children with bacterial and viral gastroenteritis. *J. Pediatr. Gastroenterol. Nutr.* **25**, 556–558.
22. Casola, A.M.K., Estes, S.E., Crawford, P.L., et al. (1995) Rotavirus infection of cultured instestinal epithelial cells induces secretion of CXC and CC chemokines. *Gastroenterology* **114**, 947–955.
23. Szajewska, H., Hoekstra, J.H., Sandhu, B.K., et al. (2000) Management of acute gastroenteritis in Europe and the impact of the new recommendations: a multicentre study. *J. Pediatr. Gastroenterol. Nutr.* **30**, 522–527.
24. Guandalini, S. (2000) Treatment of acute diarrhea in the new mellennium. *J. Pediatr. Gastroenterol. Nutr.* **30**, 486–489.
25. World Health Organization. (1992) *Management of the patient with diarrhoea*. Programme for Control of Diarrhoeal Disease. WHO, Geneva.
26. Zinc Investigators' Collaborative Group. (2002) Therapeutic effects of oral zinc in acute and persistent diarrhea in children in developing countries: pooled analysis of randomized controlled trials. *Am. J. Clin. Nutr.* **72**, 1516–1522.
27. Black, R.E., Brown, K.H., and Becker, S. (1984) Malnutrition is a determining factor in diarrhoeal duration, but not incidence, among young children in a longitudinal study in rural Bangladesh. *Am. J. Clin. Nutr.* **39**, 87–94.
28. Barclay, A.J., Foster, A., and Sommer, A. (1987) Vitamin A supplements and mortality related to measles: a randomised clinical trial. *Brit. Med. J.* 294–296.
29. Grotto, I., Mimouni, M., Gdalevich, M., and Mimouni, D. (2003) Vitamin A supplementation andchildhood morbidity form diarrhea and respiratory infections: a meta-analysis. *J. Pediatr.* **142**, 297–304.
30. Gera, T. and Sachdev, H.P.S. Effect of iron supplementation on incidence of infectious illness in children: systematic review. *Brit. Med. J.* **324**, 1142–1151.
31. Oppenheimer, S.J. (2001) Iron and its relation to immunity and infectious disease. *J. Nutr.* **131**, 616S–635S.
32. Vanderhoof, J.A. (2000) Probiotics: future directions. *Am. J. Clin. Nutr.* **73**, 1152S–1155S.

33. Brown, K.H., Black, R.E., de Romaña, G.L., et al. (1989) Infant-feeding practices and their relationship with diarrheal and other diseases in Huascar (Lima), Peru. *Pediatrics* **83**, 31–40.

34. World Health Organization. (1997) *Persistent diarrhea and breastfeeding.* WHO, Geneva.

35. Wold, A.E. and Hanson, L.A. (1994) Defense factors in human milk. *Curr. Opinion Gastroenterol.* **10**, 652–658.

36. Goldman, A.S. The immune system of human milk: antimicrobial, anti-inflammatory, and immunomodulating properties. *Breastfeeding Rev.* **2**, 422–429.

37. Glass, R.I. Commentary: reanalysis of the results of two rotavirus vaccine trials. An appraisal of the reappraisal. *Pediatr. Infect. Dis. J.* **18**, 1006–1007.

38. Nataro, J.P. and Levine, M.M. (1999) Enteric bacterial vaccines, salmonella, shigella, cholera, escherichia coli, in *Mucosal Immunology.* (Ogra, P., Mestecky, J., Lamm, M., et al., eds.) 2nd ed. Academic, San Diego, CA, pp. 851–866.

39. Davidson, G.P. (1996) Passive protection against diarrheal disease. *J. Pediatr. Gastroenterol. Nutr.* **23**, 207–212.

40. Hotez, P.J., Ghosh, K., Hawdon, J., et al. (1997) Vaccines for hookworm infection. *Pediatr. Infect. Dis. J.* **16**, 935–940.

41. Meeusen, E.N. and Maddox, J.F. (1999) Progress and expectations for helminth vaccines. *Adv. Veterin. Med.* **41**, 241–256.

42. Myaux, J.A., Unicomb, L., Besser, R.E., et al. (1996) Effect of diarrhea on the humoral response to oral polio vaccination. *Pediat. Inf. Dis. J.* **15**, 204–209.

43. Suzuki, H., Katsusuhima, N., and Konno, T. (1999) Rotavirus vaccine put on hold. *Lancet* **254**, 1390.

44. Abramson J, Baker C, Fisher M, et al. (1999) Possible association of intussusception with rotavirus vaccination. Am. Acad. Pediat. Committee on Infectious Diseases. *Pediatrics* **104**, 575.

14 HIV

Annamaria Kiure and Wafaie Fawzi

Contents

Key Points

- HIV infection is a major public health problem in many developing countries. The disease is accompanied by profound abnormalities in immune function.
- Macronutrient and micronutrient undernutrition are frequently reported among HIV-infected pregnant and lactating mothers, children, and adults.
- Observational studies have shown associations between undernutrition and a decline in immunological and virological markers of HIV-disease progression, as well as poor clinical outcomes among HIV-infected individuals.
- Randomized trials of macronutrient supplementation showed no benefit on clinical outcomes measured as weight gain among HIV-infected adults. Data on the effects of macronutrient supplements on immune and viral markers are not available. No published studies exist for macronutrient supplementation among children.

From: *Handbook of Nutrition and Immunity*
Edited by: M. E. Gershwin, P. Nestel, and C. L. Keen © Humana Press, Totowa, NJ

- Supplementing HIV-infected children with vitamin A reduced their risk of morbidity and mortality. Prenatal vitamin A supplementation to HIV-positive women reduced the risk of delivering a low-birth-weight baby in one study, but resulted in a significant increase in the overall risk of mother-to-child transmission of HIV-1.
- Multiple micronutrient supplements (vitamins B, C, or E) to mothers (during pregnancy and lactation) improved markers of disease progression (CD4$^+$ and viral load) and clinical outcomes (reduced adverse pregnancy outcomes among women and diarrhea among children). The effects of multiple micronutrients on clinical disease progression are yet to be examined.

Introduction

Human immunodeficiency virus (HIV) infection is a major public health problem worldwide. At the end of 2002, an estimated 29.4 million adults and children in sub-Saharan Africa were infected with HIV (1). Some 8.8% of adults in this region were HIV infected, of which 58% were women. Advanced HIV disease often leads to acquired immunodeficiency syndrome (AIDS). In 2002, 2.4 million people died from AIDS in sub-Saharan Africa (1). AIDS is frequently accompanied by undernutrition and progressive loss of immune function (2,3). However, the asymptomatic phase of HIV infection is also accompanied by profound abnormalities in nutritional status and immune function (4,5).

The role of nutrient supplementation to reduce HIV disease progression and transmission, and to improve nutritional status, has received attention. Micronutrient supplementation to HIV-infected individuals may be a low-cost intervention to enhance immune and nutritional status, particularly in developing countries where antiretroviral drugs are not readily available or affordable. This chapter reviews studies that examined the potential causes of undernutrition and impaired immune function among HIV-infected individuals. Macronutrients and micronutrients are discussed separately. For each nutrient, studies on the prevalence of deficiency, functions, and its potential role on immune function, viral load, and disease progression among HIV-infected individuals are reviewed. Potential mechanisms of how nutrition may slow disease progression are discussed briefly. Finally, the effects of micronutrients on HIV transmission and child health are presented.

Causes of Undernutrition in HIV-Infected Individuals

Severe undernutrition impairs the integrity of mucosal barriers, the acute-phase response, and cellular immune function thereby reducing resistance to infections (6–8). Nutritional deficiencies in HIV-infected individuals may lead to further decline in immune function and rapid HIV disease progression. Advanced disease, in turn, leads to even poorer nutritional status *(9)*. The potential causes of undernutrition in HIV-infected individuals include inadequate dietary intake *(10–12)*, nutrient malabsorption *(13–15)*, and disturbances related to weight loss and increased energy expenditure *(10,11,16)*.

Reduced food intake is common among HIV-infected individuals with undernutrition and infections: anorexia, dysphagia, and painful swallowing resulting from esophageal infections caused by *candida*, *herpes*, or *cyptomegalovirus* are some of the causes *(11,17,18)*. Energy intake was unacceptably low in HIV-infected adults in South Africa *(12)* and France *(14)* and among HIV-infected children with growth failure *(19)*. In the US-based multicenter AIDS cohort study (MACS), the total intakes of vitamins A and E (from both food and pharmaceutical supplements) among HIV-infected men were below the recommended daily allowance *(20)*. In contrast, another US-based study found the mean total intakes of vitamins A, B_6, B_{12}, E, and zinc were significantly higher in HIV^+ men having sex with men (MSM) than in the HIV^- MSM *(21)*. In South Africa, 12% of HIV-infected individuals had inadequate intakes of protein, vitamins (A, B_6, C, and D), and minerals (calcium, iron, and zinc) *(12)*.

Repeated episodes of infectious diarrhea may impair gut mucosal function and cause nutrient malabsorption. Diarrhea and fat malabsorption *(14,15,22)*, loss of intestinal absorptive surface *(23)*, and vitamin B_{12} malabsorption indicated by abnormal Schilling tests *(24,25)*, were found in HIV-infected patients with and without diarrhea. Urinary nutrient losses may exacerbate nutrient deficiencies. Renal disease is frequently reported among HIV-infected patients who develop low molecular mass proteinuria with loss of retinol, retinol-binding protein, and albumin in urine *(26,27)*.

Weight loss during disease progression often results from increased energy metabolism, particularly resting energy expenditures *(10,16,28)*, reduced food intake, infectious diarrheas and other opportunistic infections, and malabsorption *(14,15,29)*. Several studies have attributed HIV-wasting in adults *(10,11)* and growth failure in HIV-infected children *(19,30)* to low energy intake rather than increased energy expenditure. Metabolic changes in HIV-infected patients have been associated with increased levels of blood lipids and increased breakdown of carbohydrates and proteins *(10,31,32)*.

Macronutrients

Macronutrients (carbohydrates, proteins, fat, and fiber) are associated with wasting and energy balance in HIV-infected patients. Carbohydrates, the major constituent of the diet, account for up to 70% of the total energy intake *(33)*. In developing countries, however, low energy intake from carbohydrates can be related to limited food availability and sociocultural factors. The main function of carbohydrates is to provide energy for metabolic processes. Dietary fat provides up to 20% of total energy intake in Africa, whereas in the United States and Europe fat intake contributes between 30 and 45% of total energy intake *(33)*. Dietary fat is important as a source of energy and for structural components in cell membranes *(34)*. Energy stored in adipose tissue becomes available during starvation, an important feature for patients with reduced food intake. Amino acids are the building blocks for proteins required for growth and transport of nutrients in blood. Supplementation with several amino acids has been suggested as a way to reduce weight loss among HIV-infected individuals *(35)*.

Prevalence of Undernutrition Caused by Macronutrient Deficiencies

Macronutrient deficiencies, commonly defined as being wasted and/or stunted, are prevalent among HIV/AIDS-infected people. Early in the HIV epidemic, adult undernutrition in Uganda was described as "slim disease" *(36)*. Forty percent of adult AIDS patients in Burundi *(37)* and 44% of HIV$^+$ subjects in an autopsy study in Côte d'Ivoire *(38)* were wasted. Low body mass index (BMI) (<21.5 kg/m^2) was frequently reported in Côte d'Ivoire *(17)*. Twenty-three percent of the HIV-infected men participating in the MACS study had low serum albumin (<35 g/L) levels at enrolment *(20)*, whereas another US study found 83% AIDS-infected individuals had low serum albumin levels *(39)*.

Macronutrients and Progression of HIV Disease

Macronutrient undernutrition frequently accompanies disease progression to AIDS. Several studies documented the association between macronutrient deficiencies and immunological (T-lymphocytes CD4$^+$, CD8$^+$, and CD4$^+$/CD8$^+$ ratio) or virological (viral load) markers of prognosis and survival among HIV-infected individuals. Low CD4$^+$ cell counts were associated with low mean weight and low arm and muscle circumference in HIV-infected individuals in Côte d'Ivoire *(17)* and growth impairment in HIV-infected children *(30)*. An inverse association between viral load and energy intake, fat free mass, and growth velocity among children has been documented. In a cross-sectional study, high viral load, high interleukin (IL)-6 (a proinflammatory cytokine involved in HIV replication), and decreased total serum proteins were more likely to be found in HIV-infected children with growth impairment than in HIV-infected children with normal growth *(30)*. The temporal association between nutritional status and immunological and virological markers cannot be established because of the cross-sectional nature of these studies.

An association between immune status and macronutrinent deficiency was reported in a longitudinal study from Miami, in which females with advanced HIV disease (CD4$^+$ cell counts <200/mm^3) were more likely to have lower plasma prealbumin levels in the 3.5 yr of follow-up than men *(40)*. Few longitudinal studies have examined the association between macronutrient-related disorders and viral load among HIV-infected children. Low daily energy intake *(19,41)*, low fat free mass, and 12-mo growth velocity *(19)* were associated with increased plasma concentration of HIV ribonucleic acid (RNA) viral load in HIV-infected children with growth failure. Infants who had a high viral load in the first 6 mo of life were significantly more likely to have severe growth failure *(41)*.

Adverse clinical outcomes, such as advanced disease progression and mortality, are commonly observed among HIV-infected individuals with macronutrient undernutrition. Observational studies using anthropometric indicators showed a decline in BMI and depletion of body cell mass were associated with advanced disease progression among HIV-infected individuals in the United States *(5)*. In HIV-infected adults, wasting or depletion of body cell mass were associated with increased mortality *(42–44)* and susceptibility to opportunistic infections *(44)* in US-based studies. In a Rwandan study, mortality among HIV-infected individuals with a BMI $\leq$ 21 kg/m^2 was significantly higher than among those with a BMI >21 kg/m^2 *(45)*.

Perinatal HIV-infection in infants is associated with progressive growth failure followed by increased risk of mortality. Several longitudinal studies have reported associations between growth retardation among HIV-infected children and progression to AIDS or mortality. In a Ugandan study, HIV-infected infants with growth failure (average weight-for-age Z-score [WAZ] below –1.5) during the first year of life had an approx fivefold risk of mortality before 25 mo of age compared with infants with WAZ $\geq$–1.5 *(46)*. Several other studies have also reported the association between perinatal HIV infection and growth failure among children *(47–49)*. In a US study, compared with children who had low weight and height velocity, high weight and height velocity among HIV-infected children 3–15 mo old was associated with reduced mortality *(18)*.

The association between biochemical indicators of macronutrient status and mortality among HIV-infected individuals has been examined in a few longitudinal studies. Mortality risk increased threefold among HIV-infected individuals with low albumin levels compared with those with normal albumin levels in a small US-based study: the mean duration of follow-up was approx 186 d *(50)*. In another US-based study, HIV-infected women in the lowest baseline serum albumin category (<35 g/L) had a significantly threefold higher risk of mortality at 3 yr of follow-up than those in the highest category ($\geq$42 g/L) *(51)*. Both low mean BMI and C-reactive protein concentrations were significant predictors of mortality among HIV-infected individuals followed for 42 mo *(52)*. Levels of serum albumin, baseline CD4$^+$ cell counts, and HIV RNA predicted survival among HIV-1 vertically infected children *(53)*. Lower levels of serum albumin and hemoglobin were also observed in HIV-infected children who died than in the survivors.

Two intervention studies have examined the effect of macronutrient supplementation on weight gain among HIV-infected individuals with weight loss. In a randomized placebo-controlled study, 8 wk supplementation with three amino acids (β-hydroxy-β-methylbutyrate, a metabolite of leucine [L-glutamine], and L-arginine) resulted in a significant weight gain of about 3.0 kg in the treatment arm compared with 0.37 kg in the placebo arm (35). Improvements in gut function leading to absorption of the supplement and other nutrients may have contributed to this weight gain. In another randomized trial, daily supplementation with one of two diets with different energy levels or a nonenergy diet for 4 mo did not result in a significant difference in the percent change in weight among HIV-infected individuals (54). One energy diet provided 500 kcal as a supplement with peptides and medium-chain triglycerides plus a multivitamin and mineral and the other 500 kcal as a supplement with whole protein and long-chain triglycerides plus a multivitamin and mineral, whereas the nonenergy diet included multivitamin and mineral supplements only. Both of the above trials were conducted in a developed country where most patients were on antiretroviral drugs, thus generalization to developing countries cannot be made. The effects of macronutrient supplementation on HIV disease progression and clinical outcomes may warrant further studies in developing countries.

Micronutrients

Prevalence of Deficiency and Nutrient Sources

Micronutrients include fat-soluble vitamins A, D, E, and K; water-soluble B-complex vitamins such as B_1 (thiamin), B_2 (riboflavin), B_3 (niacin), B_5 (pantothenic acid), B_6 (pyridoxine), biotin, B_{12} (cobalamin), folic acid, and vitamin C; and minerals such as iron, zinc, selenium, and iodine. Micronutrient deficiencies are common among HIV-infected people. Table 1 shows both the micronutrient food sources and the frequency of deficiency (low levels of serum or plasma) among HIV-infected individuals in different locations for vitamins A, E, C, B_2, B_6, B_{12}, folate, selenium, and zinc (4,2,55–69).

Low levels of serum vitamin A (retinol levels <1.05 μmol/L) are prevalent among HIV-infected individuals (70). In a follow-up study among men in Kenya, the prevalence of low serum retinol (<0.70 Mmol/L) was 50% in HIV-1 seroconverters and 76% in those who remained seronegative (62). In South Africa, low serum retinol was reported in 39% of HIV-infected patients at World Health Organization clinical stages I and II and in 79% of those in stage IV (65). Studies from the United States reported a relatively lower prevalence of low serum vitamin A levels ranging from 3 to 15% among HIV-infected MSM and intravenous drug users (IDU) *(4,20,55)*, and from 13 to 31% among HIV-infected pregnant women *(71,72)*. Low blood levels of β-carotene *(73,74)*, vitamin C *(73)*, and vitamin E *(73,75,76)*, were reported in HIV$^+$ adults in Canada and the United States. HIV-infected children in Italy were reported to have low blood levels of β-carotene and vitamin E *(76)*.

Low blood levels of selenium were observed in HIV$^+$ individuals in Canada and the United States *(73,77)*. The prevalence of selenium deficiency was 11% in HIV-infected MSM in Miami *(68)*. Concurrent macronutrient and multiple micronutrient deficiencies are common in HIV-infected individuals, and a high prevalence of wasting and specific micronutrient deficiencies including vitamin A and carotene *(74)*, vitamin B_{12} *(67)*, folate *(74,78)*, and zinc *(79)* have been reported. A high proportion—62%—of HIV-infected children in South Africa had multiple micronutrient deficiencies *(80)*. The prevalence of anemia among asymptomatic HIV-infected pregnant women in Malawi *(81)* and Tanzania *(82)* was 73 and 83%, respectively. Some of the above studies were cross-sectional, making it impossible to establish a temporal association between HIV-related outcomes and specific nutrient deficiencies. On the one hand, HIV infection may lead to micronutrient deficiency through decreased dietary nutrient intake, malabsorption, and increased utilization and excretion of nutrients *(11–13,17,83)* but, on the other hand, micronutrient deficiencies may contribute to faster HIV disease progression to clinical AIDS by impairing immune function. Additionally, chronically HIV-infected individuals may present with low blood levels of vitamin A or other micronutrients such as zinc and selenium despite adequate body stores. For example, biochemical studies on vitamin A are limited because serum levels of vitamin A can be reduced in response to HIV infection even in the absence of liver depletion *(84)*. Therefore, vitamin A and other micronutrient levels can reflect an inflammatory response and HIV disease stage rather than micronutrient status.

Functions of Micronutrients the in Immune System

Reduced CD4$^+$ cell counts may be caused by the direct effects of the virus on the cells because HIV primarily infects CD4$^+$ cells. Low levels of antioxidant micronutrients in blood and increased levels of oxidation products may cause increased HIV replication (high viral load) *(85)*, whereby new virions infect more CD4$^+$ cells and can impair CD4$^+$ cells production. Micronutrient deficiencies are also associated with immune suppression. Potential immune response factors have been associated with vitamin A *(86,87)*, for example, deficiency was associated with impaired cell-mediated immunity presented as delayed type hypersensitivity (DTH) response in mice *(88)*. Increases in CD4$^+$

Table 1
Vitamins and Minerals: Selected Food Sources
and Prevalence of Deficiency Among HIV-Infected Individuals

Nutrient	Food sources	Study location	Prevalence (%)	Reference
Vitamin A	Preformed vitamin A, mainly from liver, fish liver oils, dairy products, eggs	US, Baltimore/Washington,	10	20
		US, Baltimore,	15	55
		US, Miami,	18	4
	Provitamin A, available in dark green leafy vegetables, and orange colored fruits, and vegetables	Kenya,	24	56
		US, New Jersey,	26	57
		US, Baltimore,	29	58
		US, New Jersey,	31	59
		Spain	36	60
		Tanzania,	34	61
		Kenya,	50	62
		Malawi,	65	63
		Germany, Berlin,	77	64
		South Africa	79	65
Vitamin E	Vegetable oils, nuts, green leafy vegetables	US, New Jersey	4	57
		US, New Jersey	12	59
		US, Baltimore/Washington	22	20
		US, Miami	27	4
Vitamin C	Citrus fruits, tomatoes, bell peppers, many berries	US, Miami	10	4
		US, New Jersey	20	57
		US, New Jersey	27	59
Riboflavin (B$_2$)	Meat, milk, dairy products, grain products, green leafy vegetables	US, Miami	26	4

310

Pyridoxine (B$_6$)	Poultry, fish, liver, eggs, whole grain products, beans, fruits, vegetables	US, New Jersey	17	59
Cobalamin (B$_{12}$)	Animal foods such as meat, poultry, milk, fish	US, Miami	53	4
		US, Miami	23	4
		Canada, Montreal	31	66
		US, Los Angeles	36	67
Folate	Green leafy vegetables, legumes, orange juice, fortified grain products, yeast	US, New Jersey	3	59
		US, New Jersey	15	57
Selenium	Mainly from vegetables and fruits, also in meat, fish, grains	US, Miami	11	68
Zinc	Meat, fish, grains	US, New Jersey	4	57
		US, California	29	69
		South Africa	45	65
		US, Miami	50	4

and CD8$^+$ cell counts following supplementation with β-carotene or vitamin A have been reported in both animal and human studies *(89–92)*. In addition, enhanced humoral immunity caused by vitamin A has been demonstrated by antibody response to other disease antigens such as tetanus *(93)* and measles *(94)* in children. In a meta-analysis, vitamin A supplementation to children whose HIV status was not determined resulted in significant reductions in the severity of measles, diarrhea, and total mortality *(95)*. The latter study estimated 60% average mortality risk reduction, which led several researchers to conduct vitamin A trials among HIV-infected women and children.

Vitamin C has been shown to decrease T-cell death and enhance natural killer (NK) cell activity *(96)*. Possible antiviral activity of vitamin C on HIV-infected human lymphocytic, myeloid, and monocytic cell lines in in vitro studies has been demonstrated *(97)*. Increased proliferation of T- and B-lymphocytes and lower rate of infections were reported following vitamin C supplementation or enhanced vitamin C status *(98,99)*. Vitamin E deficiency has been shown to impair T-cell-mediated function including DTH response, lymphocyte proliferation, and interleukin (IL)-2 production in animal and human studies *(100)*. In mice infected with murine AIDS, vitamin E supplementation was associated with significant improvements in IL-2 production and NK cell cytotoxicity, as well as reduced production of the pro-inflammatory cytokines such as tumor necrosis factor-alpha (TNF-α) and IL-6 *(101)*. Supplementation with vitamin E in healthy elderly subjects significantly improved lymphocyte proliferation, IL-2 production, DTH, and response to T-cell-dependent vaccines *(102,103)*.

The role of the B vitamins in immune function has also been documented. Vitamin B$_6$ deficiency in healthy elderly subjects significantly reduced the total number of lymphocytes, lymphocyte proliferation, and IL-2 production in response to T-cell mitogens-defects that were corrected following B$_6$ repletion *(104)*. Among HIV-infected individuals, vitamin B$_6$ deficiency was associated with reduced NK cell cytotoxicity and impaired mitogen-induced lymphocyte proliferation *(105)*. Riboflavin (vitamin B$_2$) deficiency impairs the ability to generate humoral antibodies in response to test antigens, but research on the effect of cell-mediated immunity is limited *(106)*. Clinical studies showed patients with low serum vitamin B$_{12}$ had impaired neutrophil function, whereas in vitro and animal studies indicated vitamin B$_{12}$ supplements are associated with enhanced antibody function and mitogenic responses *(106)*.

Selenium is required for proper activity of the enzyme glutathione peroxidase (GSH-Px) *(107)* that is involved in cellular antioxidant systems. Increases in GSH-Px activity following selenium supplementation has been reported in HIV-infected T-lymphocytes in in vitro studies *(108)* and in the animal murine AIDS model *(109)*. Selenium supplementation as parenteral nutrition improved immune response in patients with chronic gut failure whose HIV status was not determined *(110)*. Zinc plays an important role in the growth, development, and function of NK cells, macrophages, neutrophils, and T- and B-lymphocytes *(111)*. Zinc has been found to inhibit HIV-1 RNA transcription in an in vitro study *(112)* and possibly to slow HIV-1 replication in humans *(113)*. Zinc supplementation resulted in significant reduction in the severity of diarrhea, malaria, and acute respiratory infections among children whose HIV status was not determined in several trials *(114)*.

Micronutrients and HIV Disease Progression (see *Table 2*)

Cross-Sectional and Observational Studies

Cross-sectional studies have examined the association between biochemical markers of micronutrient status and immunologic markers of HIV-disease progression such as $CD4^+$ cell counts. First trimester HIV-1 infected pregnant Thai women with $CD4^+$ counts below 200 cells/mm^3 had mean serum vitamin A and β-carotene concentrations 37% lower than HIV-negative pregnant women *(115)*. Plasma zinc levels were significant predictors of $CD4^+$ cell counts among HIV-1-infected individuals in a cross-sectional study in the United States *(116)*. As mentioned earlier, cross-sectional studies do not provide the temporal association between low blood vitamin A levels and low $CD4^+$ cell counts.

The associations between micronutrient status, measured by biochemical markers or dietary micronutrient intakes, and immunologic markers of HIV-infection have been examined in observational studies. In longitudinal studies, low plasma vitamin A was associated with lower $CD4^+$ cell counts among HIV-infected women in Kenya *(84)* and HIV-infected MSM in the United States *(3)*. In the latter study, normalization of plasma vitamin A and zinc levels over the 18-mo period was significantly associated with higher $CD4^+$ cell counts. In Miami, HIV-1 infected women with $CD4^+$ counts below 200/mm^3 were more likely to have lower levels of plasma vitamin A, E, and selenium than men with similar $CD4^+$ cell counts *(40)*. Development of vitamin B_{12} deficiency during an 18-mo period was significantly associated with a decline in $CD4^+$ cell counts in a longitudinal study among HIV-infected MSM *(3)*. Individuals whose vitamin B_{12} level returned to normal over the same period had significantly higher $CD4^+$ cell counts.

The associations between dietary intakes of the B-vitamins and immunological markers of HIV infection have been assessed prospectively. In San Francisco, higher dietary intake of thiamine, niacin, and riboflavin were positively related to $CD4^+$ cell counts *(117)*. The same study also found higher dietary intake of zinc was positively associated with $CD4^+$ cell counts.

Table 2
Data on the Association Between Micronutrients Status and HIV Disease Progression

Nutrient	Markers of disease progression (CD4+, viral load)	Clinical outcomes (disease progression, mortality, and other morbidities)
Vitamin A	Observational studies: • Vitamin A deficiency defined by low plasma/serum retinol level associated with low CD4+ cell counts and high viral load Randomized trials: • Supplementation had no effect on CD4+ or viral load among adults	Observational studies: • Low plasma vitamin A was associated with increased mortality • Dietary intake had a U-shaped association with clinical disease progression and mortality among men Randomized trials data: • Efficacy of supplements on clinical outcomes has not been reported • Supplements given to mothers (during pregnancy and lactation) or children reduced the risk of diarrhea, pneumonia, and overall mortality among children • Reductions in the risk of low birth weight and improved neonatal growth • Antenatal supplementation to women decreased risk of anemia among children born to HIV-infected women in Malawi
Vitamins C, E, and B-vitamins (Thiamin [B₁], Riboflavin [B₂], Niacin [B₃],	Observational studies: • High biochemical levels and high dietary intakes associated with reduced risk of low CD4+ cell counts	Observational studies: • High levels of serum vitamin E and high dietary intakes of vitamin C or E associated with reduced risk of disease progression

314

Nutrient		
Pyridoxine [B$_6$], Cobalamin [B$_{12}$]	• No published data on effects on viral load Randomized trials: • Protective effect on CD4$^+$ cell counts and hemoglobin levels were reported • Effects on viral load marginally significant • Supplements given to mothers (during pregnancy and lactation) increased mean CD4$^+$ cells count	• High biochemical levels and high dietary intakes of B vitamins reduced disease progression and mortality Randomized trials: • No data on the effects on clinical outcomes in HIV-infected adults • Supplements given to mothers (during pregnancy and lactation) significantly reduced adverse pregnancy outcomes (fetal loss, low birth weight, severe preterm birth and small size for gestation age at birth) and lowered the risk of diarrhea among children in a study from Tanzania
Selenium	Observational studies: • Low biochemical levels associated with low CD4$^+$ cell counts Randomized trials: • Short duration trial with cross over design resulted in non-significant increase in CD4$^+$ cell counts • Short duration of supplementation had no effect on viral load	Observational studies: • Low plasma levels associated with increased risk of mortality among HIV-infected adults and vertically infected children Randomized trials: • No published data on effects of supplements on clinical outcomes
Zinc	Observational studies: • Normalization of zinc levels in blood and high dietary intakes increased CD4$^+$ cell counts	Observational studies: • High dietary zinc intake had harmful effects on disease progression and mortality

(continued)

Table 2 (*Continued*)
Data on the Association Between Micronutrients Status and HIV Disease Progression

Nutrient	Markers of disease progression (CD4$^+$, viral load)	Clinical outcomes (disease progression, mortality, and other morbidities)
	• No published data on effects on viral load Randomized trials: • No published data	• Low biochemical levels associated with increased disease progression Randomized trials: • No published data

Few studies have examined the association between micronutrient status and viral load. Vitamin A deficiency may be associated with an increase in HIV viral load. Longitudinal studies from Rwanda *(118)* and Kenya *(84)* found lower levels of serum retinol were associated with increased viral load among HIV-1-infected women. No studies have shown an association between the B-vitamins and viral load levels among HIV-infected individuals. The above studies were adjusted for confounding characteristics such as baseline clinical signs and symptoms that describe HIV disease stage, CD4$^+$ cell counts, and/or viral load. However, confounding caused by unmeasured factors such as the actual duration of HIV infection and time to development of nutritional deficiencies cannot be ruled out. Chronically HIV-infected individuals may present with low blood levels of vitamin A or other micronutrients such as zinc and selenium, despite adequate body stores, because many micronutrients are acute phase reactants.

Observational studies have examined the association between micronutrient status and clinical HIV disease progression. Serum retinol was significantly associated with progression to AIDS in a study from Rwanda *(118),* but not the United States. *(20).* However, baseline serum retinol was low in the study from Rwanda, and within the normal range in the US study. In a nested case-control study, HIV-infected individuals with low plasma vitamin A had an approximately fourfold higher risk of death compared with controls after adjusting for CD4$^+$ cell counts *(43).* Low serum retinol was also associated with a fourfold increased risk of mortality, after adjusting for CD4$^+$ cell counts and other clinical markers, in another longitudinal study among HIV-infected IDU in Baltimore *(55).* Presupplementation (at enrolment) serum vitamins A and E levels were strong predictors of early mortality in a cohort of HIV-infected patients with persistent diarrhea in a randomized multiple micronutrient trial in Zambia *(119).* Slower progression to AIDS and higher likelihood of survival was noted among HIV-infected women with higher serum retinol levels in Rwanda *(118).*

An association between serum levels of vitamins E and B$_{12}$, zinc, and selenium, and HIV disease progression has also been reported. In a US study, HIV-infected individuals in the highest quartile of serum vitamin E levels had a significant 35% lower risk of progression to AIDS than those in the lowest quartile *(20).* US-based HIV-infected individuals with low serum vitamin B$_{12}$ had a twofold increased risk for progression to AIDS *(120).* A case-control study nested in the MACS study found that patients who progressed to AIDS had significantly lower levels of serum zinc compared with non progressors and HIV-uninfected participants *(121).* Selenium deficiency in HIV-1-infected individuals has been associated with increased risk of mortality among adults *(122,123)* and HIV-1 infected children *(124).* As with vitamin A, serum levels of selenium and zinc may be low in response to infection, even in the absence of tissue depletion *(121)*.

The association between dietary vitamin A intake and progression to AIDS was a U-shaped in the MACS study, with poor outcomes in the lowest and highest quartiles of intake *(125)*. HIV-infected individuals in the upper-third quartile of β-carotene intake also had a higher likelihood of survival compared with those in the lowest intake quartile *(126)*. High dietary intakes of vitamin C in the MACS study *(125)* and vitamins C and E in the MSM study in San Francisco *(117)* were associated with a reduced risk of disease progression to AIDS. In both studies, high levels of thiamin or niacin intake were associated with a reduced risk of disease progression to AIDS. In addition, increased intake of riboflavin significantly reduced the hazard for AIDS *(117)*. In the MACS study, the highest quartiles of dietary intake of vitamins B_1, B_2, B_6, and niacin were associated with increased survival time of up to 1.3 yr *(126)*. Increased risk for developing AIDS was associated with higher zinc intake from dietary sources alone and from total intake (both food and pharmaceutical supplements) among HIV-infected MSM *(125)*. Higher levels of total zinc intake were also associated with poor survival *(126)*. However, the MSM study in San Francisco found no association between higher dietary zinc intake and progression to AIDS *(117)*.

Observational studies to assess the effect of dietary intake of micronutrients on HIV disease progression and mortality can be limited because of confounding from other factors such as opportunistic infections, time since seroconversion, drug treatment, and existing nutritional deficiencies. Furthermore, both dietary and biochemical studies are limited by the fact that reverse causality may partly explain the positive association between nutrient deficiencies and HIV disease progression.

Randomized Trials

Randomized trials are better suited to examining epidemiologic associations because confounding is minimized and interventions are precisely defined. Daily supplementation with 180 mg β-carotene for 4 wk in a small ($n = 21$) randomized crossover study in the U.S.A. was associated with a small increase in the total white blood cell count, change in $CD4^+$ cell count, and percentage change in $CD4^+/CD8^+$ ratio compared with subjects on placebo; these parameters decreased when the subjects in the β-carotene arm were switched to the placebo arm *(127)*. However, this effect was not observed in another study by the same investigators in which 5000 IU of vitamin A and the same dose of β-carotene were used *(128)*. Single high-dose vitamin A (200,000 IU or 60 mg of retinol equivalents) given to IDU in the United States had no significant effect on $CD4^+$ lymphocyte count measured 2 and 4 wk after treatment *(129)*.

A large double-blind placebo-controlled randomized trial of vitamins among HIV-infected pregnant women in Tanzania showed a significant increase in $CD4^+$, $CD8^+$, and CD3 cell counts in a group supplemented with vitamins B, C, and E; vitamin A alone had no effect (61). In the latter trial, the vitamin supplements were given during pregnancy and throughout the breastfeeding period. A clinical trial among children with AIDS in South Africa showed 60 mg retinol equivalents of vitamin A given on two consecutive days could increase circulating $CD4^+$ and NK cell counts one month after supplementation (130). The effects of vitamin C and/or E supplementation on $CD4^+$ cell counts have not been reported (the joint effects of the supplements on viral load will be presented in the multiple micronutrients section below). In a small randomized trial with partial cross over design ($n = 24$), a combination of N-acetylcysteine (NAC) and sodium selenite resulted in a nonsignificant increase in $CD4^+$ counts 6 wk after supplementation (131). In the latter study, HIV-infected individuals in stages I and II were randomized to receive the antioxidant combination of 600 mg NAC three times a day and 500 mg sodium selenite per day for either 24 wk (group A, $n = 13$) or from the end of week 12 (group B; control, $n = 11$) until the end of week 24. However, the effects of each nutrient could not be separated and the study was limited by a small sample size.

Few randomized trials have found a beneficial effect from micronutrient supplementation on viral load. Supplementation with retinol and β-carotene to HIV-infected pregnant women in South Africa did not change viral load (132). Single-dose vitamin A (200,000 IU) supplements given to HIV-infected IDU in the United States had no effect on viral load measured 2 and 4 wk after treatment (129). In a small trial in the United States ($n = 40$), single high oral dose of vitamin A (300,000 IU) given to HIV-infected nonpregnant women did not significantly change the viral load concentration 1, 2, 3, and 4 wk after treatment compared with baseline, and viral load concentration between the two treatment groups did not differ (133). Daily supplementation with 100 µg selenium or 30 µg β-carotene for 1 yr led to significant increases in GSH-Px activity per gram of hemoglobin at 3 and 6 mo, and was much higher in the selenium than the β-carotene group, but viral load was not measured (134). Daily supplementation with NAC and sodium selenite in a partial crossover trial had no effect on viral load at the end of 24 wk (131).

Two studies examined the effect of vitamin A or selenium supplementation on clinical outcomes among HIV-infected adults. In South Africa, vitamin A supplementation among pregnant women showed no significant benefit on HIV disease progression, as measured by reports of either HIV-1 or pregnancy-related symptoms during the prenatal or postnatal period (135). In a small randomized trial in San Diego ($n = 19$), daily supplementation with 400 mg of selenium for 70 d to HIV-infected adults with AIDS led to improved HIV-related symptoms from pulmonary, gastrointestinal, skin, and neurological disorders in 74% of patients *(136)*.

Multiple Micronutrients and HIV Disease Progression

The rationale for supplementing HIV-infected individuals with multiple micronutrients is based on their ability to enhance both humoral and cellular immune functions. Several in vitro and animal studies have shown increased immune cell proliferation and function, and inhibition of HIV replication, findings relevant to reducing disease progression. Provision of multiple micronutrient supplements may be a low-cost intervention in developing countries where micronutrient deficiency rates are high.

The effects of micronutrient supplementation on immunologic and virologic markers of disease progression among adults were reported in Canada and Tanzania. In a small randomized placebo-controlled double-blind study ($n = 49$) in Canada, large daily doses of vitamin C (1000 mg) and E (800 IU) resulted in a significant reduction in viral load after 3 mo of supplementation *(137)*. In a large randomized, double-blind placebo-controlled trial ($n = 1078$) in Tanzania, factorial design was used to examine the effects of supplementation with vitamin A (preformed vitamin A and β-carotene) and/or multivitamins (vitamins B, C, and E) during pregnancy and lactation. In Tanzania, multivitamin (vitamin B, C, E) supplements resulted in significant increases in the $CD4^+$ and $CD8^+$ cell counts among women *(61)*. Supplementation for approx 4 mo also led to significant increases in hemoglobin levels assessed at delivery. Vitamin A had no effect on these outcomes. Further analyses revealed a significantly higher mean $CD4^+$ cell count among children in the multivitamin arms than among those in the no-multivitamin arm during the first 2 yr of life *(138)*. The beneficial effects of vitamins C and E may be mediated by a mechanism whereby vitamin C regenerates vitamin E, thereby reducing reactive oxidants *(139)*.

The efficacy of multiple micronutrient supplementations on clinical outcomes among HIV-infected adults has been examined in few studies. In a randomized placebo-controlled trial ($n = 106$) in Zambia, 2 wk of daily supplementation with multiple micronutrients (vitamins A [10,500 IU], C [300 mg], and E [300 mg], selenium [150 μg], and zinc [200 mg]) among patients with persistent diarrhea did not reduce the duration of diarrhea or time to mortality during the first month of follow-up, and $CD4^+$ cell counts and hematological parameters were unaffected *(119)*. Malabsorption during persistent diarrhea and short duration of supplementation may have contributed to these results. In the trial from Tanzania referred to above, HIV-infected pregnant women who received multivitamin supplementation during pregnancy, had significant weight gain and reduced risk of low rate of weight gain during pregnancy *(140).*

Nutrition and HIV Disease Progression Among Children

Observational studies have examined the association between blood vitamin A levels and disease progression and clinical health outcomes among children. Plasma vitamin A levels and low levels of provitamin and nonprovitamin A carotenoids were related to decreased weight and height velocity among HIV-infected children in Uganda *(141).* Those with low plasma β-carotene had a significant threefold increased risk of mortality. Low serum retinol during pregnancy was associated with growth failure independent of child's HIV status *(142),* increased infant HIV disease progression *(143),* and infant mortality *(144).* In contrast, baseline vitamin A levels and vitamin A change over time had no effect on the risk of mortality among HIV-infected children in another study in North America *(145).* Low prevalence of having low plasma vitamin A levels in this cohort may partly explain the lack of association.

Vitamin A supplementation to children from populations with high deficiency rate has resulted in improved health outcomes. In a South African trial, vitamin A supplementation to children born to HIV-infected mothers reduced HIV disease progression and diarrhea by about 50% *(146).* In Tanzania, the overall reduction in mortality among HIV-infected and uninfected children was 50% and the benefits were higher among HIV+ children *(147).* In the same study, vitamin A supplementation to children admitted because of pneumonia significantly reduced morbidity from diarrhea in HIV-infected children and those with wasting disease. The risk of cough and rapid respiratory rate was also lowered, but the results were marginally significant *(148).* Vitamin A supplementation to HIV-infected women during pregnancy and lactation resulted in a significant lower risk of cough with rapid respiratory rate (proxy for pneumonia) among children *(138),* but vitamin A had no effect on diarrhea or CD4+ cell counts. In a Malawi trial, prenatal vitamin A supplementation reduced the risk of low birth weight, improved neonatal growth, and reduced the risk of anemia *(149).*

The effects of multiple micronutrients on clinical outcomes among children born to HIV-infected women has also been examined. Improvements in birth outcomes among HIV-infected pregnant women were described in Tanzania, where multivitamins supplementation significantly reduced fetal loss by 39%, low birth weight by 44%, severe preterm birth (less than 34 wk of gestation) by 39%, and small size for gestation age at birth by 43% compared with women on no multivitamins *(61).* Multivitamins had a significant effect on lowering diarrhea morbidity among children born to women receiving the supplements *(138)*.

Nutrition and HIV Transmission (*see* Table 3)

The major routes of HIV transmission in sub-Saharan Africa and other developing countries include heterosexual contact (horizontal transmission) and mother-to-child (MTCT) (vertical transmission). MTCT of HIV can occur during pregnancy, intrapartum, or lactation. The potential mechanisms through which micronutrients supplementation may reduce the risk of vertical transmission include enhancement of humoral and cellular immune function, slowing maternal disease progression, and enhanced integrity of epithelial linings of placenta, lower genital tract, and mammary ducts *(150,151)*.

The results of longitudinal studies that examined the association between biochemical levels of vitamin A and vertical transmission of HIV have been inconsistent. Low levels of serum vitamin A among HIV-infected women were associated with an increased risk of vertical transmission in Malawi and the United States *(63,71)*, and delivering a dead or HIV-positive infant in Rwanda *(152)*. These associations were not noted in studies from the Ivory Coast and Burkina Faso *(153)* and the United States *(72,154)*. In Kenya, low plasma vitamin A was associated with a higher risk of HIV shedding in secretions of the lower genital tract *(56,155)*. These findings support the hypothesis that low levels of vitamin A may be associated with increased MTCT of HIV. However, the lack of an association between vitamin A deficiency and perinatal HIV-1 transmission can be supported by results from two studies. A subset of data from the Women's Interagency HIV Study in the United States showed no association between retinol status and genital (cervical and vaginal) HIV-1-RNA load *(156)*. In Kenya, vitamin A supplementation had no effect on HIV DNA shedding in vaginal swabs and median vaginal HIV RNA concentration *(157)*.

Vitamin A deficiency and breast tissue inflammation (subclinical mastitis defined as a high sodium/potassium ratio in breast milk) may impair mucosal barrier and immunity in the mammary ducts, thus increasing permeability of blood vessels and subsequent shedding of HIV virus in breast milk. In Kenya, low plasma vitamin A levels among HIV-infected women during pregnancy was associated with a high viral shedding in breast milk *(158)*. Low serum levels of vitamin A and subclinical mastitis in Malawi *(159)* and South Africa *(160)* have been associated with high viral load in breast milk and an increased risk of HIV transmission through breast milk. However, these results need to be interpreted cautiously given that the studies were observational and serum vitamin A is not necessarily a marker of vitamin A status. Results from a randomized trial in Bangladesh showed that supplements of vitamin A alone to postpartum women did not reduce the risk of subclinical mastitis *(161)*.

Trials with vitamin A supplements have examined their association with vertical transmission of HIV. In Malawi, vitamin A supplements given to HIV-infected pregnant women had no effect on HIV transmission at 6 wk or by 12 or 24 mo compared with placebo *(149,162)*. In Tanzania, vitamin A supplementation of women during pregnancy and at delivery increased the risk of vertical transmission in utero or during the intrapartum and early breastfeeding period (up to 6 wk) *(163)*. However, these findings were not statistically significant. Further analyses from the Tanzanian study showed that vitamin A supplementation increased the risk of HIV transmission overall and through breastfeeding by 24 mo *(164)*. The risk of HIV infection in infants by three months of age were similar between treatment groups in a South African study, where HIV-infected women received preformed vitamin A and β-carotene supplements or placebo during the prenatal period *(165)*. Daily supplements of vitamins B, C, and E had no effect on the risk of vertical transmission of HIV in utero or during the intrapartum and early breastfeeding period (up to 6 wk) in Tanzania *(163)*. The latter study also found significant beneficial effects on breastfeeding transmission among subgroups of women who were nutritionally or immunologically compromised.

Data on the role of nutrition in heterosexual transmission of HIV in developing countries are scarce. In a nested case-control study among men in Kenya, serum retinol greater than 20 μg/dL (>0.70 μmol/L) was significantly associated with a 2.4-fold higher risk of seroconversion to HIV *(62)*.

Conclusion

HIV/AIDS is accompanied by profound abnormalities in nutritional status and a decline in immune function among pregnant and lactating mothers, children, and adults. Poor nutritional status and impaired immune function are further associated with poor health outcomes among HIV-infected individuals.

A decline in CD4$^+$ cell counts, increased viral load, and accelerated HIV-disease progression have been frequently reported among adults who present with wasting and among children with growth failure. There are limited data on the effect of macronutrient supplementation on weight gain, CD4$^+$ cell counts, and viral load among adults. There are no published data on the efficacy of macronutrient supplementation among HIV-infected children.

Pregnant and lactating HIV-infected women in less developed countries have been frequently found to have low plasma micronutrient levels associated with low CD4$^+$ cell counts, increased viral load in blood, and viral shedding in genital tract, and breast milk. Multiple micronutrient (vitamins B, C, and E) supplementation to HIV-infected pregnant and lactating mothers resulted in improved immunologic markers of disease progression as well as improved health outcomes including weight gain during pregnancy, improved CD4$^+$ cell

Table 3
Summary of Findings From An Association
Between Micronutrients and HIV-1 Transmission

Nutrients	Intermediate (lower genital tract, blood, breast milk)	Transmission outcome
Vitamin A	Observational studies: • Low plasma vitamin A associated with increased HIV shedding in the lower genital tract in Kenya but not in the United States • Low plasma vitamin A associated with subclinical mastitis and increased viral load in blood and breast milk Randomized trials: • No effects of supplements in reducing viral shedding in the lower genital tract (vaginal) • Supplementation during the postpartum period did not reduce subclinical mastitis	Observational studies: • Low plasma vitamin A associated with increased heterosexual and increased vertical HIV transmission. However, results are conflicting with some studies showing no effect on vertical transmission Randomized trials: • Prenatal supplements had no effect, whereas when given both prenantally and during lactation transmission increased significantly
Vitamins B, C, E	Observational studies: • No published data on the effects biochemical or dietary intakes of these vitamins on viral load in lower genital tract, or breast milk	Observational studies: • No published data

324

	Randomized trials:	Randomized trials:
	• No published data	• Daily supplements during lactation had no effect on the risk of vertical transmission of HIV overall, but decreased breastfeeding transmission in subgroups of immunologically and nutritionally compromised women
Selenium and Zinc	• No published data	• No published data

counts, improved hemoglobin status, and reductions in adverse pregnancy outcomes (such as reduced risk of low birth weight). Micronutrient supplementation to pregnant and lactating HIV-infected mothers in developing countries, where deficiency rates are high, may be a beneficial public health intervention. However, vitamin A supplementation to HIV-infected pregnant and lactating women has not been shown to be of benefit to pregnancy outcomes and markers of HIV disease progression, and resulted in increased risk of vertical transmission of HIV in a study from Tanzania.

The beneficial effects of micronutrient supplementation to HIV-infected mothers were extended to children born to these women such that there was reduced morbidity caused by diarrhea, pneumonia, and all-cause mortality. Prenatal vitamin A supplementation to HIV-infected women resulted in increased birth weight and decreased anemia among children born to these women in a trial in Malawi. Multivitamins have had no effect on the risk of vertical transmission of HIV overall, but benefits were observed in subgroups of women who were nutritionally or immunologically compromised in a trial in Tanzania. In Tanzania, multivitamin supplementation reduced HIV transmission through breastfeeding and child mortality. The use of multivitamins, zinc, and/or selenium supplements among HIV-infected children warrants additional research as these may be low-cost interventions to reduce disease progression in developing countries. Vitamin A supplementation among HIV-infected children in developing countries has had beneficial effects in reducing morbidity and mortality. There is good evidence that vitamin A supplements reduced the risk of mortality among children age 6 mo or older, compared with children receiving placebo.

Micronutrient supplementation among HIV-infected adults (nonpregnant, nonlactating) has not significantly improved immunologic markers of disease progression. Supplementation with vitamins C and E resulted in significant increases in viral load in a study from Canada. Data on clinical outcomes among HIV-infected adults are not available, thus the beneficial effects of micronutrient supplements warrant further studies. Further studies are also needed to elucidate the effects of selenium and zinc supplementation among HIV-infected individuals.

References

1. UNAIDS/WHO. (2002) AIDS epidemic update: December 2002. UNAIDS/ WHO, Geneva.
2. Seligmann, M., Pinching, A.J., Rosen, F.S., et al. (1987) Immunology of human immunodeficiency virus infection and the acquired immunodeficiency syndrome: an update. *Ann. Int. Med.* **107**, 234–232.
3. Baum, M., Shor-Posner, G., Lu, Y., et al. (1995) Micronutrients and HIV-1 disease progression. *AIDS* **9**, 1051–1056.

4. Beach, R., Mantero-Atienza, E., Shor-Posner, G., et al. (1992) Specific micronutrient abnormalities in asymptomatic HIV-1 infection. *AIDS* **6**, 701–708.

5. Maas, J., Dukers, N., Krol, A., et al. (1998) Body mass index course in asymptomatic HIV-infected homosexual men and the predictive value of a decrease of body mass index for progression to AIDS. *J. AIDS Hum. Retrovirol.* **19**, 254–259.

6. Chandra, R. (1991) Nutrition and immunity: lessons from the past and new insights into the future. *Am. J. Clin. Nutr.* **53**, 1087–1101.

7. Doherty, J., Golden, M.H.N., Raynes, J.G., Griffin, G.E., and McAdam, K.P.W.J. (1993) Acute-phase protein response is impaired in severely malnourished children. *Clin. Sci.* **84**, 169–175.

8. Scrimshaw, N. and SanGiovanni, J.P. (1997) Synergism of nutrition, infection, and immunity: an overview. *Am. J. Clin. Nutr.* **66**, 464S–477S.

9. Semba, R. and Tang, A.M. (1999) Micronutrients and the pathogenesis of human immunodeficiency virus infection. *Br. J. Nutr.* **81**, 181–189.

10. Grunfeld, C., Pang, M., Schimizu, L., Shigenaga, J.K., Jensen, P., Feingold, K.R. (1992) Resting energy expenditure, caloric intake, and short-term weight change in human immunodeficiency virus infection and the acquired immunodeficiency syndrome. *Am. J. Clin. Nutr.* **55**, 455–460.

11. Macallan, D., Noble, C., Baldwin, C., et al. (1995) Energy expenditure and wasting syndrome in human immunodeficiency virus infection. *New Engl. J. Med.* **333**, 83–88.

12. Dannhauser, A., van Staden, A.M., van der Ryst, E., et al. (1995) Nutritional status of HIV-1 seropositive patients in Free State Province of South Africa: Anthropometric and dietary profile. *Eur. J. Clin. Nutr.* **53**, 165–173.

13. Gillin, J., Shike, M., Alock, N., et al. (1985) Malabsorption and mucosal abnormalities of the small intestine in the Acquired Immunodeficiency Syndrome. *Ann. Int. Med.* **102**, 619–622.

14. Carbonnel, F., Beaugerie, L., Abou Rached, A., et al. (1997) Macronutrient intake and malabsorption in HIV infection: a comparison with other malabsorptive states. *Gut* **41**, 805–810.

15. Beaugerie, L., Carbonnel, F., Carrat, F., et al. (1998) Factors of weight loss in patients with HIV and chronic diarrhea. *J. AIDS Hum. Retrovirol.* **19**, 34–39.

16. Melchior, J., Salmon, D., Rigaud, D., et al. (1991) Resting energy expenditure is increased in stable, malnourished HIV-infected patients. *Am. J. Clin. Nutr.* **53**, 437–441.

17. Castetbon, K., Kadio, A., Bondurand, A., et al. (1997) Nutritional status and dietary intakes in human immunodeficiency virus (HIV)-infected outpatients in Abidjan, Côte D'Ivoire, 1995. *Eur. J. Clin. Nutr.* **51**, 81–86.

18. Carey, V., Yong, F.H., Frenkel, L.M., McKinney, R.E., Jr. (1998) Pediatric AIDS prognosis using somatic growth velocity. *AIDS* **12**, 1361–1369.

19. Arpadi, S., Cuff, P.A., Kotler, D.P., et al. (2000) Growth velocity, fat-free mass and energy intake are inversely related to viral load in HIV-infected children. *J. Nutr.* **130**, 2498–2502.

20. Tang, A., Graham, N.M.H., Semba, R.D., and Saah, A.J. (1997) Association between serum vitamin A and E levels and HIV-1 disease progression. *AIDS* **11**, 613–620.
21. Baum, M., Cassetti, L., Bonvehi, P., Shor-Posner, G., Lu, Y., and Sauberlich, H. (1994) Inadequate dietary intake and altered nutrition status in early HIV-1 infection. *Nutr* **10**, 16–20.
22. Koch, J., Garcia-Shelton, Y.L., Neal, E.A., Chan, M.F., Weaver, K.E., and Cello, J.P. (1996) Steatorrhea: a common manifestation in patients with HIV/AIDS. *Nutr* **12**, 507–510.
23. Pernet, P., Vittecoq, D., Kodjo, A., et al. (1999) Intestinal absorption and permeability in human immunodeficiency virus-infected patients. *Scand. J. Gastroenterol.* **34**, 29–34.
24. Harriman, G., Smith, P.D., Horne, M.K., et al. (1989) Vitamin B12 malabsorption in patients with acquired immunodeficiency syndrome. *Arch. Int. Med.* **149**, 2039–2041.
25. Ehrenpreis, E., Carlson, S.J., Boorstein, H.L., and Craig, R.M. (1994) Malabsorption and deficiency of vitamin B12 in HIV-infected patients with chronic diarrhea. *Digestive Dis. Sci.* **39**, 2159–2162.
26. Kabanda, A., Vandercam, B., Bernad, A., Lauwerys, R., and van Ypersele de Strihou, C. (1996) Low molecular weight proteinuria in human immunodeficiency virus-infected patients. *Am. J. Kidney Dis.* **27**, 803–808.
27. Jolly, P., Moon, T.D., Mitra, A.K., del Rosario, G.R., Blount, S., and Clemons, T.E. (1997) Vitamin A depletion in hospital and clinic patients with acquired immunodeficiency syndrome—a preliminary report. *Nutr. Res.* **17**, 1427–1441.
28. Melchior, J., Raguin, G., and Boulier, A. (1993) Resting energy expenditure in human immunodeficiency virus-infected patients: comparison between patients with and without secondary infections. *Am. J. Clin. Nutr.* **57**, 614–619.
29. Macallan, D., Noble, C., Baldwin, C., Fosket, M., McManus, M., and Griffin, GE. (1993) Prospective analysis of patterns of weight change in stage IV human immunodeficiency virus infection. *Am. J. Clin. Nutr.* **58**, 417–424.
30. Johann-Liang, R., O'Neill, L., Cervia, J., et al. (2000) Energy balance, viral burden, insulin-like growth factor-1, interleukin-6 and growth impairment in children infected with human immunodeficiency virus. *AIDS* **14**, 683–690.
31. Coodley, G., Loveless, M.O., and Merrill, T.M. (1992) The HIV wasting syndrome: A review. *J. AIDS* **7**, 681–694.
32. Grunfeld, C., Kotler, D.P., Hamadeh, R., Tierney, A., Wang, J., and Pierson, R.N. (1998) Hypertriglyceridemia in the acquired immunodeficiency syndrome. *Am. J. Med.* **86**, 27–31.
33. Ziegler, E. and Filer, L.J. (1996) Present knowledge in nutrition. Washington, DC. International Life Sciences Institute.
34. Murray, R., Granner, D.K., Mayes, P.A., and Rodwell, V.W. (2000) *Harper's Biochemistry*. Appleton & Lange, CT.
35. Clark, R., Feleke, G., Din, M., et al. (2000) Nutritional treatment for acquired immunodeficiency virus-associated wasting using beta-hydroxy beta-methyl-

butyrate, glutamine, and arginine: a randomized, double-blind, placebo-controlled study. *J. Parenteral. Enteral. Nutr.* **24**, 133–139.

36. Serwadda, D., Mugerwa, R.D., and Sewankambo, N.K. (1985) Slim disease: a new disease in Uganda and its association with HTLV-III infection. *Lancet* **2**, 849–852.

37. Niyongabo, T., Henzel, D., Ndayishimyie, J.M., et al. (1999) Nutritional status of adult inpatients in Bujumbura, Burundi (impact of HIV infection). *Eur. J. Clin. Nutr.* **53**, 579–582.

38. Lucas, S., De Cock, K.M., Hounnou, A., et al. (1994) Contribution of tuberculosis to slim disease in Africa. *Br. Med. J.* **308**, 1531–1533.

39. Chlebowski, R., Grosvenor, M.B., Bernhard, N.H., Morales, L.S., and Bulcavage, L.M. (1989) Nutritional status, gastrointestinal dysfunction, and survival in patients with AIDS. *Am. J. Gastroenterol.* **84**, 1288–1293.

40. Baum, M., Shor-Posner, G., Zhang, G., et al. (1997) HIV-1 infection in women is associated with severe nutritional deficiencies. *J. AIDS Hum. Retrovirol.* **16**, 272–278.

41. Pollack, H., Glasberg, H., Lee, E., et al. (1997) Impaired early growth of infants perinatally infected with human immunodeficiency virus: Correlation with viral load. *J. Pediatr.* **130**, 915–922.

42. Kotler, D., Tierney, A.R., Wang, J., and Pierson, R.N. (1989) Magnitude of body-cell-mass depletion and the timing of death from wasting in AIDS. *Am. J. Clin. Nutr.* **50**, 444–447.

43. Semba, R., Caiaffa, W.T., Graham, N.M.H., Cohn, S., and Vlahov, D. (1995) Vitamin A deficiency and wasting as predictors of mortality in human immunodeficiency virus-infected injection drug users. *J. Inf. Dis.* **171**, 1196–1202.

44. Wheeler, D., Gilbert, C.L., Launer, C.A., et al. (1998) Weight loss as a predictor of survival and disease progression in HIV infection. Terry Beirn Community Programs for Clinical Research on AIDS. *J. AIDS Hum. Retrovirol.* **18**, 80–85.

45. Lindan, C., Allen, S., and Serufilira, A. (1992) Predictors of mortality among HIV-infected women in Kigali, Rwanda. *Ann. Intern. Med.* **116**, 320–328.

46. Berhane, R., Bagenda, D., Marum, L., et al. (1997) Growth failure as a prognostic indicator of mortality in pediatric HIV infection. *Pediatr.* **100**, e7(pp 1–4).

47. McKinney, R. and Robertson, W.R. (1993) Effect of human immunodeficiency virus infection on the growth of young children. *J. Pediatr.* **123**, 579–582.

48. Miller, T., Evan, S.J., Orav, E.J., Morris, V., McIntosh, K., and Winter, H.S. (1993) Growth and body composition in children infected with the human immunodeficiency virus-1. *Am. J. Clin. Nutr.* **57**, 588–592.

49. Saavedra, J., Henderson, R.A., Perman, J.A., et al. (1995) Longitudinal assessment of growth in children born to mothers with human immunodeficiency virus infection. *Arch. Pediatr. Adolesc. Med.* **149**, 497–502.

50. Guenter, P., Muurahainen, N., Simons, G., et al. (1993) Relationships among nutritional status, disease progression, and survival in HIV infection. *J. AIDS* **6**, 1130–1138.

51. Feldman, J., Burns, D.N., Gange, S.J., et al. (2000) Serum albumin as a predictor of survival in HIV-infected women in the Women's Interagency HIV study. *AIDS* **14**, 863–870.

52. Melchior, J., Niyongabo, T., Henzel, D., Durack Bown, I., Henri, S.C., and Boulier, A. (1999) Malnutrition and wasting, immunodeficiency, and chronic inflammation as independent predictors of survival in HIV-infected patients. *Nutrition* **15**, 865–869.

53. Shearer, W., Easley, K.A., Goldfarb, J., et al. (2000) Evaluation of immune survival factors in pediatric HIV-1 infection. *Ann. NY Acad. Sci.* **918**, 298–312.

54. Gibert, C., Wheeler, D.A., Collins, G., et al. (1999) Randomized, controlled trial of caloric supplements in HIV infection. Terry Beirn Community Programs for Clinical Research on AIDS. *J. AIDS* **22**, 253–259.

55. Semba, R., Graham, N.M.H., Caiaffa, W.T., Margolick, J.B., Clement, L., and Vlahov, D. (1993) Increased mortality associated with vitamin A deficiency during human immunodeficiency virus type 1 infection. *Arch. Int. Med.* **153**, 2149–2154.

56. John, G., Nduati, R.W., Mbori-Ngacha, D., et al. (1997) Genital shedding of human immunodeficiency virus type 1 DNA during pregnancy: association with immunosuppression, abnormal cervical or vaginal discharge, and severe vitamin A deficiency. *J. Inf. Dis.* **175**, 57–62.

57. Skurnick, J., Bogden, J.D., Baker, H., et al. (1996) Micronutrient profiles in HIV-1-infected heterosexual adults. *J. AIDS Hum. Retrovirol.* **12**, 75–83.

58. Semba, R., Farzadegan, H., and Vlahov, D. (1997) Vitamin A levels and human immunodeficiency virus load in injection drug users. *Clin. Diag. Lab. Immunol.* **4**, 93–95.

59. Bogden, J., Baker, H., Frank, O., et al. (1990) Micronutrient status and human immunodeficiency virus infection. *Ann. NY Acad. Sci.* **587**, 189–195.

60. Jimenez-Exposito, M., Bullo Bonet, M., Alonso-Villaverde, C., et al. (2002) Micronutrients in HIV-infection and the relationship with the inflammatory response. *Med. Clin. (Barc.)* **119**, 765–769.

61. Fawzi, W., Msamanga, G.I., Spiegelman, D., et al. (1998) Randomized trial of effects of vitamin supplements on pregnancy outcomes and T cell counts in HIV-1-infected women in Tanzania. *Lancet* **351**, 1477–1482.

62. MacDonald, K., Malonza, I., Chen, D.K., et al. (2001) Vitamin A and risk of HIV-1 seroconversion among Kenyan men with genital ulcers. *AIDS* **15**, 635–639.

63. Semba, R., Miotti, P.G., Chiphangwi, J.D., et al. (1994) Maternal vitamin A deficiency and mother-to-child transmission of HIV-1. *Lancet* **343**, 1593–1597.

64. Ullrich, R., Schneider, T., Heise, W., et al. (1994) Serum carotene deficiency in HIV-infected patients. Berlin diarrhoea/wasting syndrome study group. *AIDS* **8**, 661–665.

65. Visser, M., Maartens, G., Kossew, G., and Hussey, G.D. (2003) Plasma vitamin A and zinc levels in HIV-infected adults in Cape Town, South Africa. *Br. J. Nutr.* **89**, 475–482.

66. Paltiel, O., Falutz, J., Veilleux, M., Rosenblatt, D.S., and Gordon, K. (1995) Clinical correlates of subnormal vitamin B12 levels in patients infected with the human immunodeficiency virus. *Am. J. Hematol.* **49**, 318–322.

67. Burkes, R., Cohen, H., Krailo, M., Sinow, R.M., and Carmel, R. (1987) Low serum cobalamin level occur frequently in the acquired immune deficiency syndrome and related disorders. *Eur. J. Haematol.* **38**, 141–147.

68. Mantero-Atienza, E., Sotomayor, M.G., Shor-Posner, G., et al. (1991) Selenium status and immune function in asymptomatic HIV-1 seropositive men. *Nutr. Res.* **11**, 1237–1250.

69. Koch, J., Neal, E.A., Schlott, M.J., et al. (1996) Zinc levels and infections in hospitalized patients with HIV/AIDS. *Nutrition* **12**, 515–518.

70. Semba, R. (1997) Vitamin A and human immuno-deficiency virus infection. *Proc. Nutr. Soc.* **57**, 459–469.

71. Greenberg, B., Semba, R.D., Vink, P.E., et al. (1997) Vitamin A deficiency and maternal infant transmission of HIV in two metropolitan areas in the United States. *AIDS* **11**, 325–332.

72. Burger, H., Kovacs, A., Weiser, B., et al. (1997) Maternal serum vitamin A levels are not associated with mother-to-child transmission of HIV-1 in the United States. *J. AIDS Hum. Retrovirol.* **14**, 321–326.

73. Allard, J., Aghdassi, E., Chau, J., Salit, I., and Walmsley, S. (1998) Oxidative stress and plasma antioxidant micronutrients in humans with HIV infection. *Am. J. Clin. Nutr.* **67**, 143–147.

74. Coodley, G., Coodley, M.K., Nelson, H.D., and Loveless, M.O. (1993) Micronutrient concentrations in the HIV wasting syndrome. *AIDS* **7**, 1595–1600.

75. Pacht, E., Diaz, P., Clanton, T., Hart, J., and Gadek, J.E. (1997) Serum vitamin E decreases in HIV-seropositive subjects over time. *J. Lab. Clin. Med.* **130**, 293–296.

76. Mastroiacovo, P., Ajassa, C., Berardelli, G., et al. (1996) Antioxidant vitamins and immunodeficiency. *Int. J. Vit. Nutr. Res.* **66**, 141–145.

77. Look, M., Rockstroh, J.K., Rao, G.S., et al. (1997) Serum selenium, plasma glutathione (GSH) and erythrocyte glutathione peroxidase (GSH-Px)-levels in asymptomatic versus symptomatic human immunodeficiency virus-1 (HIV-1)-infection. *Eur. J. Clin. Nutr.* **51**, 266–272.

78. Smith, J., Howells, D.W., Kendall, B., Levinsky, R., and Hyland, K. (1987) Folate deficiency and demyelination in AIDS. *Lancet* **2**, 215.

79. Falutz, J., Tsoukas, C., and Gold, P. (1998) Zinc as a cofactor in human immunodeficiency virus-induced immunosuppression. *JAMA* **259**, 2850–2851.

80. Eley, B., Sive, A.A., Abelse, L., et al. (2002) Growth and micronutrient disturbances in stable, HIV-infected children in Cape Town. *Ann. Trop. Paediatr.* **22**, 19–23.

81. Semba, R., Kumwenda, N., Hoover, D.R., et al. (2000) Assessment of iron status using plasma transferring receptor in pregnant women with and without human immunodeficiency virus infection in Malawi. *Eur. J. Clin. Nutr.* **54**, 872–877.

82. Antelman, G., Msamanga, G.I., Spiegelman, D., et al. (2000) Nutritional factors and infectious disease contribute to anemia among pregnant women with Human Immunodeficiency Virus in Tanzania. *J. Nutr.* **130**, 1950–1957.

83. Kcusch, G. and Farthing, M.J.G. (1990) Nutritional aspects of AIDS. *Ann. Rev. Nutr.* **10**, 475–501.

84. Baeten, J., McClelland, R.S., Richardson, B.A., et al. (2002) Vitamin A deficiency and the acute phase response among HIV-1-infected and -uninfected women in Kenya. *J. AIDS* **31**, 243–249.

85. Pace, G. and Leaf, C.D. (1995) The role of oxidative stress in HIV disease. *Free Rad. Biol. Med.* **19**, 523–528.

86. Semba, R. (1998) The role of vitamin A and related retinoids in immune function. *Nutr. Rev.* **56**, S38–S48.

87. Semba, R. (1999) Vitamin A and immunity to viral, bacterial and protozoan infections. *Proc. Nutr. Soc.* **58**, 719–727.

88. Smith, S., Levy, N.S., and Hayes, C.E. (1987) Impaired immunity in vitamin A-deficient mice. *J. Nutr.* **117**, 857–865.

89. Alexander, M., Newmark, H., and Miller, R.G. (1985) Oral beta-carotene can increase the number of OKT4+ cells in human blood. *Immunol. Lett.* **9**, 221–224.

90. Watson, R., Prabhala, R.H., Plezia, P.M., and Alberts, D.S. (1991) Effect of β-carotene on lymphocyte subpopulations in elderly humans: evidence for a dose-response relationship. *Am. J. Clin. Nutr.* **53**, 90–94.

91. Semba, R., Muhilal, Ward, B.J., et al. (1993) Abnormal T-cell proportions in vitamin A-deficient children. *Lancet* **341**, 5–8.

92. Prabhala, R., Garewal, H.S., Hicks, M.J., Sampliner, R.E., and Watson, R.R. The effects of 13-cis-retinoic acid and beta-carotene on cellular immunity on humans. *Cancer* **67**, 1556–1560.

93. Semba, R., Muhilal, Scott, A.L., et al. (1992) Depressed immune response to tetanus in children with vitamin A deficiency. *J. Nutr.* **122**, 101–107.

94. Coutsoudis, A., Kiepiela, P., Coovadia, H., and Broughton, M. (1992) Vitamin A supplementation enhances specific IgG antibody levels and total lymphocyte numbers while improving morbidity in measles. *Ped. Inf. Dis. J.* **11**, 203–209.

95. Fawzi, W., Chalmers, T.C., Herrera, M.G., and Mosteller, F. (1993) Vitamin A supplementation and child mortality: a meta-analysis. *J. Am. Med. Assoc.* **269**, 898–903.

96. Field, C., Johnson, I.R., and Schley, P.D. (2002) Nutrients and their role in host resistance to infection. *J. Leuokocyte Biol.* **71**, 16–32.

97. Rivas, C., Vera, J.C., Guaiquil, V.H., et al. (1997) Increased uptake and accumulation of vitamin C in human immunodeficiency virus 1-infected hematopoietic cell lines. *J. Biol. Chem.* **272**, 5814–5820.

98. Bendich, A. (1988) Antioxidant vitamins and immune responses, in *Nutrition and Immunology*. (Chandra, R.K. and Alan, R., eds.) Liss, New York, pp. 125–147.

99. Hemila, H. (1997) Vitamin C and infectious diseases, in *Vitamin C in Health and Disease*. (Pacler, L. and Fuchs, J., eds.) Marcel Dekker, New York.

100. Meydani, S., Wu, D., Santos, M.S., and Hayek, M.G. (1995) Antioxidants and immune response in the aged: overview of present evidence. *Am. J. Clin. Nutr.* **62**, 1462S–1476S.
101. Wang, Y., Huang, D.S., Lian, B., and Watson, R.R. (1994) Nutritional status and immune response in mice with murine AIDS are normalized by vitamin E supplementation. *J. Nutr.* **124**, 2024–2032.
102. Meydani, S., Barklund, P.M., Liu, S., et al. (1990) Vitamin E supplementation enhances cell-mediated immunity in healthy elderly subjects. *Am. J. Clin. Nutr.* **52**, 557–563.
103. Meydani, S., Meydani, M., Blumberg, J.B., et al. (1997) Vitamin E supplementation enhances in vivo immune response in healthy elderly: A dose-response study. *J. Am. Med. Assoc.* **277**, 1380–1386.
104. Meydani, S., Ribaya-Mercado, J.D., Russell, R.M., Sahyoun, N., Morrow, F.D., and Gershoff, S.N. (1991) Vitamin B-6 deficiency impairs interleukin 2 production and lymphocyte proliferation in elderly adults. *Am. J. Clin. Nutr.* **53**, 1275–1280.
105. Baum, M., Mantero-Atienza, E., Shor-Posner, G., et al. (1991) Association of vitamin B-6 status with parameters of immune function in early HIV-1 infection. *J. AIDS* **4**, 1122–1132.
106. Bendich, A. and Cohen, M. (1988) B vitamins: effects on specific and non-specific immune responses, in *Nutrition and Immunology*. (Chandra, R.K. and Alan, R., eds.) Liss, New York, 101–123.
107. Rotruck, J., Pope, A.L., Ganther, H.E., Swanson, A.B., Hafeman, D.G., and Hoekstra, W.G. (1973) Selenium: biochemical role as a component of glutathione peroxidase. *Science* **179**, 588–590.
108. Sappey, C., Legrand-Poels, S., Best-Belpomme, M., Favie,r A., Rentier, B., and Piette, J. (1994) Stimulation of glutathione peroxidase activity decreases HIV type 1 activation after oxidative stress. *J. AIDS Res. Hum. Retroviruses* **10**, 1451–1461.
109. Chen, C., Zhou, J., Xu, H., Jiang, Y., and Zhu, G. (1997) Effect of selenium supplementation on mice infected with LP-BM5 MuLV, a murine AIDS model. *Biol. Tr. Elem. Res.* **59**, 187–193.
110. Peretz, A., Neve, J., Duchateau, J., et al. (1991) Effects of selenium supplementation on immune parameters in gut failure patients on home parenteral nutrition. *Nutr.* **7**, 215–221.
111. Shankar, A. and Prasad, A.S. (1998) Zinc and immune function: the biological basis of altered resistance to infection. *Am. J. Clin. Nutr.* **68**, 447S–463S.
112. Haraguchi, Y., Sakurai, H., Hussain, S., Anner, B.M., and Hoshino, H. (1999) Inhibition of HIV-1 infection by zinc group metal compounds. *Antiviral Res.* **43**, 132–133.
113. Baum, M., Shor-Posner, G., and Campa, A. (2000) Zinc status in human immunodeficiency virus infection. *J. Nutr.* **130**, 1421S–1423S.
114. Black, R. (1998) Therapeutic and preventive effects of zinc on serious childhood infectious diseases in developing countries. *Am. J. Clin. Nutr.* **68**, 476S–479S.

115. Phuapradit, W., Chaturachinda, K., Taneepanichskul, S., Sirivarasry, J., Khupulsup, K., and Lerdvuthisopon, N. (1996) Serum vitamin A and beta-carotene levels in pregnant women infected with human immunodeficiency virus-1. *Obstetr. Gynecol.* **87**, 564–567.

116. Bogden, J., Kemp, F.W., Han, S., et al. (2000) Status of selected nutrients and progression of human immunodeficiency virus type 1 infection. *Am. J. Clin. Nutr.* **72**, 809–815.

117. Abrams, B., Duncan, D., and Hertz-Picciotto, I. (1993) A prospective study of dietary intake and acquired immune deficiency syndrome in HIV-seropositive homosexual men. *J. AIDS* **6**, 949–958.

118. Camp, W., Allen, S., Alvarez, J.O., et al. (1998) Serum retinol and HIV-1 RNA viral load in rapid and slow progressors. *J. AIDS Hum. Retrovirol.* **18**, 401–406.

119. Kelly, P., Musonda, R., Kafwembe, E., Kaetano, L., Keane, E., and Farthing, M. (1999) Micronutrient supplementation in the AIDS diarrhoea wasting syndrome in Zambia: A randomized controlled trial. *AIDS* **13**, 495–500.

120. Tang, A., Graham, N.M.H., Chandra, R.K., and Saah, A.J. (1997) Low serum vitamin B-12 concentrations are associated with faster human immunodeficiency virus type 1 (HIV-1) disease progression. *J. Nutr.* **127**,345–351.

121. Graham, N., Sorenson, D., Odaka, N., et al. (1991) Relationship of serum copper and zinc levels to HIV seropositivity and progression to AIDS. *J. AIDS* **4**, 976–980.

122. Allavena, C., Dousset, B., May, T., Dubois, F., Canton, P.F.B. (1999) Relationship of trace element, immunological markers, and HIV-1 infection progression. *Biol. Tr. Elem. Res.* **47**, 133–138.

123. Baum, M., Shor-Posner, G., Lai, S., et al. (1997) High risk of HIV-related mortality is associated with selenium deficiency. *J. AIDS Hum. Retrovirol.* **15**, 370–374.

124. Campa, A., Shor-Posner, G., Indacochea, F., et al. (1999) Mortality risk in selenium-deficient HIV-positive children. *J. AIDS Hum. Retrovirol.* **20**, 508–513.

125. Tang, A., Graham, N.M.H., Kirby, A.J., McCall, L.D., Willett, W.C., and Saah, A.J. (1993) Dietary micronutrient intake and risk of progression to Acquired Immunodeficiency Syndrome (AIDS) in Human Immunodeficiency Virus type 1 (HIV-1)-infected homosexual men. *Am. J. Epidemiol.* **138**, 937–951.

126. Tang, A., Graham, N.M.H., and Saah, A.J. (1996) Effects of micronutient intake on survival in human immunodeficiency virus type 1 infection. *Am. J. Epidemiol.* **143**, 1244–1256.

127. Coodley, G., Nelson, H.D., Loveless, M.O., and Folk, C. (1993) Beta-carotene in HIV infection. *J. AIDS* **6**, 272–276.

128. Coodley, G., Coodley, M.K., Lusk, R., et al. (1996) Beta-carotene in HIV infection: an extended evaluation. *AIDS* **10**, 967–973.

129. Semba, R., Lyles, C.M., Margolick, J.B., et al. (1998) Vitamin A supplementation and human immunodeficiency virus load in injection drug users. *J. Inf. Dis.* **177**, 611–616.

130. Hussey, G., Hughes, J., Potgieter, S., et al. (1996) Vitamin A status and supplementation and its effects on immunity in children with AIDS, XVII International Vitamin A Consultative Group Meeting, Guatemala City, Guatemala, 1996. International Life Sciences Institute, Washington, DC.

131. Look, M., Rockstroh, J.K., Rao, G.S., et al. (1998) Sodium selenite and N-acetylcysteine in antiretroviral-naive HIV-1-infected patients: a randomized, controlled pilot study. *Eur. J. Clin. Invest.* **28**, 389–397.

132. Coutsoudis, A., Moodley, D., Pillay, K., et al. (1997) Effects of vitamin A supplementation on viral load in HIV-1-infected pregnant women. *J. AIDS Hum. Retrovirol.* **15**, 86–87.

133. Humphrey, J., Quinn, T., Fine, D., et al. (1999) Short-term effects of large-dose vitamin A supplementation on viral load and immune response in HIV-infected women. *J AIDS Hum. Retrovirol.* **20**, 44–51.

134. Delmas-Beauvieux, M., Peuchant, E., Couchrouron, A., et al. (1996) The enzymatic antioxidant system in blood and glutathione status in human immunodeficiency virus (HIV)-infected patients: effects of supplementation with selenium or β-carotene. *Am. J. Clin. Nutr.* **64**, 101–107.

135. Kennedy, C., Coutsoudis, A., Kuhn, L., et al. (2000) Randomized controlled trial assessing the effect of vitamin A supplementation on maternal morbidity during pregnancy and postpartum among HIV-infected women. *J. AIDS* **24**, 37–44.

136. Olmsted, L., Schrauzer, G.N., Flores-Arce, M., and Dowd, J. (1989) Selenium supplementation of symptomatic human immunodeficiency virus infected patients. *Biol. Tr. Elem. Res.* **20**, 59–65.

137. Allard, J., Aghdassi, E., Chau, J., et al. (1998) Effects of vitamin E and C supplementation on oxidative stress and viral load in HIV-infected subjects. *AIDS* **12**, 1653–1659.

138. Fawzim W., Msamangam G.I., Weim R., et al. (2003) Effect of providing vitamin supplements to human immunodeficiency virus-infected, lactating mothers on the child's morbidity and CD4+ cell counts. *Clin. Inf. Dis.* **36**, 1053–1062.

139. Niki, E., Noguchi, N., Tsuchihashi, H., and Gotoh, N. (1995) Interaction among vitamin C, vitamin E, and beta-carotene. *Am. J. Clin. Nutr.* **62**, 1322S–1326S.

140. Villamor, E., Msamanga, G., Spiegelman, D., Antelman, G., Peterson, K.E., and Hunter, D.J. (2002) Effect of multivitamin and vitamin A supplementation on weight gain during pregnancy among HIV-1-infected women. *Am. J. Clin. Nutr.* **76**, 1082–1090.

141. Melikian, G., Mmiro, F., Ndugwa, C., et al. (2001) Relation of vitamin A and carotenoid status to growth failure and mortality among Ugandan infants with human immunodeficiency virus. *Nutrition* **17**, 567–572.

142. Semba, R., Miotti, P.G., Chiphangwi, J.D., et al. (1997) Maternal vitamin A deficiency and child growth failure during human immunodeficiency virus infection. *J. AIDS Hum. Retrovirol.* **14**, 219–222.

143. Rich, K., Fowler, M.G., Mofenson, L.M., et al. (2000) Maternal and infant factors predicting disease progression in human immunodeficiency virus type 1-infected infants. Women and Infants Transmission Study Group. *Pediatr.* **105**, e8.

144. Semba, R., Miotti, P.G., Chiphangwi, J.D., et al. (1995) Infant mortality and maternal vitamin A deficiency during human immunodeficiency virus infection. *Clin. Infect. Dis.* **21**, 966–972.

145. Read, J., Bethel, J., Harris, D.R., et al. (1999) Serum vitamin A concentrations in a North American cohort of human immunodeficiency virus type 1-infected children. National Institute of Child Health and Human Development Intravenous Immunoglobulin Clinical Trial Study Group. *Pediatr. Inf. Dis. J.* **18**, 134–142.

146. Coutsoudis, A., Bobat, R.A., Coovadia, H.M., Kuhn, L., Tsai, W.Y., and Stein, Z.A. (1995) The effects of vitamin A supplementation on the morbidity of children born to HIV-infected women. *Am. J. Pub. Hlth.* **85**, 1076–1081.

147. Fawzi, W., Mbise, R.L., Hertzmark, E., et al. (1999) A randomized trial of vitamin A supplements in relation to mortality among human immunodeficiency virus-infected and uninfected children in Tanzania. *Pediatr. Inf. Dis. J.* **18**, 127–133.

148. Fawzi, W., Mbise, R., Spiegelman, D., Fataki, M., Hertzmark, E., and Ndossi, G. (2000) Vitamin A supplements and diarrheal and respiratory tract infections among children in Dar es Salaam, Tanzania. *J. Pediatr.* **137**, 660–667.

149. Kumwenda, N., Miotti, P.G., Taha, T.E., et al. (2002) Antenatal vitamin A supplementation increases birth weight and decreases anemia among infants born to human immunodeficiency virus-infected women in Malawi. *Clin. Infect. Dis.* **35**, 618–624.

150. Fawzi, W. and Hunter, D.J. (1998) Vitamins in HIV disease progression and vertical transmission. *Epidemiol.* **9**, 457–466.

151. Fawzi, W. (2000) Nutritional factors and vertical transmission of HIV-1. Epidemiology and potential mechanisms. *Ann. NY Acad. Sci.* **918**, 99–114.

152. Graham, N., Bulterys, M., Chao, A., et al. (1993) Effect of maternal vitamin A deficiency on infant mortality and perinatal HIV transmission, Paper presented at the National Conference on Human Retroviruses and Related Infection; December 12–16, Baltimore, Maryland, USA.

153. Castetbon, K., Manigart, O., Bonard, D., et al. (2000) Maternal vitamin A status and mother-to-child transmission of HIV in West Africa. *DITRAME Study Group. AIDS* **14**, 908–910.

154. Burns, D., FitzGerald, G., Semba, R., et al. (1999) Vitamin A deficiency and other nutritional indices during pregnancy in human immunodeficiency virus infection: prevalence, clinical correlates, and outcome. Women and Infants Transmission Study Group. *Clin. Inf. Dis.* **29**, 328–334.

155. Mostad, S., Overbaugh, J., De Vange, D.M., et al. (1997) Hormonal contraception, vitamin A deficiency, and other risk factors for shedding of HIV-1 infected cells from the cervix and vagina. *Lancet* **350**, 922–927.

156. French, A., Cohen, M.H., Gange, S.J., et al. (2002) Vitamin A deficiency and genital viral burden in women infected with HIV-1. *Lancet* **359**, 1210–1212.

157. Baeten, J., McClelland, R.S., Overbaugh, J., et al. (2002) Vitamin A supplementation and human immunodeficiency virus type 1 shedding in women: results of a randomized clinical trial. *J. Inf. Dis.* **185**, 1187–1191.

158. Nduati, R., John, G.C., Richardson, B.A., et al. (1995) Human immunodeficiency virus type 1-infected cells in breast milk: association with immunosuppression and vitamin A deficiency. *J. Inf. Dis.* **172**,1461–1468.

159. Semba, R., Kumwenda, N., Hoover, D.R., et al. (1999) Human immunodeficiency virus load in breast milk, mastitis, and mother-to-child transmission of human immunodeficiency virus type 1. *J. Inf. Dis.* **180**, 93–98.

160. Willumsen, J., Filteau, S.M., Coutsoudis, A., Uebel, K.E., Newell, M.L., and Tomkins, A.M. (2000) Subclinical mastitis as a risk factor for mother-infant HIV transmission. Advances in *Exp. Med. Biol.* **478**, 211–223.

161. Filteau, S., Rice, A.L., Ball, J.J., et al. (1999) Breast milk immune factors in Bangladeshi women supplemented postpartum with retinol or beta-carotene. *Am. J. Clin. Nutr.* **69**, 953–958.

162. Semba, R. (1998) Nutritional interventions: vitamin A and breastfeeding, Paper presented at the III International Symposium on Global strategies to Prevent Perinatal HIV Transmission; November, 9–10, Valencia, Spain.

163. Fawzi, W., Msamanga, G.I., Hunter, D., et al. (2000) Randomized trial of vitamin supplements in relation to vertical transmission of HIV-1 in Tanzania. *J. AIDS* **23**, 246–254.

164. Fawzi, W., Msamanga, G., Hunter, D., et al. (2002) Randomized trial of vitamin supplements in relation to transmission of HIV through breastfeeding and early child mortality. *AIDS* **16**,1935–1944.

165. Coutsoudis, A., Pillay, K., Spooner, E., Kuhn, L., and Coovadia, H.M. (1999) Randomized trial testing the effect of vitamin A supplementation on pregnancy outcomes and early mother-to-child HIV-1 transmission in Durban, South Africa. South African Vitamin A Study Group. *AIDS* **13**, 1517–1524.

15 Summary and Future Directions

PENELOPE NESTEL AND RITU NALUBOLA

CONTENTS

KEY POINTS

- Overnutrition and undernutrition can impair immunity. Micronutrients are important immunomodulators, and deficiencies are associated with impaired responses and immune functions.
- A flexible immunological investigative system that can be adapted to different situations is needed. Validated miniaturized assays that are field friendly, safe, and cold chain-free using dried whole blood or dried serum spots are also needed.
- Well accepted indices of nutritional status, and cutoff points defining under and over nutrition, are available for infants and young children, nonpregnant women, and adult men. Cutoff points are also available for adolescents, but the applicability of cutoffs based on data in developing countries is not yet completely certain.
- Micronutrient blood levels often do not reflect true tissue stores because they are acute phase reactants that can be altered in the presence of fever as a result of acute and chronic infections. A better understanding of how biochemical markers are related to intake and what else affects their levels

From: *Handbook of Nutrition and Immunity*
Edited by: M. E. Gershwin, P. Nestel, and C. L. Keen © Humana Press, Totowa, NJ

needs to be determined. Functional markers for micronutrients status need to be developed.

- Nutrition plays an important role in the onset, severity, and duration of diarrheal diseases in childhood. Nutrition also strongly influences the disease burden of malaria with undernutrition being associated with increased malaria mortality and more severe malaria-associated anemia. Whether multiple or repeated exposures boost the immune response to common infections under different nutritional status remains unknown.
- Micronutrients occur together in food and do not act in isolation; they probably exert a synergistic effect within the body to promote optimal health. However, little work has been done on multiple micronutrients and immunity. More research is needed to determine which nutrients to include in multiple micronutrient supplements for nonpregnant and nonlactating women and for children in HIV endemic and nonendemic areas.
- The effects of dietary fats and fatty acids on immune responses appear to be dependent on many factors. Fish oils and n-3 fatty acids appear to selectively affect specific immune functions in humans.
- The full biological significance of most of the nutritional antioxidants is poorly understood or unknown and is an important area for research. The mechanisms of oxidative stress and the role of dietary components in the modulation of processes associated with aging also need to expand in future years.
- Increasingly, consumers are looking at food not only for nutritional purposes, but also for health benefits in such areas as cardiovascular disease, vision, cognitive function, diabetes, and obesity. However, further insight and debate is needed on the marketing of these foods and whether they can, in fact, produce the claimed health benefits.

Introduction

Malnutrition, be it overnutrition or undernutrition, can impair immunity among specific groups of people including low-income groups who may not consume an adequate amount of a good-quality diet, the elderly, the chronically ill, and low birth weight infants. Specific conditions such as alcoholism, eating disorders, and gastrointestinal diseases cause physiological and pathological conditions that disrupt the immune system. Severe undernutrition impairs the integrity of mucosal barriers, the acute phase response, and the cellular immune function, thereby reducing resistance to infections (1–3).

Micronutrients are important immunomodulaters and deficiencies are associated with impaired responses and immune functions. Vitamin A deficiency is the most recognized vitamin deficiency in developing countries (4). Vitamin A supplementation reduces child mortality (5) and may reduce maternal mortality *(6)*. Other common vitamin deficiencies include the B vitamins, especially folic acid, B_6, B_{12}, thiamin (B_1), riboflavin (B_2), although reliable data on the extent of these deficiencies are limited. Deficiencies of vitamin C and the other fat-soluble vitamins, namely D, E, and K are less common, although specific subgroups may be at risk.

Iodine, iron, selenium, and zinc deficiencies are prevalent in many developing countries *(8)*. Low intakes of these trace elements can markedly affect multiple components of the immune system, resulting in greater susceptibility to infectious disease. Whereas deficiencies in copper, magnesium, and manganese are rare, certain population groups may be susceptible to marginal deficiencies or secondary deficiencies, such as copper deficiency resulting from zinc supplementation. Marginal deficiencies can also affect an individual's overall risk of infection and contribute to chronic immune-associated disorders, such as asthma and chronic obstructive pulmonary disease.

Advances in Assessment Technology

Most immunodeficiencies can be diagnosed using tests that can be carried out in many clinical laboratories, with more precise evaluations of immunologic function and treatment being referred to specialized centers. Because most primary and secondary health care facilities in developing countries do not have a regular and/or reliable supply of electricity, sometimes even water, and the cadre of staff can vary enormously, a flexible immunological investigative system that can be adapted to different situations is needed. Selmi et al. (*see* Chapter 1) propose the establishment of a three-tier network between centers whereby biological samples can be sent to a higher tier facility where tests can be carried out in a more controlled environment or additional immunologic parameters can be determined using methods that are not possible in the lower tier facility or facilities. For the tier system to be effective, however, the practicality of preserving and transporting biological samples and ways to communicate and share information between the three levels must be known. Testing the implementation of the proposed tier system is important because an ideal method to study an at-risk population's response to common infections, thereby enabling the monitoring and evaluation of preventive strategies, requires an efficient system for collecting blood samples before and after energy and/or nutrient supplementation. Ultimately, it may be possible to operate with a one- or two-tier system as methods for assessing immunological status and function, such as the use of recombinant antigens, develop further.

Nutritional status is conventionally determined from dietary intakes and clinical signs and symptoms *(9,10)*. Measures of body composition and nutritional biochemistry can also be used. Various methods of different complexity, hence cost, are used to estimate dietary intake. Their reliability is dependent on the respondent's memory and cooperation, the intraindividual variation in usual food intake, and the appropriateness and/or accuracy of the food composition tables used. Physical assessments require trained and competent health care providers as the signs and symptoms of undernutrition are invariably multi-causal.

Assessing nutritional status from anthropometric measurements is much simpler than using dietary and clinical methods and can be carried out reliably by unskilled workers with good training. Although weight and height reflect both recent and long-term nutritional status, they can be influenced by non nutritional factors, notably illness, and they do not indicate specific nutrient deficiencies. Circumferences such as the mid-arm, which reflect the amount of subcutaneous fat and muscle, can also be appropriate for specific age groups. Skinfold thickness measurements can provide an estimate of the amount of subcutaneous and total body fat. Well-accepted indices of nutritional status, and cutoff points defining under- and overnutrition, are available for infants and young children as well as for nonpregnant women and adult men *(11,12)*. New growth standards for infants and young children are currently under development *(13)*. Cutoff points are also available for adolescents, although few reference data are available for developing countries *(11)* and the applicability of cutoffs based on developed countries data is not yet completely certain.

Body composition is usually expressed as the percentage of body fat. Skinfold thickness, body mass index, densitometry, bioelectrical impedance, and total body electrical conductivity are used to measure body composition based on fat and fat-free mass. Neutron activation analysis, isotope dilution, and dual-energy X-ray absorptiometry measure body composition based on water, protein, mineral, and fat, but can also be used to measure fat mass and fat-free mass. Each method has its limitations as discussed by Hendricks and Hussey (*see* Chapter 2). Clearly, methods that use skinfold thickness and weight and height have more applicability in epidemiological studies. Research is needed to validate indices that use these measures against the more sensitive and complex techniques that measure body composition, which is important for measuring obesity and for monitoring and evaluating interventions.

Biochemical indicators of nutritional status are either static, whereby they measure a nutrient or related metabolite in blood or another body fluid, or functional reflecting a specific physiological or biochemical reaction, for example, enzymatic. Micronutrient blood levels, however, often do not reflect true tissue stores because they are acute phase reactants that can be altered in the presence of fever caused by acute and chronic infections. The functional significance of the change in serum concentrations during the early phase of infection is not always unknown, but its understanding is important for micronutrients such as selenium that is essential for both innate and acquired immunity *(14)*. Moreover, a persistent acute phase response-induced alteration in micronutrient concentrations, such as hypozincemia, may represent a significant risk to the individual if it occurs during pregnancy *(15)*. Measuring aspects of the immune system and its active state can help interpret serum concentrations of micronutrients affected by acute phase responses. Functional indicators are less affected by recent changes in food and fluid intake, but they can be influenced by a number of nutrient abnormalities and may not be nutrient specific. Functional markers for the status of micronutrients such as zinc, iron, or vitamin A need to be developed.

Because of the limitations associated with dietary assessment methods and the fact that biochemical markers do not always reflect nutritional status, the correlation between blood levels and the intake of a specific nutrient is often not high *(9)*. Some biomarkers may have a role in clinical practice as surrogate measures of intake, for example, lutein for β-carotene *(17)*, or of nutritional status for example, the plasma-soluble transferrin receptor for iron deficiency *(17)*. For biochemical markers to be useful, however, a better understanding of how they are related to intake and what else affects their levels needs to be determined. Finally, pregnancy hemodilution appears to decrease plasma micronutrient levels, but a formal allowance for this effect has not been made for all micronutrients—as it has been for hemoglobin—and further work is needed in this area.

Relatively low technological immunoassay methods are continually being developed. Most of the new laboratory assays require smaller volumes of blood samples that can be obtained from capillary blood *(18)* by minimally trained nonclinical staff. The challenge is how to make the available miniaturized assays field-friendly, safe, and cold chain-free using dried whole blood or dried serum spots. Many analytes are stable at ambient temperature in dried blood spots and filter papers can be easily sent to a higher tier laboratory for analysis. However, as Gitau and Filteau (*see* Chapter 3) note, the collection of finger prick blood can include variable amounts of extracellular fluid depending on the collection technique. Additionally, the spread of the spot on filter paper is not completely uniform consequently the variability in results from these samples can be greater than that from plasma. Blood spots are currently most useful for qualitative analyses, such as the presence or absence of a specific antibody, or semiquantitative analyses where large differences are expected between normal and abnormal levels, such as with thyroid stimulating hormone. A second limitation to using the new and ever-expanding number of low technology immunoassay methods is that reference standards for interlaboratory comparisons are often not available. There is also no general agreement on the cutoff for deficiency for some biomarkers such as retinol binding protein. Cutoffs are also needed for many acute phase proteins such as α1-antichymotrypsin, α1-acid-glycoprotein, and C-reactive protein, indicating that additional work is needed in this area. Finally, determining the functional significance, in terms of important maternal and infant outcomes, of the newly developed methods and their indicators need is essential.

The advent of validated miniaturized assays for both immune and nutritional status and good access to laboratories with effective quality control procedures will facilitate the testing of nutritional interventions using challenge formats—that is, vaccinations—to explore adaptive responses. They will also enable the testing of theoretical associations between the vaccination challenges used and the expected deficits from specific micronutrient deficiency states.

Advances in the Understanding of Nutritional Effects on Immunity

Significant progress has been made in the area of nutrition and immune response and, as discussed in the preceding chapters, the roles of different nutrients and dietary components in immune function are now better understood. Nevertheless, there are a number of gaps in both our understanding of the complex interaction between immune function and nutritional status, and in the implementation of this understanding into effective public health interventions.

The synergism between nutrition and immunity depends on the extent to which adequate nutrition provides the body with the capacity to maintain its function and to protect itself. Nutrient deficiencies are often associated with a poor diet, but they are also often brought about or made worse by increased losses of specific nutrients during periods of stress such as infection. Jackson and Calder (*see* Chapter 4) highlight that in severe undernutrition, both the generalized response—for example, the presence of fever, increased pulse, increased respiratory rate, feeling unwell, or the loss of appetite—and localized response that is indicated by the activation of an immune response and the presence of an inflammatory infiltrate are often diminished. In some cases, they may be completely absent. Consequently, affected individuals are severely immunocompromised. Indeed, Jackson and Calder emphasize that for a treatment regimen to be successful it is essential to assume that most, if not all, severely undernourished children have an infection. In the meantime, much more work is needed to understand how best to treat severe undernutrition effectively.

Ramakrishnan et al. (*see* Chapter 5) summarize the evidence base for the associations between infection, immunity, and vitamins. They focus on vitamin A because this is the most extensively studied vitamin. Recent in vitro research suggests that retinoic acid may promote the development of specialized helper-T (Th)-type cells, such as Th2 cells, rather than Th1 cells *(19)*. It is currently hypothesized that vitamin A supplementation to normal or well-nourished children may increase the normal inflammatory response and exacerbate damage to the respiratory tract, for example, whereas large doses of vitamin A to deficient children may normalize the Th1 response and restore an optimal Th2 response, in addition to improving gut integrity in the case of diarrhea *(20,21)*. Additional research is needed to determine the specialized functions and roles of the different Th-type cells to elucidate why vitamin A may produces varying effects with different infections.

Few well-designed human studies have looked at the effect of other vitamins on morbidities or immunity. Researchers hypothesize that vitamin B_6 deficiency may suppress Th1 activity, whereas repletion enables a proper Th2 response; vitamin B_{12} deficiency may suppress the Th2 response, although the role of vitamin B_{12} in the Th2/Th1 response is not known; and folate deficiency may act mechanistically by inducing suppression of the Th1 response, but few have examined the benefits of improving folate status in reducing morbidity *(22)*.

Keen et al. (*see* Chapter 6) describe the important roles that minerals play in all components of the immune system. A deficiency of an essential mineral such as zinc, copper, iron, or magnesium can have severe immunomodulatory effects. Mineral deficiencies can arise through a variety of mechanisms as either primary deficiencies caused by an inadequate intake, or as secondary or conditioned deficiencies arising from genetic factors that can create a higher than normal requirement for a nutrient. The extent to which multiple gene abnormalities contribute to altered mineral metabolism in humans is unknown. However, based on rates among animals, it is reasonable to speculate that they may occur with relatively high frequency. Conditioned deficiencies may also occur from three other situations. First, mineral interactions—although the extent to which an excess concentration of nonessential minerals contributes to the immune system abnormalities observed in individuals with a deficiency of an essential mineral is unknown. Second, chemicals or drugs that can alter the metabolism of numerous minerals through the acute phase response, but the extent to which acute phase response-induced changes in the metabolism of zinc, copper, iron, and selenium attenuates or augments the disease process is unclear. Third, through stressor-induced physiological changes in mineral metabolism, excessive loss of a mineral or altered metabolism through the acute phase response. Mineral deficiency-induced abnormalities in the immune system can be particularly profound when they occur during fetal and early postnatal development.

Copper is essential for normal functioning of the immune system. Copper deficiency inhibits the production of interleukin (IL)-2, a cytokine essential for normal T-cell metabolism. Marginal, subclinical copper deficiency may occur because of infection, inflammation, exercise, or chronic disease conditions such as diabetes and hypertension. Not enough, however, is known about how these factors alter immune function. The mechanism(s) by which iodine deficiency compromises immune function is also not well established. Although excessive iodine intake has been reported to impair immune activity (23), the underlying mechanisms are not understood. Magnesium deficiency may be higher than previously thought; it results in an increase in both reactive oxygen and reactive nitrogen species (24). Studies on the effects of magnesium deficiency on all aspects of the immune system are needed. Data on the effects of manganese on the immune system are lacking.

Significant progress has been made in the area of nutrition and immunity as it relates to malarial infection. Menéndez and Dobaño note that recent controlled studies have demonstrated that nutrition strongly influences the disease burden of malaria with undernutrition being associated with increased malaria mortality and more severe malaria-associated anemia (see Chapter 11). Nevertheless, a better understanding of the molecular and cellular events related to naturally acquired immunity is needed to determine how they influence the role of nutrition in malarial onset, progression, and recovery. Low plasma retinol levels have been observed with infection; however, whether the low plasma retinol levels indicate true vitamin A depletion or are caused by the acute phase response is not yet known. Supplementation with vitamin A has produced inconsistent results (25,26). High-dose riboflavin supplementation can suppress malaria parasite growth (27), but the mechanisms are yet to be determined. Vitamin E is hypothesized to suppress the parasite-damaging oxidative stress reaction generated by the immune system, thus increasing survival of the P. falciparum parasite (28). Vitamin E is known to modify the protective effects of fish oil in malaria although the mechanisms are not well understood (29). Controlled intervention trials in adults and children in malaria endemic areas and in individuals of varying stages of nutritional deficit are needed. The role of iron in malaria appears to be clearer than that of the other micronutrients and agreed upon guidelines are needed for the administration of iron in a malarial infection. Future research will determine the need for, and appropriateness of, including other micronutrients in a therapeutic regimen.

Zinc deficiency and protein-energy malnutrition are known to influence humoral and cell-mediated immunity (30) and supplementation with zinc reduces the incidence of pneumonia by more than 40% (31). However, as Riley notes, its effect on mortality from acute lower respiratory infection is not known (see Chapter 12). Vitamin A supplementation has no effect on recovery from acute respiratory infections such as bacterial pneumonia. The role of other micronutrients in respiratory infections, however, is unclear. Vitamin E offers a promising role because of its antioxidant function and the mechanisms of vitamin E-induced protection against the influenza virus and other respiratory infections are being explored (*see* Chapter 9). Several observational studies have suggested a role of vitamin D deficiency in various respiratory infections including tuberculosis and, to a lesser extent, pneumonia although whether it is causal is not yet clear *(32)*.

As Taren notes (*see* Chapter 13), nutrition plays an important role in the onset, severity, and duration of diarrheal diseases in childhood. Several nutrition interventions are now being studied as adjuvants to conventional therapies during diarrheal episodes. Zinc and vitamin A supplementation have proven promising *(33–35)* although the benefits of vitamin A supplementation in cases where diarrhea is not severe are not conclusive *(36)*. Whether other nutrients, such as iron, may be beneficial as adjuvants to diarrheal treatments is not yet known. Borchers et al. (*see* Chapter 10) discuss the use of probiotics, that is, live microorganisms to manage diarrheal disease. Some lactic acid producing bacteria have been reported to reduce the incidence of diarrheal episodes in infants and children *(37)*. More work is required as the use of other probiotics and the mechanisms need to be elucidated. Vaccines against common diarrheal agents are also being developed and progress has been made against rotavirus and cholera, although their effectiveness and efficacy under different nutritional status or concomitant infections is not fully determined. Studies are also underway to develop vaccines against Shigella and *Escherichia coli* (*E. coli*) *(38)*.

Whether multiple or repeated exposures boost the immune response to common infections under different nutritional status remains unknown. A recent study reported that children with apparent biochemical micronutrient deficiencies (based on hemoglobin, ferritin, and serum zinc and retinol levels) and stunting had significant and protective levels of antibodies to the *H. pylori*, hepatitis A virus, rotavirus, (and malaria) pathogens *(39)*. The same study found infection with *H. pylori* may be associated with anemia. However, the actual route of transmission of *H. pylori* and the immune response to *H. pylori* under conditions of nutritional deficiencies is yet unknown.

Chang (*see* Chapter 8) in his discussion on allergies and nutrition notes that gastrointestinal pathogens such as Toxoplasma, Helicobacter, and Shistosoma may protect against the development of food sensitivities and lead to a decrease in the incidence of atopic dermatitis in the young child. However, the association between overall hygiene, food intake, bacterial colonization of the gastrointestinal tract, exposure to environmental allergens, and the balance between Th1 and Th2 subsets is still not completely clear and requires further investigation.

Kiure and Fawzi (*see* Chapter 14) focus on HIV infection, immunity, and nutrition. Vitamin A supplementation had no effect on disease progression

(CD4$^+$ or viral load among adults); the efficacy of supplements on clinical outcomes has not been reported. Vitamin A supplementation also had no effect on HIV-1 transmission during pregnancy (viral shedding in the lower genital tract) or postpartum (subclinical mastitis), but transmission was significantly increased when given both pre- and postpartum (40). In vitro experiments using HIV-infected human cell lines showed exposure to high doses of vitamin C decreased proliferation and survival of the infected cells and reduced viral production (41). In humans, supplementation with both vitamins C and E decreased lipid peroxidation and showed a trend toward a reduced HIV viral load, which appears to confirm a role for vitamin C independent of vitamin E, but additional studies are needed. Vitamin E may protect against HIV progression in infected subjects (42). Iron supplementation has been reported to be a potential risk factor for HIV progression and morbidity (43,44) although others suggest more evidence is needed (45). A short-term selenium intervention trial showed a small, but nonsignificant, effect on slowing HIV disease progression (increased CD4$^+$ cell counts) (46), but no effect on viral load (47). Intervention trials using zinc have not been carried out, but observational data show high dietary intakes of zinc may delay HIV disease progression (increased CD4$^+$ cell counts) (48). The efficacy of zinc and/or selenium supplements to reduce HIV disease progression and transmission in HIV-infected individuals warrants further research as these may be low-cost interventions in developing countries. As Harbige and Gershwin discuss (see Chapter 9), the use of antioxidant supplements along with n-6 fatty acids in HIV-infected individuals also needs to be investigated.

Micronutrients do not act in isolation; they probably exert a synergestic effect within the body to promote optimal health. Harbige and Gershwin (see Chapter 9) point out that nutritional antioxidants occur together in food, rather than in isolation, and, particularly when taken together, enhance both adaptive and innate immunity. For example, vitamins C and E have been reported to produce synergistic effects on immune functions. Vitamins C and E, given together to healthy adults, improved blood mononuclear cell production of IL-1β and Tumor Necrosis Factor-α and levels of IgG and complement C3, compared with either vitamin given alone (49,50). Studies with other antioxidant combinations, including vitamin E and β-carotene, have also been reported to increase CD4 T-cell count (51). Micronutrient deficiencies, too, rarely occur in isolation. Subclinical deficiencies of multiple micronutrients, rather than single micronutrient deficiencies, are likely to be highly prevalent in developing countries where access to high-quality food is limited and the majority of household income is spent on a few simple staples.

Little work has been done on multiple micronutrients and immunity. Multiple micronutrient supplementation was associated with improved immune function and delayed disease progression in HIV/AIDS-infected children *(52)*. However, multiple vitamins alone had no effect on the risk of vertical transmission of HIV overall, although benefits were observed in subgroups of women who were nutritionally or immunologically compromised *(40)*. The beneficial effects of multiple vitamin supplementation to HIV-infected mothers were extended to children born to these women and morbidity, as a result of diarrhea and pneumonia, as well as all-cause mortality were reduced *(53,54)*. More research is needed to determine which nutrients to include in multiple micronutrient supplements for nonpregnant and nonlactating women and for children in HIV endemic—to delay disease progression and clinical outcomes—and in nonendemic areas—to improve immune status and reduce the risk of adverse outcomes. Studies are also needed on the dose and method of delivery that will be most effective in developing countries. Additionally, investigations on issues such as micronutrient interactions, safety, cost, accessibility, and quality are required.

New concepts in the understanding of nutritional effects on immunology may emerge in the future. For example, the current evidence base does not support a role for minerals or vitamins in the development of atopy. However, as Chang discusses (*see* Chapter 8), it is hypothesized that an allergic response to antigen challenge, including inflammatory cell infiltration, results in the generation and release of reactive oxygen species (superoxide and hydrogen peroxide), which are further metabolized to oxygen free radicals that lead to bronchoconstriction, increased mucus secretion, and microvascular leakage *(55)*. Thus, the association between the development of allergies and asthma and the presence of oxygen free radicals is an important area that is being explored. Currently, avoidance or elimination of the allergenic food(s) appear to be the primary modes of treatment; however, immunotherapy strategies such as immunomodulatory agents *(56)* and anti-IgE treatments *(57)* have shown promise and may provide an effective treatment in the future.

Another area of active research is the role of the arachidonic acid pathway intermediates in asthma and atopic dermatitis. Arachidonic acid is metabolized to a class of compounds known as leukotrienes, which are mediators of inflammation, or to various prostaglandins and thromboxane that also have inflammatory effects. A potential treatment for both allergies and asthma is the use of leukotriene pathway inhibitors. Fish oils are rich in eicosapentanoic acid, a competitor of arachidonic acid, which is metabolized into metabolites that do not possess the same inflammatory activity as the leukotrienes. Some studies have demonstrated the benefits of fish oil consumption in decreasing the risk of asthmatic responses *(58,59)*. However, whether these benefits extend to the treatment of atopic dermatitis or other allergic inflammations is not clear *(59,60)*. As Erickson et al. discuss (*see* Chapter 7), the effects of dietary fats and fatty acids on immune responses appear to be dependent on many factors, including the concentration and type of fat or fatty acid, duration of study, assay methods, gender, age, the antioxidant status of the individual, and, in some cases, the levels of supplemental vitamin E provided. Consequently, studies investigating the role of fish oils and the fatty acids most commonly found in fish oils, eicosapentanoic acid (EPA), and docasahexanoic acid (DHA), in immune responses among humans have produced varying results. Although some of these discrepancies in results will need to be resolved, fish oils and omega-3 (n-3) fatty acids appear to selectively affect specific immune functions in humans.

Harbige and Gershwin in their discussion on the role of antioxidant nutrition and immunity (*see* Chapter 9) note that the full biological significance of most of the nutritional antioxidants (vitamin E, β-carotene [provitamin A], vitamin C, manganese, copper, zinc, and selenium) is poorly understood or unknown. Animal models have demonstrated beneficial effects and studies in humans are needed to fully understand the role of antioxidants in viral, bacterial, and parasitic infections. Some antioxidants interact with polyunsaturated fatty acids (PUFA), for example, vitamin E often reverses PUFA's immunologic effects particularly the n-3 forms *(29)* and selenium and vitamin E may spare each other's effects *(61,62)*. Flavonoids may mask the effects of the classical antioxidants (vitamin E, β-carotene, vitamin C) and some appear to have opposing functions. Thus flavonoids may have different effects on immune functions and understanding these additional interacting nutritional factors when investigating antioxidants, immune functions, and infection is important. Nutritional antioxidants may also have a role in lymphopoiesis—another area that is poorly understood. Studies in mice have shown that β-carotene and lycopene increased the T- and B-cell counts and β-carotene enhanced serum IgG levels in neonate mice *(63)*. Human studies, however, are lacking.

Ageing is associated with dysregulation of the immune response and changes in the antioxidant/oxidant balance. These differences contribute to the development of various age-associated diseases such as infections, cancers, and atherosclerosis, as well as to prolonged illness recovery time. Epidemiological studies suggest that consumption of antioxidant-rich fruits and vegetables reduces the risk of certain chronic diseases such as cardiovascular disease and cancer, and may contribute to longevity and quality of life. Dietary antioxidants such as vitamin E, carotenoids, and flavonoids can affect the development of atherosclerosis and tumors *(64,65)*. However, the role of these nutrients and their interaction with ageing during these processes has not been well studied. Knowledge of the mechanisms of oxidative stress and the role of dietary components in the modulation of these processes associated with ageing needs to expand in future years.

Novel Approaches to Food: Functional Foods

In recent years, consumers in developed countries have begun to look at food not only for nutritional purposes, but also for health benefits. This trend is now starting to take hold in developing countries such as Brasil, India, and South Africa. As the beneficial role of specific nutrients in reducing the risk of disease has become apparent, so has the awareness and demand from consumers for individual nutrients or other dietary components in the form of the so-called "functional foods." The term "functional foods" is generally used to refer to foods that provide a health benefit beyond basic nutrition, such as a reduction in the risk of chronic disease or promotion of well-being. These, foods include fruits and vegetables such as tomatoes, spinach, broccoli, blueberries, garlic, soy beans, red wine, green tea, fish, nuts, and oats. For example, lycopene in tomatoes is linked to preventing conditions such as cancer, heart disease, osteoporosis, and macular degeneration *(66)*. Similarly, epidemiologic studies have found reduced overall risk of vascular disease associated with drinking red wine *(67)*.

Functional foods target a range of health conditions, including reducing the risk of hypercholesterolemia, cardiovascular disease, osteoporosis, poor child health and development, high blood pressure, diabetes, gastrointestinal disorders, menopausal problems, and lactose intolerance. Those in the US market include prune juice with lutein; complete nutritional beverages with lutein; cranberry juice with the label claim "may help maintain urinary tract health"; fermented dairy beverages with probiotic bacteria; tomato products with the label claim "lycopene may help reduce the risk of prostate and cervical cancer"; oat grain breakfast cereals with the label claim "may help reduce your cholesterol"; and garlic extract supplements and green teas with claims about health benefits.

The focus of scientific research in this area has shifted in the past few years from the benefits of the whole food itself to the benefits of combinations of bioactive components isolated from such foods. The efficacy of providing isolated components or mixtures, rather than the whole food, and the effective dose of such a medicinal approach is also being investigated. Although most previous research focused on the effects of foods and dietary components on cardiovascular disease, whether these foods extend benefits to other health outcomes such as eye health, cognitive function, diabetes, and obesity is now being explored.

The market for functional foods is large, continues to grow, and is driven by a growing consumer understanding of diet-disease relationships, aging populations, and advances in food technology and nutrition *(68)*. Although governments and the research community are enthusiastic about the potential for these food applications to improve public health, there is rising concern about the proliferation and marketing of these foods. In some cases, labeling claims are made that are not scientifically supported or accurate, the biological efficacy is not known, or the functional ingredient is not present in meaningful amounts. In other cases, there are safety concerns associated with their use. In the coming years, consumer awareness and demand for such foods is expected to grow as more evidence about the importance of diet in health becomes available. However, further insight and debate is also needed on the marketing of these foods and whether they can, in fact, produce the claimed health benefits.

Conclusion

As the roles and mechanisms of nutrients and dietary components become clearer, and investigators determine the appropriate forms and levels of nutrients and dietary components necessary for maintaining optimal immune response, appropriate public health interventions can be designed and dietary recommendations developed to maintain optimum immunity and enhance overall health.

References

1. Chandra, R. (1991) Nutrition and immunity: lessons from the past and new insights into the future. *Am. J. Clin. Nutr.* **53**, 1087–1101.
2. Doherty, J., Golden, M.H.N., Raynes, J.G., Griffin, G.E., and McAdam, K.P.W.J. (1993) Acute-phase protein response is impaired in severely malnourished children. *Clin. Sci.* **84**, 169–175.
3. Scrimshaw, N. and SanGiovanni, J.P. (1997) Synergism of nutrition, infection, and immunity: an overview. *Am. J. Clin. Nutr.* **66**, 464S–477S.
4. World Health Organization. (1995) Global prevalence of vitamin A deficiency. Micronutrient deficiency information system working paper no. 2. WHO, Geneva. (WHO/NUT/95.3).
5. Beaton, G.H., Martorell, R., Aronson, K.J., et al. (1993) Effectiveness of vitamin A supplementation in the control of young child mortality in developing countries. Nutrition policy discussion paper no. 13. ACC/SCN: Geneva.
6. West, K.P., Jr., Katz, J., Khatry, S.K., et al. (1999) Double blind, cluster randomised trial of low dose supplementation with vitamin A or beta carotene on mortality related to pregnancy in Nepal. The NNIPS–2 Study Group. *Br. Med. J.* **318**, 570–575.
7. Ramakrishnan, U. (2002) Prevalence of micronutrient malnutrition worldwide. *Nutr. Rev.* **60**, S46–S52.
8. World Health Organization. (2002) Nutrition for health and development: A global agenda for combating malnutrition. WHO, Geneva. (WHO/NHD/00.6).
9. Gibson R.S. (1990) Principles of nutritional assessment. Oxford University Press, New York.
10. Lee, R.D. and Nieman, D.C. (1996) *Nutritional Assessment.* 2nd ed. Library of Congress Cataloging in Publication Data. Mosby, St. Louis, MO.

11. World Health Organization. (1995) *The use and interpretation of anthropometry; report of the WHO expert committee on physical status.* WHO, Geneva. (WHO Technical Report Series, 854).

12. Beaton, G., Kelly, A., Kevany, J., Martorell, R., and Mason, J. (1990) *Appropriate uses of anthropometric indices in children.* Nutrition policy discussion paper no. 7. United Nations ACC/SCN: Geneva.

13. De Onis, M., Garza, C., and Habicht, J.P. (1997) Time for a new growth reference. *Pediatr.* **100**, E8.

14. Maehira, F., Luyo, G.A., Miyagi, I., et al. (2002) Alterations of serum selenium concentrations in the acute phase of pathological conditions. *Clin. Chim. Acta* **316**, 137–146.

15. Keen, C.L., Clegg, M.S., Hanna, L.A., et al. (2003) The plausibility of micronutrient deficiencies being a significant contributing factor to the occurrence of pregnancy complications. *J. Nutr.* **133**, 1597S–1605S.

16. Thurnham, D.I., Northrop-Clewes, C.A., and Chopra, M. (1998) Biomarkers of vegetable and fruit intakes. *Am. J. Clin. Nutr.* **68**, 756–758.

17. Hambidge, M. (2003) Biomarkers of trace mineral intake and status. *J. Nutr.* **133 Suppl 3**, 948S–955S.

18. Steinberg, K., Beck, J., Nickerson, D., et al. (2002) DNA banking for epidemiologic studies: a review of current practices. *Epidemiology* **13**, 246–254.

19. Stephensen, C.B., Rasooly, R., Jiang, X., et al. (2002) Vitamin A enhances in vitro Th2 development via retinoid X receptor pathway. *J. Immunol.* **168**, 4495–503.

20. Stephenson, C.B. (2001) Vitamin A, infection, and immune function. *Annu. Rev. Nutr.* **21**, 167–192.

21. Erickson, K.L., Medina, E.A., and Hubbard, N.E. (2000) Micronutrients and innate immunity. *J. Infect. Dis.* **182**, 5–10.

22. Long, K.Z. and Santos, J.I. (1999) Vitamins and the regulation of the immune response. *Ped. Infect. Dis. J.* 283–90.

23. Wenzel, B.E., Chow, A., Baur, R., Schleusener, H., and Wall, J.R. (1998) Natural killer cell activity in patients with Graves' disease and Hashimoto's thyroiditis. *Thyroid* **8**, 1019–1022.

24. Kramer, J.H., Mak, I.T., Phillips, T.M., and Weglicki, W.B. (2003) Dietary magnesium intake influences circulating pro-inflammatory neuropeptide levels and loss of myocardial tolerance to postischemic stress. *Exp. Biol. Med. (Maywood)* **228**, 665–673.

25. Binka, F.N., Ross, D.A., Morris, S.S., et al. (1995) Vitamin A supplementation and childhood malaria in northern Ghana. *Am. J. Clin. Nutr.* **61**, 853–859.

26. Shankar, A.H., Genton, B., Semba, R.D., et al. (1999) Effect of vitamin A supplementation on morbidity due to *Plasmodium falciparum* in young children in Papua New Guinea: a randomised trial. *Lancet* **354**, 203–209.

27. Akompong, T., Ghori, N., and Haldar, K. (2000) In vitro activity of riboflavin against the human malaria parasite *Plasmodium falciparum. Antimicrob. Agents Chemother.* **44**, 88–96.

28. Levander, O.A. and Ager, A.L., Jr. (1993) Malarial parasites and antioxidant nutrients. *Parasitol.* **107**, S95–S106.
29. Harbige, L.S. (2003) Fatty acids, the immune response, and autoimmunity: a question of n–6 essentiality and the balance between n–6 and n–3. *Lipids* **38**, 323–341.
30. Fraker, P. (2000) Impact of nutritional status on immune integrity, in *Nutrition and Immunology: Principles and Practice.* (Gershwin, M.E., German, J.B., Keen, C.L., eds.) Humana, Totowa, NJ, pp. 147–156.
31. Zinc Investigators' Collaborative Group. (1999) Prevention of diarrhea and pneumonia by zinc supplementation in children in developing countries: pooled analysis of randomized controlled trials. *J. Pediatr.* **135**, 689–697.
32. Sasidharan, P.K., Rajeev, E., and Vijayakumari, V. (2002) Tuberculosis and vitamin D deficiency. *J. Ass. Phys. India* **50**, 554–558.
33. Zinc Investigators' Collaborative Group. (2002) Therapeutic effects of oral zinc in acute and persistent diarrhea in children in developing countries: pooled analysis of randomized controlled trials. *Am. J. Clin. Nutr.* **72**, 1516–1522.
34. Black, R.E., Brown, K.H., and Becker, S. (1984) Malnutrition is a determining factor in diarrhoeal duration, but not incidence, among young children in a longitudinal study in rural Bangladesh. *Am. J. Clin. Nutr.* **39**, 87–94.
35. Barclay, A.J., Foster, A., and Sommer, A. (1987) Vitamin A supplements and mortality related to measles: a randomised clinical trial. *Br. Med. J.* 294–296.
36. Grotto, I., Mimouni, M., Gdalevich, M., and Mimouni, D. (2003) Vitamin A supplementation andchildhood morbidity form diarrhea and respiratory infections: a meta-analysis. *J. Pediatr.* **142**, 297–304.
37. Vanderhoof, J.A. (2000) Probiotics: future directions. *Am. J. Clin. Nutr.* **73**, 1152S–1155S.
38. Nataro, J.P. and Levine, M.M. (1999) Enteric bacterial vaccines, salmonella, shigella, cholera, escherichia coli, in *Mucosal Immunology.* (Ogra, P., Mestecky, J., Lamm, M., et al., eds.) 2nd ed. Academic, San Diego, CA, pp. 851–866.
39. Siekmann, J.H., Allen, L.H., Watnik, M.R., et al. (2003) Titers of antibody to common pathogens: relation to food-based interventions in rural Kenyan school-children. *Am. J. Clin. Nutr.* **77**, 242–249.
40. Fawzi, W., Msamanga, G.I., Spiegelman, D., et al. (1998) Randomized trial of effects of vitamin supplements on pregnancy outcomes and T cell counts in HIV-1-infected women in Tanzania. *Lancet* **351**, 1477–1482.
41. Rivas, C.I., Vera, J.C., Guaiquil, V.H., et al. (1997) Increased uptake and accumulation of vitamin C in human immunodeficiency virus 1-infected hematopoietic cell lines. *J. Biol.* **272**, 5814–5820.
42. Patrick. L. (2000) Nutrients and HIV: Part two-vitamins A and E, zinc, B-vitamins, and magnesium. *Altern. Med. Rev.* **5**, 39–51.
43. Afacan, Y.E., Hasan, M.S., and Omene, J.A. (2002) Iron deficiency anemia in HIV infection: immunologic and virologic response. *J. Natl. Med. Assoc.* **94**, 73–77.
44. Gordeuk, V.R., Delanghe, J.R., Langlois, M.R., and Boelaert, J.R. (2001) Iron status and the outcome of HIV infection: an overview. *J. Clin. Virol.* **20**, 111–115.

45. Totin, D., Ndugwa, C., Mmiro, F., Perry, R.T., Jackson, J.B., and Semba, R.D. (2002) Iron deficiency anemia is highly prevalent among human immunodeficiency virus-infected and uninfected infants in Uganda. *J. Nutr.* **132**, 423–429.

46. Delmas-Beauvieux, M., Peuchant, E., Couchrouron, A., et al. (1996) The enzymatic antioxidant system in blood and glutathione status in human immunodeficiency virus (HIV)-infected patients: effects of supplementation with selenium or β-carotene. *Am. J. Clin. Nutr.* **64**, 101–107.

47. Look, M., Rockstroh, J.K., Rao, G.S., et al. (1998) Sodium selenite and N-acetylcysteine in antiretroviral-naive HIV–1–infected patients: a randomized, controlled pilot study. *Eur. J. Clin. Invest.* **28**, 389–397.

48. Graham, N., Sorenson, D., Odaka, N., et al. (1991) Relationship of serum copper and zinc levels to HIV seropositivity and progression to AIDS. *J. AIDS* **4**, 976–980.

49. Jeng, K.C., Yang, C.S., Siu, W.Y., Tsai, Y.S., Liao, W.J., and Kuo, J.S. (1996) Supplementation with vitamins C and E enhances cytokine production by peripheral blood mononuclear cells in healthy adults. *Am. J. Clin. Nutr.* **64**, 960–965.

50. Ziemianski, S., Wartanowicz, M., Klos, A., Raczka, A., and Klos, M. (1986) The effect of ascorbic acid and alpha-tocopherol supplementation on serum proteins and immunoglobulin concentration in the elderly. *Nutr. Int.* **2**, 1–5.

51. Alexander, M., Newmark, H., and Miller, R.G. (1985) Oral beta-carotene can increase the number of OKT4+ cells in human blood. *Immunol. Lett.* **9**, 221–224.

52. Buys, H., Hendricks, M., Eley, B., and Hussey, G. (2002) The role of nutrition and micronutrients in paediatric HIV infection. *S. Afr. Dis. J.* **57**, 454–456.

53. Fawzi, W., Mbise, R.L., Hertzmark, E., et al. (1999) A randomized trial of vitamin A supplements in relation to mortality among human immunodeficiency virus-infected and uninfected children in Tanzania. *Pediatr. Inf. Dis. J.* **18**, 127–133.

54. Fawzi, W.W., Msamanga, G.I., Wei, R., et al. (2003) Effect of providing vitamin supplements to human immunodeficiency virus-infected, lactating mothers on the child's morbidity and CD4+ cell counts. *Clin. Inf. Dis.* **36**, 1053–1062.

55. Doleman, C. and Bast, A. (1990) Oxygen radical in lung pathology. *Free Radical Biol. Med.* **9**, 381–400.

56. Paller, A., Eichenfield, L., Leung, D., Stewart, D., and Appell, M. (2001) A 12-week study of tacrolimus ointment for the treatment of atopic dermatitis in pediatric patients. *J. Am. Acad. Dermatol.* **44**, S47–S57.

57. Fahy, J., Fleming, H., Wong, H., et al. (1997) The effect of an anti-IgE monoclonal antibody on the early- and late-phase responses to allergen inhalation in asthmatic subjects. *Am. J. Respir. Crit. Care Med.* **155**, 1828–1834.

58. Hodge, L., Salome, C., Peat, J., Haby, M., Xuan, W., and Woolcock, A. (1996) Consumption of oily fish and childhood asthma risk. *Med. J. Aust.* **164**, 137–140.

59. Arm, J., Horton, C., Spur, B., Mencia-Huerta, J., and Lee, T. (1989) The effects of dietary supplementation with fish oil lipids on the airway response to inhaled allergen in bronchial asthma. *Am. Rev. Respir. Dis.* **139**, 1395–1400.

60. Soyland, E., Funk, J., Rajka, G., et al. (1994) Dietary supplementation with very long-chain n–3 fatty acids in patients with atopic dermatitis. A double-blind, multicentre study. *Br. J. Dermatol.* **130**, 757–764.
61. Beck, M.A. (1999) Selenium and host defence towards viruses. *Proc. Nutr. Soc.* **58**, 707–711.
62. Levander, O.A., Ager, A.L., Jr., and Beck, M.A. (1995) Vitamin E and selenium: contrasting and interacting nutritional determinants of host resistance to parasitic and viral infections. *Proc. Nutr. Soc.* **54**, 475–487.
63. Garcia, A.L., Ruhl, R., Herz, U., Koebnick, C., Schweigert, F.J., and Worm, M. (2003) Retinoid and carotenoid enriched diets influence the ontogenesis of the immune system in mice. *Immunology* **110**, 180–187.
64. Block, G., Patterson, B., and Subar, A. (1992) Fruit, vegetables, and cancer prevention: a review of the epidemiological evidence. *Nutr. Cancer* **18**, 1–29.
65. Ross, R. (1999) Atherosclerosis—an inflammatory disease. *N. Engl. J. Med.* **340**, 115–126.
66. Giovannucci, E. (1999) Tomatoes, tomato-based products, lycopene, and cancer: a review of the epidemiologic literature. *J. Natl. Cancer Inst.* **91**, 317–331.
67. de Gaetano, G., De Curtis, A., di Castelnuovo, A., et al. (2002) Antithrombotic effect of polyphenols in experimental models: a mechanism of reduced vascular risk by moderate wine consumption. *Ann. NY Acad. Sci.* **957**, 174–188.
68. Hasler, C.M. (2003) Functional foods: benefits, concerns and challenges-a position paper from the american council on science and health. *J. Nutr.* **132**, 3772–3781.

INDEX

357